HARRY'S COSMETICOLOGY 9TH EDITION

FOCUS BOOKS

The Hair: Testing, Process and Repair for the Cosmetic Industry

ISBN: 978-0-8206-0405-3

Harry's Cosmeticology

9th Edition

Volume One - ISBN: 978-0-8206-01762
Volume Two - ISBN: 978-0-8206-01779
Volume Three - ISBN: 978-0-8206-01786
eBook - ISBN: 978-0-8206-01793

First Edition

Chemical Publishing Company

www.chemical-publishing.com

Printed in the United States of America

A Note from the Publisher:

The new 9th edition of Harry's Cosmeticology is available as a 3 volume set containing over 2600 pages of new information on the recent changes in the cosmetic and personal care products industry.

Chemical Publishing is now offering key parts of the title for those interested in a particular subject area covered in the book.

Harry's Cosmeticology 9th Edition has developed a new line of titles called "Focus Books" for this purpose.

"Focus Books" are a series of selected chapters that can be used as a reference guide for partial subject areas covered in the parent text.

Because the chapters have been taken from the original individual volumes, the reader will find that the pages have not been renumbered in standard order starting from page one, moving forward, but rather they have been left in the original format so that the information will flow chronologically, although the pages may in fact not be numbered as so.

The benefit of leaving the page numbers as they were taken from the original text is that the reader will be able to use the Table of Contents and page numbers referenced within the Focus Book to find the desired content and we have tried to keep the chapter segments in the same order in which you would find them in the master text.

The full 3 volume Trilogy of Harry's Cosmeticology 9th Edition can be purchased through Chemical Publishing Company at www.chemical-publishing.com or through any major online retailer. It is also available in Ebook format through Kindle or as mobi, or ePub available directly from the publisher.

www.chemical-publishing.com

Our webpage featuring Authors, Reviews and other information about the 9th edition:

www.harryscosmeticology.com

About the Editor-in-Chief

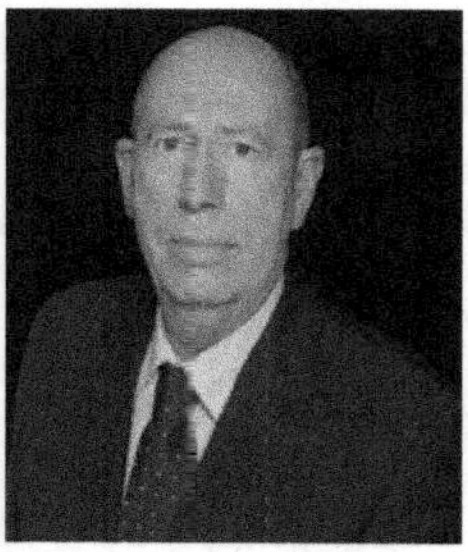

Meyer R. Rosen

CChem, CPC, CChE, CFEI, DABFE, DABFET, FAIC

Meyer R. Rosen is President of Interactive Consulting, Inc. (www.chemicalconsult.com). He is a Thought-Leader and expert in the field of Technical Marketing and multi-industry Technology Transfer Applications including, but not limited to: cosmetics and personal care, applied rheology, applied surface and interfacial chemistry, polymers, organosilicones, professional editing and custom preparation of Mind-Maps® for the organization and presentation of complex information.

Mr. Rosen is a Chartered Chemist and Fellow of the Royal Society of Chemistry (London); a Fellow of the American Institute of Chemists and both a Nationally Certified Professional Chemist and Certified Professional Chemical Engineer. He is a member of the U.S. Society of Cosmetic Chemists (SCC) & the American Institute of Chemical Engineers. Meyer serves as an Advisor for David Smith, Executive Director of the SCC Advisory Committee. He is also Editor for U.S. & Canada and Editor-in-Chief for North and Latin America for Euro Cosmetics Magazine in Germany. Mr. Rosen is Editor of the Delivery System Handbook for Personal Care and Cosmetic Products and Editor-in-Chief of Harry's Cosmeticology, 9th Ed.

Meyer served for six years as the Chief Scientific Advisor and Director of Technical Programming for United Business Media's (UBM) HBA Technical Conferences. He a former Director of the American Institute of Chemists, past Vice President of the Association of Consulting Chemists and has served on the Scientific Advisory Board of Supply Side West/East: Virgo Publications. Mr. Rosen is also the Founder, Organizer and co-moderator for HBA's Annual International Safety, Regulatory and Certification Symposia.

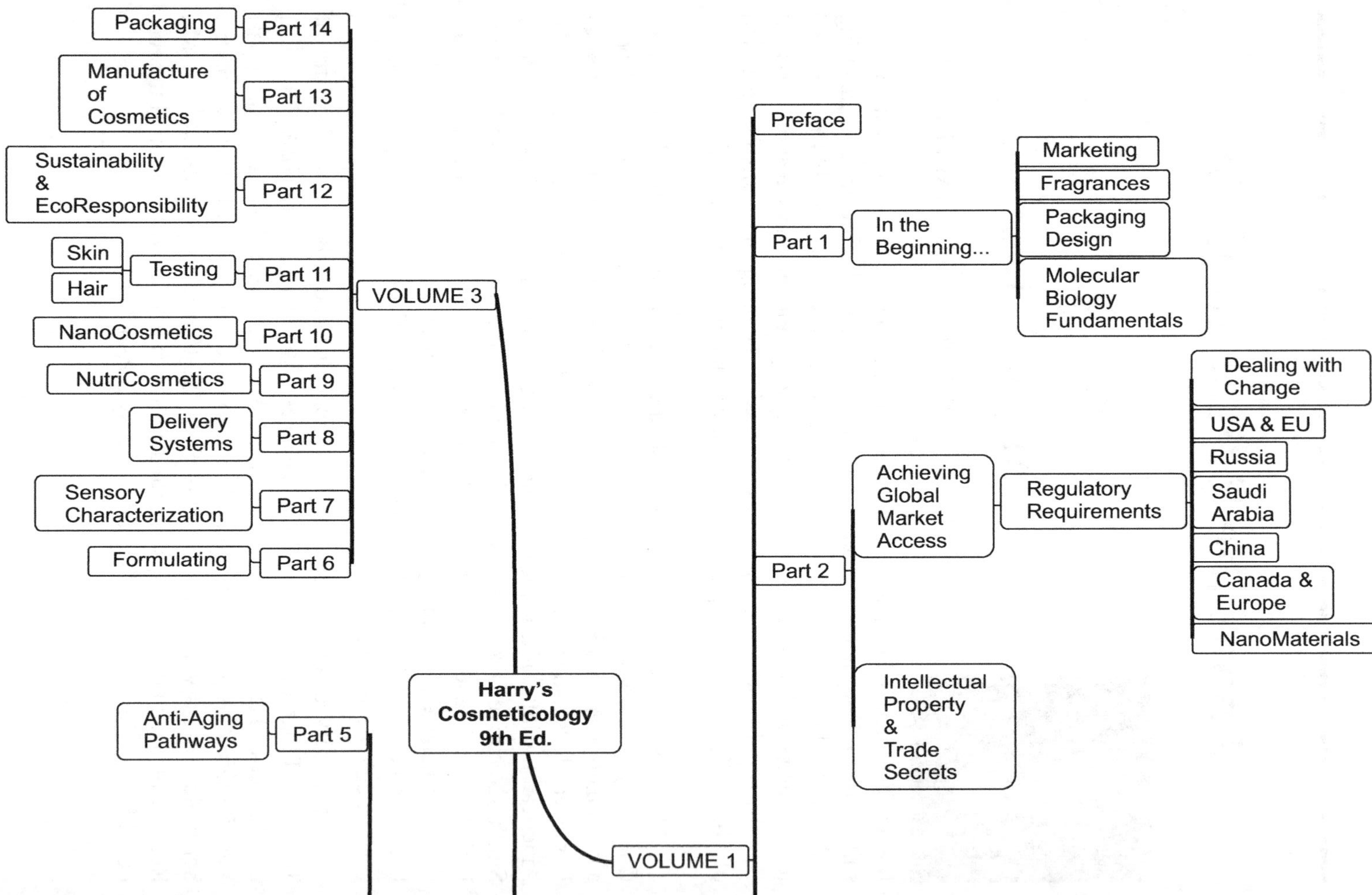

Harry's Cosmeticology 9th Ed.
VOLUME 1
Preface
Part 1
In the Beginning...
Marketing
Fragrances
Packaging Design
Molecular Biology Fundamentals
Part 2
Achieving Global Market Access
Regulatory Requirements
Dealing with Change
USA & EU
Russia
Saudi Arabia
China
Canada & Europe
NanoMaterials
Intellectual Property & Trade Secrets
Part 5
Anti-Aging Pathways
VOLUME 3
Part 6
Formulating
Part 7
Sensory Characterization
Part 8
Delivery Systems
Part 9
NutriCosmetics
Part 10
NanoCosmetics
Part 11
Testing
Skin
Hair
Part 12
Sustainability & EcoResponsibility
Part 13
Manufacture of Cosmetics
Part 14
Packaging

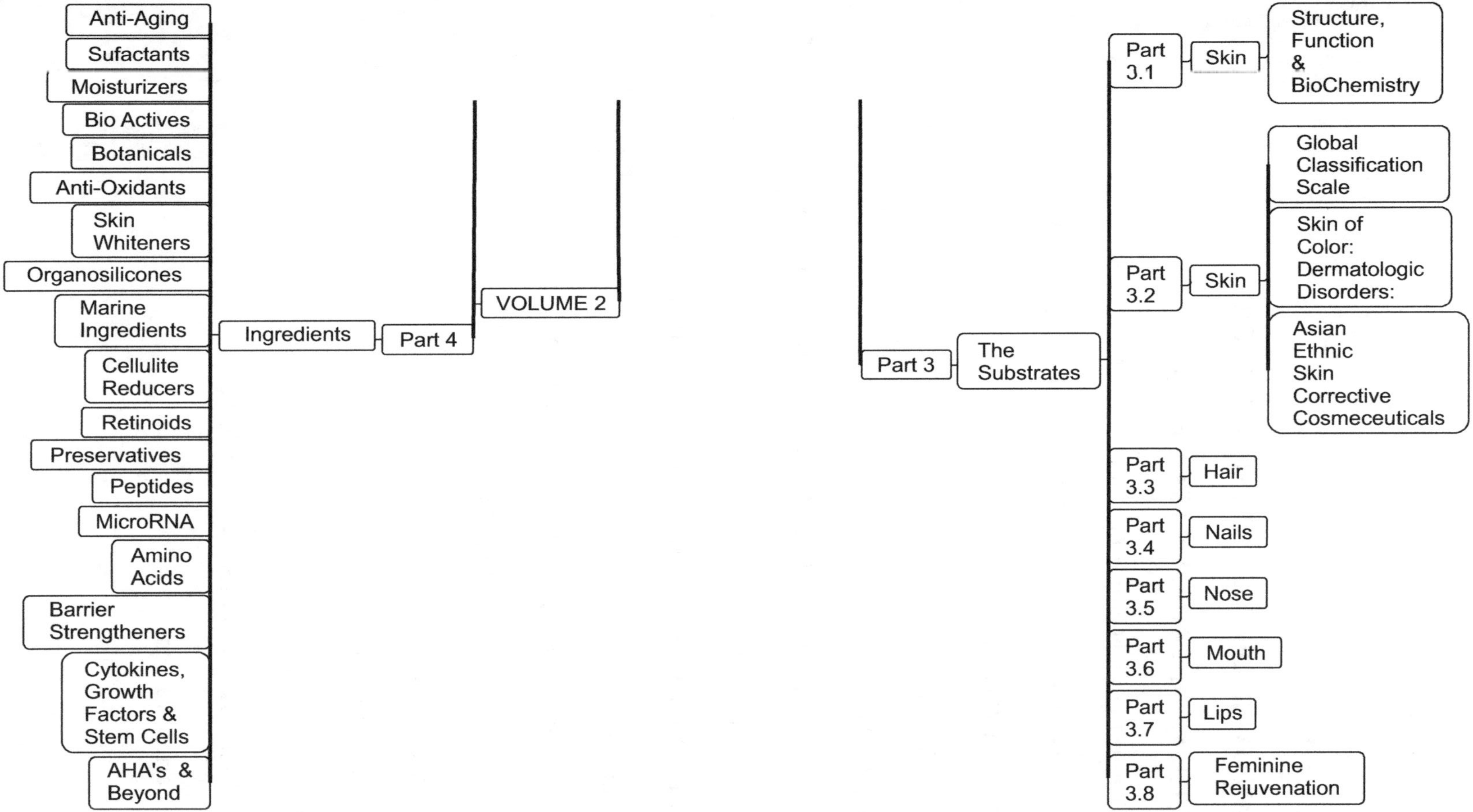

VOLUME 2
Part 4
Ingredients
Anti-Aging
Sufactants
Moisturizers
Bio Actives
Botanicals
Anti-Oxidants
Skin Whiteners
Organosilicones
Marine Ingredients
Cellulite Reducers
Retinoids
Preservatives
Peptides
MicroRNA
Amino Acids
Barrier Strengtheners
Cytokines, Growth Factors & Stem Cells
AHA's & Beyond
Part 3
The Substrates
Part 3.1
Skin
Structure, Function & BioChemistry
Part 3.2
Skin
Global Classification Scale
Skin of Color: Dermatologic Disorders:
Asian Ethnic Skin Corrective Cosmeceuticals
Part 3.3
Hair
Part 3.4
Nails
Part 3.5
Nose
Part 3.6
Mouth
Part 3.7
Lips
Part 3.8
Feminine Rejuvenation

AUTHORS

AN OVERVIEW OF THE PHYSICAL AND CHEMICAL PROPERTIES OF HAIR

Editor: Manuel Gamez-Garcia

AN OVERVIEW OF HAIR FOLLICLE ANATOMY AND BIOLOGY

Paul Mouser

HAIR AGING: FUNDAMENTALS, PROTECTION AND REPAIR

Padmaja Prem

MECHANISMS OF CHANGES IN HAIR SHAPE

Manuel Gamez-Garcia

SHAMPOOS INGREDIENTS, FORMULATION AND EFFICACY EVALUATION

Carrie Shipley

HAIR STYLING

Charles Warren

SPECIALTY STYLING PRODUCTS

Charles Warren

AUTHORS

WAVING

Charles Warren

CONDITIONERS/TREATMENTS

Charles Warren

HAIR COLORANTS AND PROTECTION

Padmaja Prem

REACTIVE HAIR CARE PRODUCTS

Charles Warren

A SURVEY OF TEST METHODOLOGY USED IN EVALUATING THE DAMAGE, PROTECTION AND REPAIR OF HAIR

Ray Rigoletto

PART 3.3.1

AN OVERVIEW OF THE PHYSICAL AND CHEMICAL PROPERTIES OF HAIR AND THEIR RELATION TO COSMETIC NEEDS, PERFORMANCE AND PROPERTIES

Manuel Gamez-Garcia
Ashland Specialty Ingredients

TABLE OF CONTENTS

PART 3.3.2

AN OVERVIEW OF HAIR FOLLICLE ANATOMY AND BIOLOGY

Paul Mouser Ph.D.
Ashland, Inc., Ashland Specialty Ingredients, Bridgewater, NJ, United States

TABLE OF CONTENTS:

PART 3.3.3

HAIR AGING: FUNDAMENTALS, PROTECTION AND REPAIR

Padmaja Prem, Ph.D
Vice President, Research & Development
Combe Incorporated, 1101 Westchester Avenue
White Plains, NY 10604

TABLE OF CONTENTS

PART 3.3.4

MECHANISMS OF CHANGES IN HAIR SHAPE

Manuel Gamez-Garcia
Ashland Specialty Ingredients

TABLE OF CONTENTS:

HAIR CARE

PART 6.10

SHAMPOOS INGREDIENTS, FORMULATION AND EFFICACY EVALUATION

Author Carrie Shipley, Applications Scientist, Grain Processing Corporation

TABLE OF CONTENTS

PART 6.15

HAIR COLORANTS AND PROTECTION

Author: Padmaja Prem Vice President, Research & Development
Combe Incorporated, 1101 Westchester Avenue
White Plains, NY 10604

TABLE OF CONTENTS

PART 6.16

REACTIVE HAIR CARE PRODUCTS

Author Charles Warren

TABLE OF CONTENTS

PART 11.4

A SURVEY OF TEST METHODOLOGY USED IN EVALUATING THE DAMAGE, PROTECTION AND REPAIR OF HAIR

Authors:
Ray Rigoletto Sr. Manager,
Global R&D Applications Care Specialties: Hair Care; Home Care
Ashland, Inc.
1005 US Hwy No. 202/206 Bridgewater, NJ 08807

Tim Gillece
Ashland, Inc.

TABLE OF CONTENTS:

PART 3.3.1

AN OVERVIEW OF THE PHYSICAL AND CHEMICAL PROPERTIES OF HAIR AND THEIR RELATION TO COSMETIC NEEDS, PERFORMANCE AND PROPERTIES

Author

Dr. Manuel Gamez-Garcia, Ph.D.,
Research Fellow,
Ashland Specialty Ingredients

ABSTRACT

In this chapter we present an unusual approach to the subject wherein we consider the system of hair structure and its relation to hair function. The approach used for this purpose consists in reviewing the most recent and advanced hair structural concepts derived from the fields of chemistry and biology, while providing a strong emphasis on the physical, social, and cosmetic aspects of hair function.

The chapter is divided into six parts:

- The four first sections describe the chemical and biological composition of hair, which forms the foundation for its complex physical architecture. Through these sections a detailed analysis is made of the hair internal structure, its viscoelastic and optical properties, and its response to moisture. Wherever possible an effort is made to always connect physical properties and related processes with the functional aspects of hair.
- In the last two sections, a review is made of the various processes taking place in the follicle to create hair. We point out that the follicle is *alive*, and that the native proteins in mature hair still have biological activity and a function to play. This provides access to cosmetic approaches to improve its beauty, and of course, it is a relatively new concept since the hair protein architecture has long been considered as a structure with no biological activity. There a description is made of the main biological activities occurring in the various zones and phases of the follicle to assemble cells and produce hair. As this description is made, special attention is given

to the follicular activities that create, from its inception, the foundations that correlate hair architectural structure with hair function. We assert that this unique approach and a true understanding of the relationship between hair architecture and functional biology opens an entirely new field for the development of new concepts and products for the cosmetic and personal care industry catering to both men and women.

TABLE OF CONTENTS

3.3.1.1 INTRODUCTION

It is a general principle of nature that any living organism, or biological material created by nature, is made and structured in such a way that its properties are optimized to perform a specific function. In this sense, hair is not different from any other biomaterial found in the organs of our body. Contrary to the common belief that hair is a dead material and of little or no importance, hair is an optimized assembly of proteins, lipids, and polysaccharides organized into units or cells for a specific function. All cells in our body undergo a life cycle and are created to fulfill a function. However, in this respect there is a considerable difference between hair cells and other organ cells. Cells from other parts of the body undergo a programmed form of cell death, known also as "apoptosis," once they have fulfilled their function. After this event, the cells are discarded and eliminated from the body. In contrast, when hair cells die by "apoptosis" in the follicle, their function is not finished; rather, it has just begun. Thus, when hair cells die, they are not discarded by the body because it is then that they are needed the most for their specialized biological function of scalp/skin protection and aesthetic purposes. The short-lived period of hair cells in the follicle is just a preparatory stage for their final function.

Another common belief is that since hair cells are inanimate or lifeless, their structure has no biological activity. This statement is somewhat incorrect because the protein structure of inanimate hair cells still possesses biological activity that is crucial for our living organism. Even when hair cells are dead and inanimate, if their protein structure is damaged, as in the case of enzyme structures, their biological function is compromised. Let us remember that enzymes are lifeless protein structures whose activity plays a critical role in many of our biological processes. Enzymes are not living organisms, and they lose their biological activity when their natural conformations are lost by denaturation due to harsh stresses, either thermal, chemical, or mechanical (1).

Likewise, the proteins composing our hair cells also lose their biological function/activity when they are subjected to harsh stresses, i.e., heat, chemical treatments, mechanical fatigue, or excessive mechanical elongations. Hair treatments with hot irons and with other chemical processes such as perm waving, bleaching, and alkali straightening are known to cause denaturation and bond breakage in hair's native proteins (2). As a consequence, many hair properties are compromised, i.e., hair loses the ability to control moisture absorption. Its mechanical/thermal/optical response is compromised, and ultimately it loses its aesthetic purpose and ability to protect the scalp. Thus, the chemical composition and protein architecture of inanimate hair cells still possess biological activity enabling hair to fulfill the biological function for which it was created.

3.3.1.2 STRUCTURE AND CHEMICAL COMPOSITION OF HAIR

Hair is composed of proteins and a very small quantity of lipids and polysaccharides. These biomaterials form the hair cells, which are spatially separated and sequentially organized in a brick-and-mortar fashion in the cylindrical hair body. Consequently, they form membranes, amorphous and crystalline protein regions that extend all along the hair fiber, giving rise to the complex architecture of hair (see Figure 1). As will be seen later, these structures are the foundation of hair's remarkable physical properties. Table 1 displays the overall amino acid chemical composition of hair (3); the data in this table clearly show that hair is rich in half-cystine, serine, glutamic acid, and proline, i.e., the amino acids characteristic of a protein known as keratin. The next most abundant materials in hair, although at a smaller scale compared to the amount of protein, are lipids and polysaccharides, which account for 2–10% of the fiber weight. These materials, as will be discussed later, mainly appear in the cement layer gluing cortical and cuticle cells, as well as on the hair surface.

Another substance that is always present in hair is water. Incidentally, water is never considered part of the hair composition. Surprisingly, many scientists consider water to be an integral part of most biologically active proteins and, therefore, for all practical purposes water is also part of the hair composition. Native proteins contain a substantial amount of water in two forms, namely bound and free water. Free water, also referred to as "bulk water" or "loose water," has only a minor influence in the native structure of proteins. In contrast, "bound water," with its strong binding physical forces, attaches to specific protein groups stabilizing the protein secondary structure (4). Bound water plays an important role in the conformation of exposed side chains, and because of its role on protein stabilization many scientists consider it to be part of the protein structure. Water is thus also part of the hair keratin composition (5) because it is needed for its stability. The role of water on hair behavior will be discussed in further detail later in this chapter.

Percentages amino acids in hair:

Alanine	4.6
Arginine	5.8
Aspartic acid	4.9
Half-cystine	17.8
Glutamic acid	11.4
Glycine	6.4
Histidine	0.9
Isoleucine	2.6
Leucine	5.8
Methionine	0.6

Phenylalanine	1.6
Proline	8.4
Serine	11.7
Threonine	6.8
Tyrosine	2.0
Valine	5.8

Table 1) Amino acid composition of unaltered human hair (3)

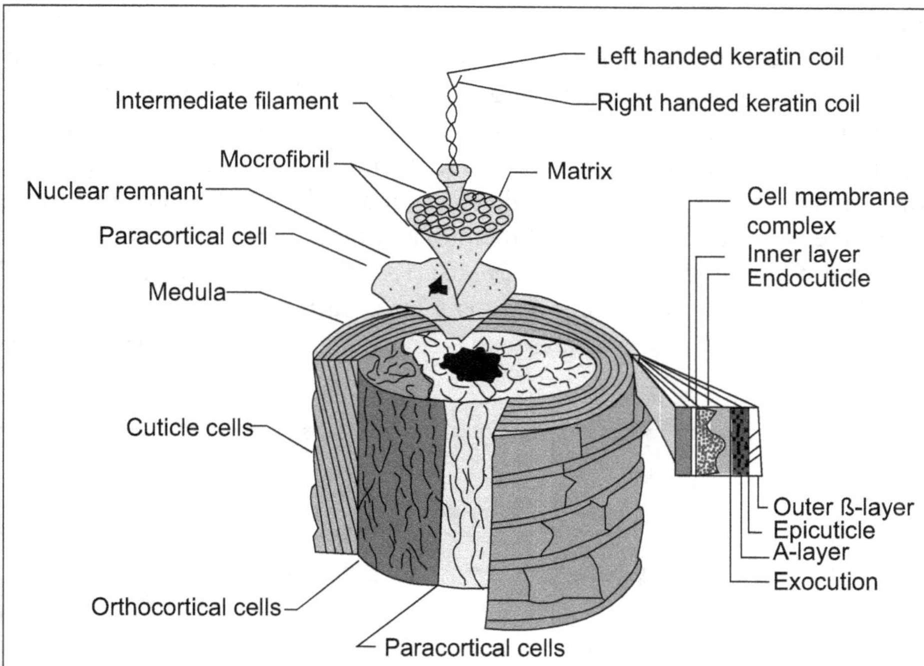

Figure 1: Diagram of a hair fiber showing its various components (60).

3.3.1.3 MAIN TYPES OF CELLS IN HAIR

A hair fiber is mainly composed of three types of cells, namely, cortical, cuticle, and medulla cells (see Figure 2). These three types of cells are made, organized, and assembled to form hair fibers by a tiny organ called the follicle (see Figure 3). This small organ sits on the scalp, and there are as many follicles as hair fibers. While hair cells are still alive in the follicle, they acquire a protein structure, composition, and architecture that prepare them for their final function. Before the hair cells undergo apoptosis the follicle carefully feeds and instructs them so they can arrange their internal protein structures into highly specialized conformations. For instance, a large percentage of the proteins found in the cortical cells of hair are arranged into a type of peptide sequence and conformation that is unique among all proteins. This unique protein is called keratin and its helical structure is such that, later, it allows hair to attain a high degree of mechanical strength (see Figure 4).

Keratin is a protein designed by nature to provide mechanical strength wherever needed in living organisms (6). Keratin proteins are usually coiled into filaments and constitute the micro-skeleton that gives mechanical stability to many cells. Without keratin filaments, many living cells would burst or collapse under the action of fluid pressure; i.e., in the liver they act as scaffolding structures that provide mechanical strength to the hepatocytes (7). Depending on their mechanical characteristics, keratins can be divided into alpha and beta keratins, or soft and hard keratins, respectively. Alpha or soft keratins are mostly found in hair, nails, skin, other body cells, wool, and the fur of other mammals, while the hard beta keratins are typical of reptile claws, the shell of turtles, etc. (8). Alpha keratins are also classified as type I (acidic) and type II (basic) keratins, and, in hair they are always coiled in pairs (9–10). Keratins can vary in structure and molecular weight, and therefore, there is a large variety of them; however, regardless of their type, nature always uses them when there is need for mechanical strength.

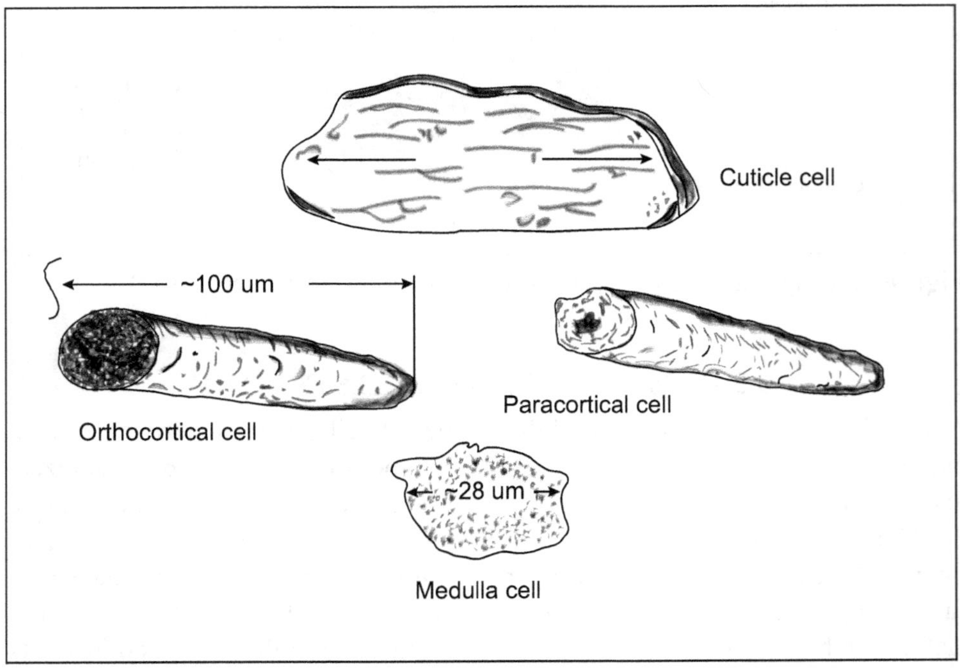

Figure 2: Pictographic representation of three types of cells in hair (60).

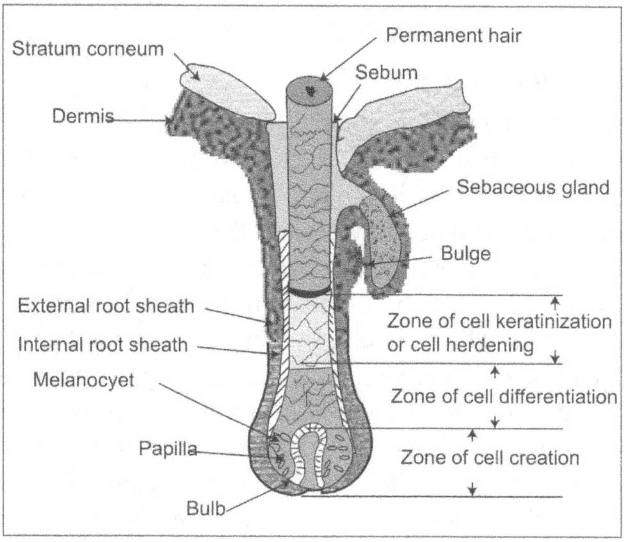

Figure 3: Diagrammatic representation of hair follicle with its main general components and the lipid gland (62).

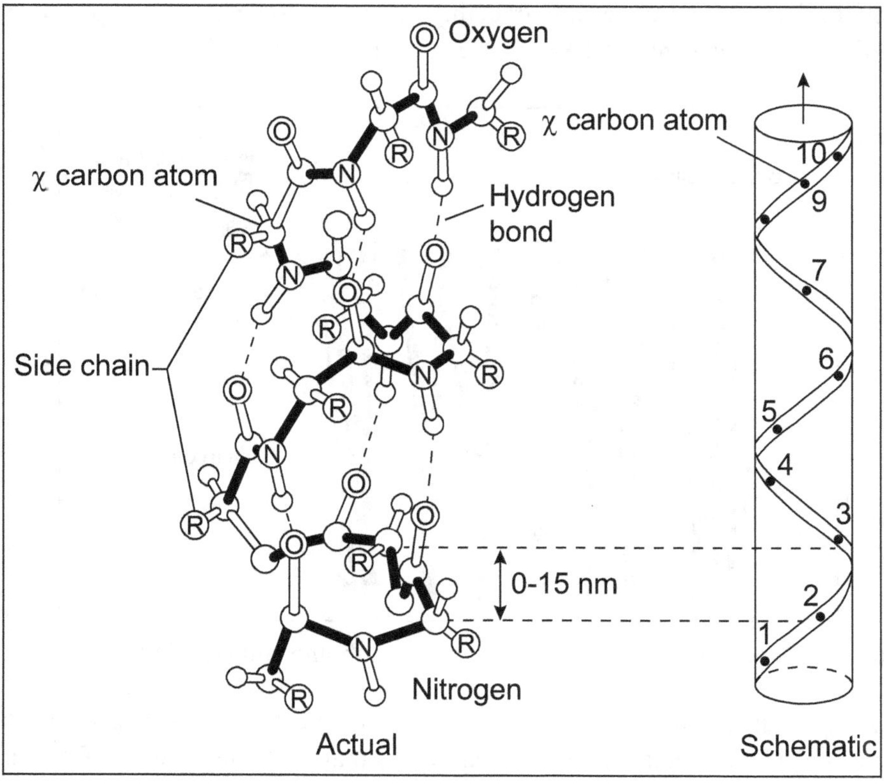

Figure 4: Helical structure of alpha helix in keratin.

3.3.1.4 CORTICAL CELLS AND THEIR ROLE IN HAIR PROPERTIES

a. Cortical cell structure and composition

The cortical cells are elongated and spindle-like in shape; they constitute the major cellular component of hair fibers and are responsible for most of the mechanical properties of hair (10–11). Their irregular circular shape in a grown hair fiber has an average diameter of approximately 20 μm; their entire body length is approximately 100 μm long (see Figure 2). The cortical cells in grown hair fibers are not alive. However, before the hair fibers emerge from their follicles there is a point at which they are still alive. The main task of these cells during their life period is to synthesize keratin proteins in their bodies by assembling key amino acids into helical structures, strand them into filaments—also called intermediate filaments (IFs), and finally, bind them via disulfide bonds to an amorphous protein matrix to form macrofibrils (11–14). The amorphous protein matrix gluing the microfibrils will then be cross-linked with disulfide bonds and hardened as the cells die. The keratin filaments are crystalline in nature and are known to possess remarkable mechanical strength. To further maximize the mechanical resistance of the nascent hair fiber, the follicle facilitates the creation of hundreds of cortical cells and instructs them to interdigitate and produce an extracellular material, the cell membrane complex (CMC), which glues them all together in a cylindrical shape (Figure 5).

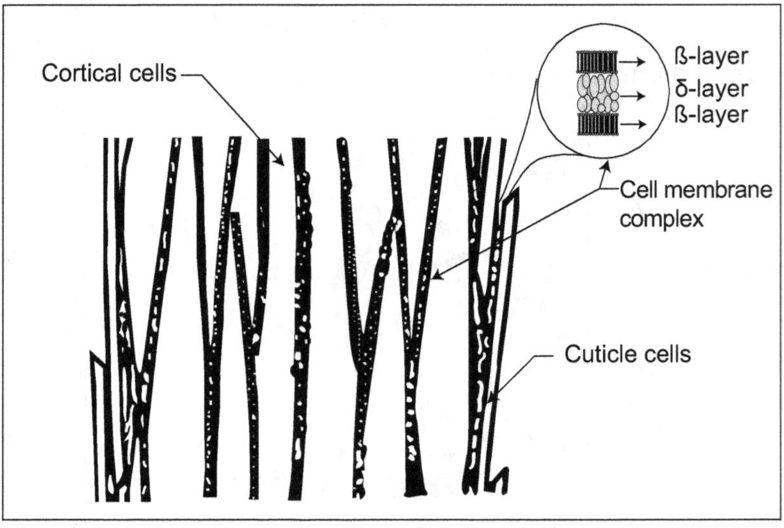

Figure 5: Schematic representation of cell membrane complex in hair fiber.

Because the cortical cells contain high levels of keratin, the resistance of a hair fiber to mechanical breakage is comparable to that of a copper wire of the same diameter. Yet, in spite of this remarkable mechanical strength, the hair fibers do not behave like rigid metallic wires. We all know that hair fibers on the scalp are rather soft and easy to bend and move. This motion allows them to separate and create inter-fiber pockets of air needed for sweat transfer, thermal insulation, scalp protection, and aesthetic purposes (15, 16). Unlike a bundle of copper wires, hair is known for exchanging moisture with the environment by a physical process of absorption and desorption that involves heat transfer with the environment. This process, which occurs also in wool fibers, allows them not only to act as insulating materials, but also as heat buffers that effectively regulate skin/scalp temperature (17, 18). Furthermore, from a cosmetic point of view, hair fibers do not behave like copper fibers since an assembly of hair fibers can be deformed or styled into any desired shape with the aid of water, and it can later recover its original shape.

This particular behavior of hair, which combines mechanical strength with softness and moisture absorption/desorption with heat exchange, is at the base of its biological and cosmetic function. This combination of properties results from the biological activity of hair proteins with their unique architecture within both cortical and cuticle cells. The biggest contribution to this behavior comes, however, from hundreds of keratin micro-fibrils embedded in a protein-amorphous matrix in the cortical cells. The keratin micro-fibrils have a high degree of molecular order. Being crystalline, they do not swell in water, while the amorphous phase has no order, and a part of its structure is highly swellable by water. In terms of strength, the combination of keratin micro-fibrils embedded in an amorphous phase is akin to that of an epoxy composite material reinforced with glass fibers. In this sense a single hair fiber can be considered as an amorphous protein matrix reinforced with keratin micro-fibrils.

b. Viscoelasticity in hair and cortical cells

In 1959 a mechanical model was proposed by Max Feughelman (15, 20, 21) to explain the remarkable relationship existing between elasticity, softness, strength, and moisture displayed by wool and hair. This scientist considered that the outstanding mechanical behavior of hair and wool and, in general, of most keratin fibers, results mainly from the mechanical response of keratin micro-fibrils, or intermediate filaments (Ifs), embedded in an amorphous protein matrix forming macro-fibrils in the cortical cells.

In order to explain the time-delayed elasticity associated with hair softness and its dependence on moisture, Max Feughelman introduced the concept of viscoelasticity to keratin fibers. He proposed a two-phase mechanical model that didn't take into account the discrete nature of cortical cells, cell membrane complex (CMC), and cuticle cells. He thus generated a model of the hair fiber as if it were a continuum material—made only of keratin micro-fibrils embedded in an amorphous protein matrix (see Figure 6). In this model, now supported by a large amount of experimental evidence, the keratin micro-fibrils (C phase) are considered to act mechanically like rods in parallel with the amorphous phase (M phase M in which they are embedded) (15).

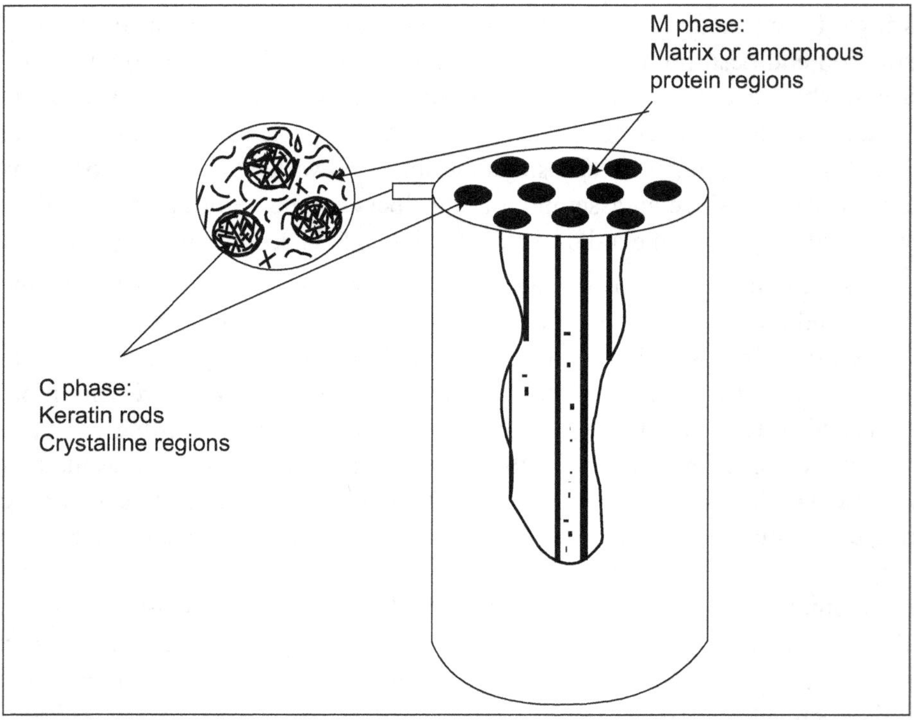

Figure 6: Representation of Max Feughelman mechanical model of keratin fibers showing keratin rods embedded in an amorphous matrix (20).

Since the introduction of the Max Feughelman model, three other models have been proposed to explain the mechanical behavior of keratin fibers. The main differences among all them seem to center on the way the amorphous phase interacts with the crystalline phase. A more detailed discussion of these differences can be found elsewhere (21). For the purpose of this chapter it suffices to emphasize, however, that all of these models recognize the existence of the amorphous and crystalline phases as two separate entities with different mechanical behavior. In all these models it is agreed that the amorphous protein phase corresponds to the zone of scrambled proteins surrounding the keratin micro-fibrils. The proteins in this zone constitute the "cement" that supports and interconnects, via disulfide bond cross-linking, hundreds of micro-fibrils to form the macro-fibrils we know as "hair."

Within the amorphous matrix, the two-phase mechanical model recognizes the existence of two regions with different cystine content, namely, the high- and low-sulfur regions. The low-sulfur amorphous region is considered to be in close proximity to the micro-fibrils, while the high-sulfur region is further away from them. Furthermore, the amorphous phase contains hydrophilic and hydrophobic protein groups that form extended structures all along the cortical cells. Because of these two structures, the amorphous phase can display two distinct patterns of physical behavior. The first one consists of a softening effect usually observed when the amorphous phase interacts with water. The softening effect is due to the hydrophilic extended structure of the amorphous phase and is also referred to as the "gel structure" by Max Fueghelman (20). This structure absorbs large amounts of water, is susceptible to plasticization by moisture, and its viscoelastic response is moisture dependent. In contrast, the non-gel structure of the amorphous phase is hydrophobic, highly cross-linked, and softens at very high temperatures.

Phase C comprises the crystalline keratin rods forming the macro-fibrils. As a result of their crystalline character, these rods do not to absorb water, and therefore, cannot be plasticized by water. The macro-fibrils thus act like strong micro-springs that respond only elastically to mechanical stresses. Thus, macro-fibrils and amorphous phases combine their mechanical and water absorbing/desorbing properties to make hair a viscoelastic material. Because the content of crystalline keratin macro-fibril protein in hair is approximately 95%, a hair fiber has a melting temperature (Tm) of ~ 156°C. Hair has also a glass transition temperature (Tg) of ~ 144°C, and it is primarily related to the noncrystalline amorphous matrix (23). Let us not forget that the Tg in polymers or biopolymers is nothing but the temperature at which a hard amorphous polymer becomes softer (24). Therefore polymers that are very hard and brittle at room temperatures can be softened, by raising their temperature to their respective Tg. They can also be softened by adding a plasticizer. In fact, hair fibers are biopolymers, which under dry and room-temperature conditions are mechanically hard but can become softer, either, by raising their temperature above 174°C, or by adding a plasticizer. We are all familiar with the fact that water is the natural plasticizer for proteins. Thus, hair without moisture is hard and brittle, but when it absorbs moisture it becomes softer because the gel structure of the amorphous phase becomes plasticized by water. This plasticization effect by water is clearly shown in Figure 7, where it can be seen that the amount of force needed to deform a hair fiber is always lower when it has higher levels of moisture.

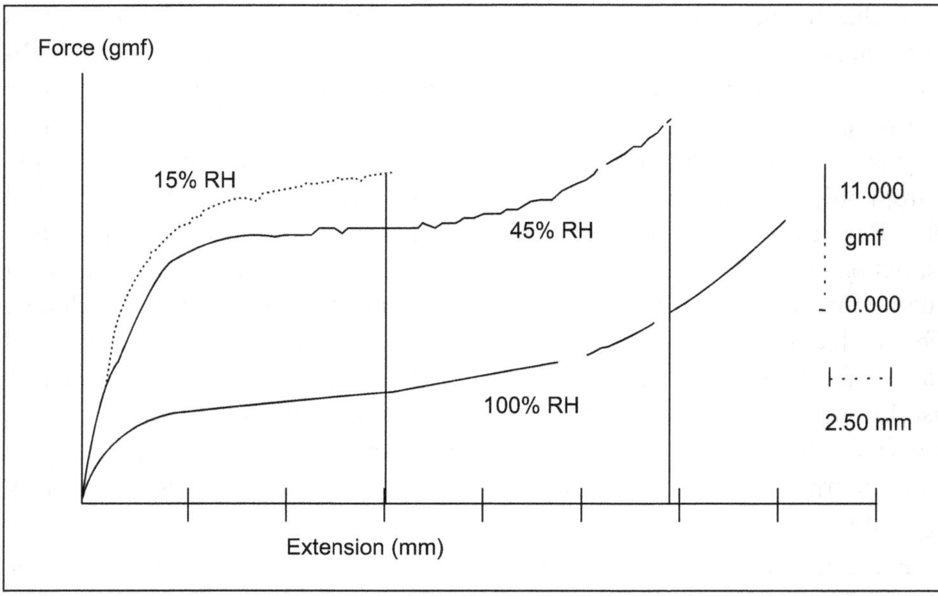

Figure 7: Typical stress-strain deformation curves of hair fibers obtained at three different moisture conditions (60).

The effects of water plasticization/softening in hair are more significant when hair fibers are deformed below 2% water level. The reason for this is that the main hair component that responds to low deformations is the gel structure of the amorphous phase with its large number of hydrogen bonds. At deformations (d), 2% > d < 40% the mechanical response of the fiber is not influenced by the presence of water. Rather, it is mainly controlled by the unfolding of the alpha-keratin into the beta-keratin configuration. Unfolding of the alpha helical keratin in the micro-fibrils thus allows for larger deformations in the hair fiber, thereby preventing it from immediately breaking in the yield region. The transformation of keratin from the alpha to beta configuration is a thermodynamic phase transition and can be induced in hair by many processes other than mechanical extension. When it is produced by heat or chemical damage, it is usually irreversible; however, when it is induced mechanically it is fully reversible. The beta configuration of keratin sometimes is also called the "ladder or platelet" keratin structure (22, 23). Deformations larger than 5%, giving rise to keratin unfolding, occur in hair in daily grooming practices. They occur mostly upon repetitive combing, in particular, when the hair is wet or when the hair is still wet and is being detangled.

The stress/strain curve of hair is shown in Figure 8, where it can be seen that when we deform a single hair fiber from 0 to approximately 40% in length, the hair displays three different slope regions of force versus deformation. The first line is comprised between 0 and 2 or 5% deformation depending on the relative humidity of the environment (segment A). It is known as the Hookean region and has the steepest slope. This region represents the stress/strain mechanical response of the amorphous and crystalline (alpha keratin) phases. In particular, it represents the mechanical response of protein region with hydrogen bonds. Since these levels of deformation are easily attained with everyday combing and grooming practices, we stress the amorphous and macro-fibril phases of our hair almost everyday. If we continue to deform the hair fiber between 2 and 35% (segment B), the slope stress/strain changes because it is produced by a different phenomenon, namely, the opening of keratin coils in the macro-fibrils. This section of the stress-strain curve of hair is known as the yield region. Hair deformations falling in this range are typical during excessive tangling when the hair is wet. Deformations higher than 35% cause the final change in slope before the fiber breaks; the physical phenomenon associated with these deformations seems to be a process of recrystallization of the amorphous phase (segment C) (11).

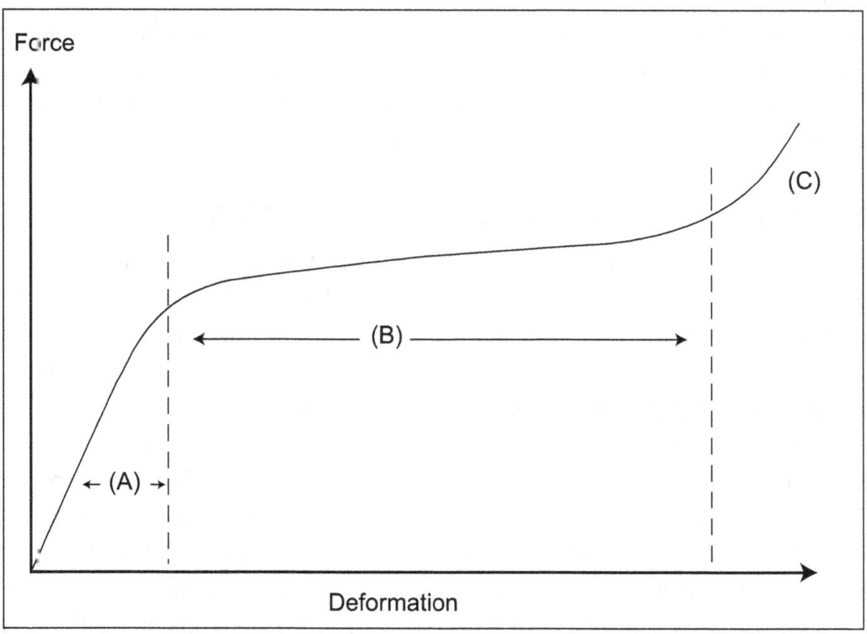

Figure 8: Stress strain curve for hair up to 30% deformation.

c. Shape-memory properties of hair

It is known from the field of polymer science that the mechanical behavior of polymers can be characterized as either being of the thermoset or thermoplastic type. Thermoset characteristics are those that do not respond to temperature changes, while thermoplastic characteristics refer to those materials that soften when heat is applied.

When polymers contain a high level of cross-linking bonds, they are usually of the thermoset type. In many cases these materials behave also as "smart" materials displaying shape-memory properties (24, 25). Since approximately 90% of the hair is composed of cortical cells filled with crystalline and amorphous proteins cross-linked by disulfide bonds, hair like any other polymeric cross-linked material behaves also as a thermoset, viscoelastic, shape-memory biopolymer. Thus, hair has a permanent shape that may be temporarily changed, but can also be reversed later under the appropriate conditions. For instance, whether the hair is limp, wavy, curly, or extremely curly, it will always remember its native shape regardless of what type of styling shape has been imposed on it. Furthermore, the fact that the hair geometry can successfully be changed after styling, and held there for a certain period of time without the hair immediately recovering its shape, is by far one of the most important cosmetically useful examples of hair viscoelasticity and memory-shape properties. If the behavior of hair were purely elastic, hair would not be able to easily deform and accommodate for deformations needed for fiber separation, air pocket formation, thermal insulation, scalp protection, and aesthetic purposes. Also, hair would not be able to transiently change its shape during styling for cosmetic purposes. Thus, hair is a viscoelastic shape-memory material, *and failure to comprehend this will hamper our understanding of one of the most fundamental properties of hair's biological and cosmetic behavior.*

d. Viscoelasticity and the shape-memory properties of hair

Because of the great importance of viscoelasticity in the shape-memory properties of hair, a brief review of this concept will be helpful. We are all familiar with the fact that when a small force is applied to a pure elastic material, for instance, to a rubber band, it will deform a certain short distance. Then, when we release the force, the rubber band will recover almost instantaneously to its original shape. In this process it is obvious that the energy applied to deform the rubber band is stored as mechanical tension energy, and then returned when the force is released. In contrast, in a pure viscous material this does not happen. Rather, when we apply a similar force to a viscous material, for instance, to a string of chewing gum, a small deformation is also produced. However, contrary to the elastic material, the string of chewing gum will not recover its original shape once the force is released and it will stay deformed forever. Furthermore, the energy spent to deform a viscous material like the string of chewing gum is not returned but rather, it is dissipated as heat (26). In summary, an elastic material—when deformed—recovers its shape instantaneously when the force causing the deformation is released, while a viscous material does not.

A viscoelastic material, like hair, displays both behaviors simultaneously, namely, viscous and elastic. In fact, we all have daily encounters with materials that behave viscoelastically. For instance, when we apply a force for a short period of time, i.e., for one second, to a piece of plastic film from a sandwich bag, it will deform slightly. The shape of the film will be recovered instantaneously again when we release the force. However, if we now apply the same force, but for a longer period of time, let's say five minutes, we will still produce the same deformation, but we will notice that when we release the force, the plastic film does not recover its original shape right away. If we wait for some time and pay careful attention to the plastic film, we will notice that it slowly crawls back and eventually recovers its original shape.

In the above example, with a one-second force application, the piece of film displayed typical elastic behavior; yet in the case of a five-minute force application the same plastic film showed initially a viscous behavior followed by a delayed, gradual, and slow elastic recovery. Thus, depending on the time period of force application, the plastic film displayed either pure elastic behavior or a combination of a viscous and elastic behavior. This is the universal characteristic of viscoelastic materials, namely, they either display elastic behavior in response to rapid deformations, or display a combination of viscous and elastic behavior in response to very slow deformations, or to deformations produced by forces applied for long time (27). Hair displays exactly the same behavior. When we deform it rapidly, as in a rapid head movement; or when we pass our fingers between the hair fibers, it behaves elastically, yet, the hair displays viscoelastic behavior when we deform it for long time. For instance, when we sleep with our hair bent or uncombed in an unwanted geometry, or in the morning when we wake up, our hair seems to stay bent and uncombed for long time, i.e., it does not recover immediately; but if we give it enough time it will remember its shape and recover gradually.

In summary, this remarkable mechanical behavior of hair is essentially due to the viscoelastic and shape-memory properties resulting from the disulfide cross-linked amorphous matrix and the keratin crystalline structure in the cortical cells. This behavior has been put in place by nature to provide an optimized assortment of mechanical properties for scalp protection and social communication—perhaps even as a part of the attractive mechanism between members of the opposite sex to facilitate propagation of the species.

The optimum mechanical and biological function of hair is thus achieved by a combination of an amorphous protein phase containing a gel and a non-gel structure, attached to the strong-coiled elastic keratin macro-fibrils. For hair to maintain this optimum combination of softness, elasticity, strength, and shape recovery, it is necessary that we keep the biological activity of its proteins unchanged. We can achieve this, first, by helping hair to keep its amorphous proteins moisturized so they are plasticized; and second, by keeping as long as possible the primary, secondary, and tertiary structure of the proteins in its native structure. We are all familiar with the fact that hair becomes hard and brittle when it lacks moisture, or with the fact that hair becomes weaker when its proteins oxidize or become brittle under the action of heat or prolonged UV radiation. We also know that hair becomes mechanically weaker after chemical treatments that we blithely apply in an attempt to look more beautiful, yet destroy strong hydrogen and covalent disulfide bonds that stabilize its tertiary structure, i.e., its crystalline structure (28, 29).

e. Water and moisture absorption/desorption by cortical cells

As in any other protein biomaterial, hair most of the time contains water, even at very low relative humidities. Water in general plays a crucial role on protein structure and function. It can be found in two states, namely, strongly bound and free or unbound water (30). In the case of hair, strongly bound water is critical for the conformation and mechanical stability of the helicoidal keratin fibrils that strand and form the macro-fibrils in the cortical cells (31). This type of water is therefore critical in maintaining the mechanical properties of hair, and it can be found in hair even after it is subjected to zero relative humidity. This behavior is found even with a few water molecules that are strongly attached to protein functional groups and can only be removed from the hair by applying high temperatures close to its denaturation temperature (32). In fact, in the case of hair, denaturation of its proteins is caused by both losses of strongly bound water *and* breakage of disulfide bonds in the protein-amorphous regions.

In most cases, protein plasticization is ascribed to water molecules whose bond strength is weaker and can be broken by the movement of thermal motions of protein chains. This type of water molecule adsorbs onto the protein chains in multilayers and, at high moisture content, takes the form of bulk water. It is the water that causes swelling in hair and in other natural biopolymers (33–36). A great deal of information on the formation of water molecule multilayers and bulk water absorbed can be obtained by looking at the shape of the water absorption isotherm of a specific material. Figure 9 shows the water absorption isotherm corresponding to hair. One can see it is sigmoidal in shape and presents a hysteresis effect (37, 38). Namely, the amount of water content in hair depends on whether we moisturize it from a dried state or whether we dry it from a wet state. In very dry hair there are a few water monolayer or nucleating sites for multilayers to form by a process of condensation, therefore, the amount of water absorption is low (line A). However, when hair is fully wet, water multilayers are already formed *inside* the hair. Under these conditions the desorption of water occurs by an evaporative process (line B).

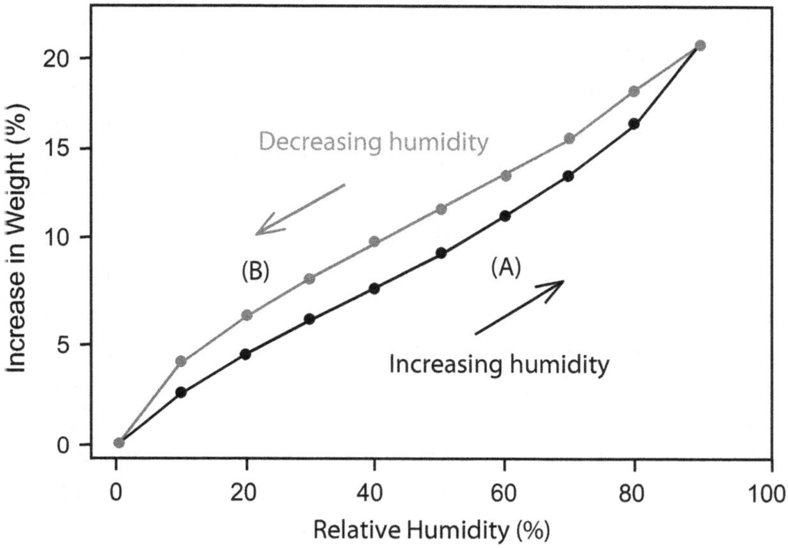

Figure 9: Water absorption isotherm of hair (37).

In total, at 100% relative humidity hair absorbs up to approximately 30% of water, and even when moisture is also absorbed by the cuticle cells and the cell membrane complex, most of the moisture is absorbed by the cortical cells (19). Many other synthetic fibers also have the ability to absorb and desorb moisture.

Surprisingly, the process of water absorption/desorption by human hair has an ulterior natural function and it is not like any other ordinary process of moisture interaction with solid matter. It is part of the physiological phenomena used by nature to provide for hair softness, thermal regulation, and sweat transport. Hair interacts with moisture in ways that no other fiber can emulate. Incidentally, wool is the only other fiber that performs like hair, but this is so because wool is also a keratin fiber with a cellular and protein architecture similar to that found in hair. Hair and wool both have water properties that, in principle, appear antagonistic, i.e., they have a hydrophobic exterior that repels water and a hydrophilic protein interior that allows it to absorb and retain water depending on the environmental moisture conditions. These unique and paradoxical properties are not shared by other synthetic fibers. This analogical behavior is at the root of why so much research in developing cosmetic hair products begins in literature reviews of wool.

Because of their cross-linked structure, hair and wool have the ability to absorb large amounts of moisture and sweat without changing their mechanical integrity. The absorption of large amounts of water by hair occurs without the hair feeling wet and soaked and without excessive weakening of its protein structure. These properties of keratin in hair contrast with those found in keratin of the skin. If we simultaneously submerge a piece of *stratum corneum* and a hair fiber in water we will observe, after a few hours, that cornoecytes in the *stratum corneum* swell without limit and lose their mechanical integrity. In contrast, the cortical and cuticle cells in the hair do not swell without limit and keep their integrity. Furthermore, as the amorphous protein matrix in hair absorbs and desorbs moisture it is able to release and gain heat depending on temperature differences between scalp and external environment. This particular behavior allows it to act as a heat buffer against rapid environmental temperature changes.

The effects of heat release upon moisture absorption by hair and wool, and their ability to keep warm surfaces is well documented (39). For instance, it is considered that if 1 kg of dry wool absorbs moisture from 40 to 70% RH it will release approximately 164 kJ (18, 32). If the wool is dried and absorbs approximately 35% of water it will release ~960 kJ of heat; this is as much heat as an electric blanket will release during eight hours. For these heat effects to take place, the wool or hair has to be dried and absorb moisture from low to higher moisture conditions. Then, as the wool or hair absorbs moisture the temperature will increase due to heat release. The water absorption isotherm of hair associated to this remarkable behavior was already shown in Figure 9; the points in this curve represent equilibrium states. The proteins in the amorphous matrix of cortical cells have various active sites for water adsorption. They are amino, carboxyl, and other hydrogen-bonding groups (40, 41). These proteins also act as nucleation centers for water multilayer adsorption. It has been reported that most of the heat released by wool or hair occurs when their hydrophilic groups absorb moisture in multilayer form at low relative humidities. At high relative humidities, moisture condensation and bulk water formation take place and there is less heat released.

3.3.1.5 DIFFERENT TYPES OF CORTICAL CELLS AND HAIR SHAPE

There are two types of cortical cells in hair; these are the ortho- and para-cortical cells (see Figure 10). Hair fibers from other mammals contain also a third type of cortical cells, namely, the meso-cortical cell, but this type of cell does not seem to be part of the human hair. There must be a reason for nature to have created two different types of cortical cells and confining them in two different sections of the cortex within the same hair fiber. Existing data, whose interpretation is still controversial, suggest that the presence of ortho- and para-cortical cells is associated to the creation and stabilization of hair shape (42–44). It appears that by creating these two types of cells, nature can control hair shape by making it straight, curly, or extremely curly as a response to environmental adaptation. For instance, the cortical cells of hair fibers that are straight and limp have been found to be mostly of the para type. In contrast, the cortical cells found in hair that is curly are of two types, namely para and ortho, and their location in the cortex is such that they fill two distinct separate regions within the cortex of the same fiber (see Figure 10). Furthermore, the ratio of para to ortho type cells varies with the degree of curliness, i.e., the higher the content of ortho-cortical cells the curlier the hair is.

In spite of their differences, the ortho- and para-cortical cells are still made mostly of keratin filaments embedded in an amorphous matrix. However, because of their different packing density, the viscoelastic response of the hair section filled with para-cortical cells should be different from the section filled with ortho-cortical cells. Furthermore, the ortho-cortical cells seem to absorb less moisture than the para-cortical cells and this should result in a lower degree of water plasticization for this type of cell. This difference in moisture plasticization and viscoelastic response between the two inner sections of a single fiber has been evoked to explain the curliness enhancement seen in wavy and curly hair when moisturized.

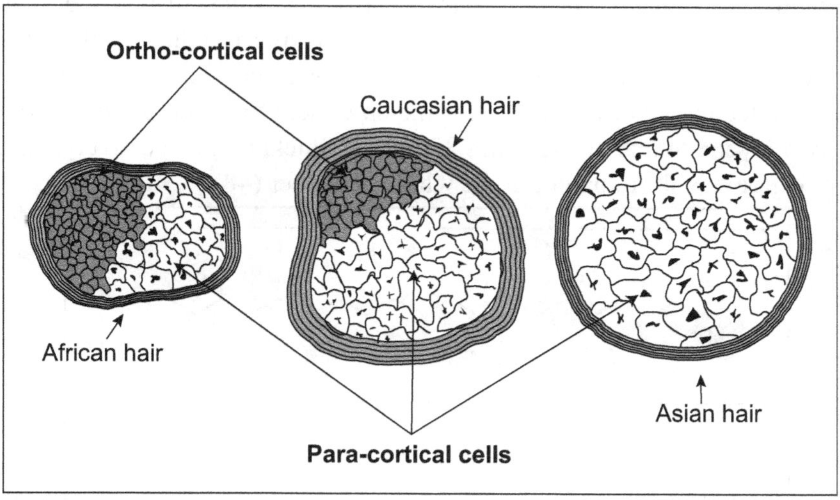

Figure 10: Schematic representation of different ratios of ortho- and para-cortical cells in African, Caucasian, and Asian hair (60).

3.3.1.6 CUTICLE CELLS AND THEIR ROLE IN HAIR PROPERTIES

a. Cuticle cell structure and composition

As the follicle produces the cortical cells from stem cells, it also creates the cuticle cells. Like the cortical cells, the activity of the living cuticle cells is also highly specialized. In the process of differentiation they are instructed to become layered and flat in shape, with a final thickness of approximately 0.5 μm (see Figure 1). Subsequently, the follicle arranges them in stacks of 5 to 11 cuticle cells like shingles on a roof all around the cortical cells to create a strong protective shield. Their flat and layered structure organized in ordered stacks allows them to form the cuticle sheath. This form of cellular envelope acts as an effective shield that protects the cortical cells against friction, mechanical abrasion, impact, and other environmental stresses. It has been put there by nature to extend the life of hair to fulfill its function. Without the cuticle sheath around the hair fibers, the cortical cells will fray out and become rapidly damaged by friction. The cuticle sheath acts also as a gate to control incoming and outgoing light from the cortex to provide protection against radiation and color for aesthetic and social communication.

All of these important property/functions of the cuticle cells would not be possible without the unique architecture of their various layers and their specific chemical composition. For instance, the very top layer of a hair fiber, called the F layer, is made up of a fatty-acid chain, the 18-methyl eicosanioc acid or 18-MEA (see Figure 11). This fatty acid chain is attached covalently to an ultra-high sulfur-rich protein on the epicuticle surface (45–47). The attachment is made in such a way that the waxy part of the 18 MEA protrudes away from the epicuticle surface to provide the highly needed lubricity and hydrophobicity of hair fibers. Beneath the monomolecular layer of 18-MEA is the epicuticle followed by the exocuticle. These two layers, which are 120 and 250 nm in thickness, respectively, have the highest degree of sulfur content in the whole hair fiber (48).

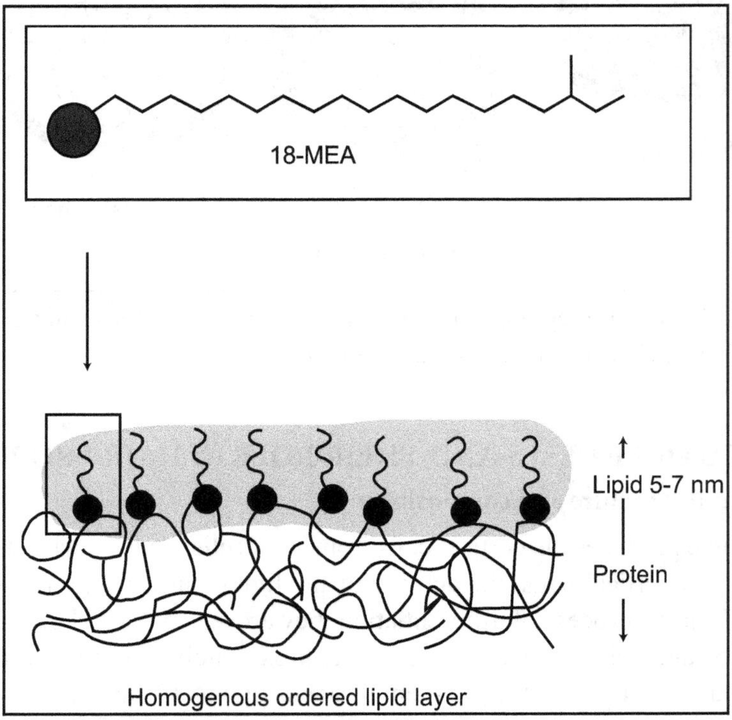

Figure 11: Representation of F layer on cuticle cell surface showing 18-MEA attached covalently to the epicuticle (47).

The high sulfur content in these layers is testimony to the high degree of cross-linking bonds needed by the proteins at the surface so that the cuticle sheath can become hard and strong in order to resist mechanical abrasion. Then, beneath the exocuticle we find the endocuticle, this layer is composed of a non-cross-linked negatively charged protein, which is very susceptible to water swelling (49). The absence of cross-linked and crystalline proteins in this layer makes it highly deformable, very soft, and somewhat weak to mechanical stresses. It has been speculated that the soft nature of this layer allows it to act as a soft viscoelastic cushion to protect the hair against mechanical impact.

Below the endocuticle one can find the cell membrane complex (CMC), which is also the extracellular material used by the cuticle cells to bind and cement together. The structure of this cementing substance is very important because it not only glues cuticle and cortical cells but also plays a crucial role in the diffusion of moisture and other chemicals into the hair cortex.

The cell membrane complex is essentially composed of three layers: the upper beta layer, the delta layer, and the lower beta layer (see Figure 12). The beta layers are made of lipid chains arranged in palisades and attached on one side covalently to their immediate near protein network on the epicuticle. The other side of the lipid palisade is not covalently bound to the proteins in the delta layer; it is rather attached by physical forces also called dispersion forces. For this reason, many researchers consider this junction to be the weakest mechanical link in the whole fiber assembly (49–52). Cuticle and cortical cells fail at this junction when hair fibers are elongated to their breaking point and when the cuticle cells chip away during dry combing. When wet, the cuticle cell fails rather at the soft protein zones in the endocuticle and not at the cell membrane complex (CMC).

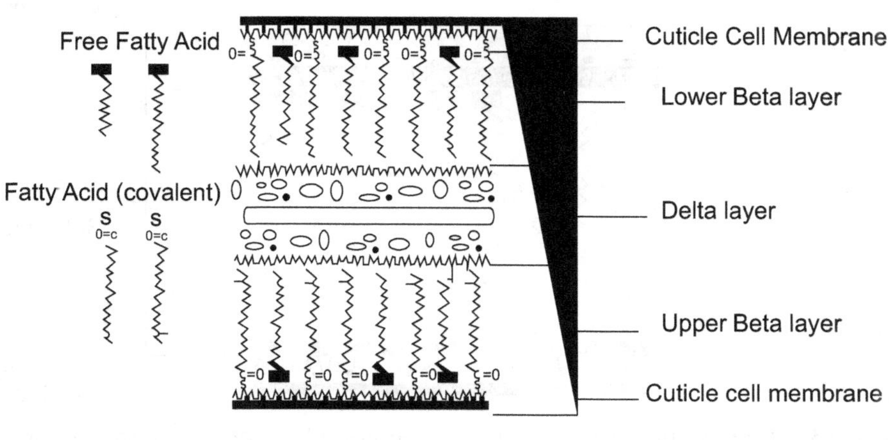

Figure 12: Representation of cell membrane complex between cuticle cells (53).

The delta layer in the CMC appears to be made of proteins that are partially hydrophilic and partially hydrophobic. This layer is considered to contribute, in great part, to the diffusion of many liquids into the cortex. In the past, it was thought that the overall composition of the CMC, with its delta layer forming a sandwich between the two beta layers, was uniform all across the hair fiber. However, recent analyses made by C. Robbins and others appear to suggest that its composition changes depending on whether the CMC is cementing the cuticle cells, the cortical cells, or the cuticle/cortical cells interface (53) (see Figure 13). It has been proposed that the beta layers in the CMC gluing the cuticle cells are made of a monolayer of 18-MEA. As it was previously explained, this fatty acid is attached covalently to the epicuticle and physically attached to the delta layer. In contrast, the beta layers gluing the cortical cells are made of bi-layers of fatty acids, cholesterol, and ceramides, all of which are only physically attached on both sides. This important proposition suggests that the lipid of choice by nature to provide for high levels of hydrophobicity and lubricity to the hair surface is 18-methyl eicosanoic acid (18-MEA).

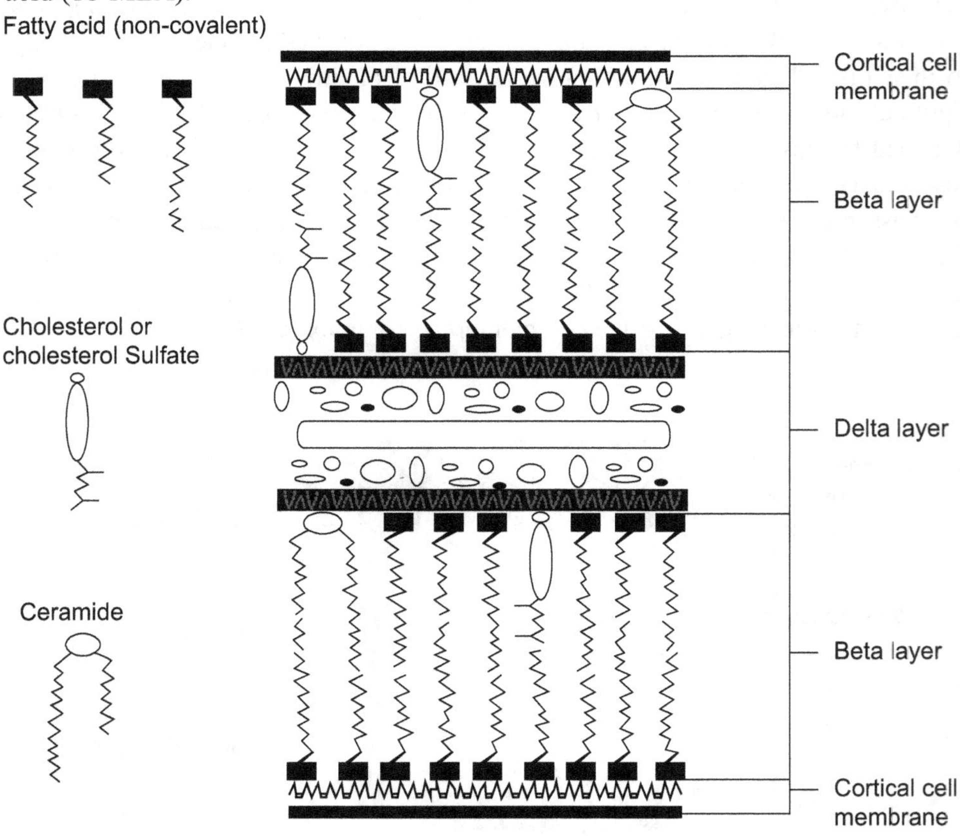

Figure 13: Representation of cell membrane complex between cortical cells of hair (53).

b. Viscoelasticity in hair and cuticle cells

The mechanical properties of the cuticle cells are just as important, if not more important, than those of the cortical cells for the function of hair. In fact, since hair is made of fibers whose length is comparably larger than their diameter, the fiber surface becomes predominant in controlling the mechanical properties of a hair assembly. Inter-fiber separation and air pocket formation for thermal regulation and aesthetic appearance are, therefore, mainly controlled by the mechanical behavior of the hair surface at the cuticle cells. Further, the integrity and mechanical stability of the cortical cells depends on the cuticle cells. Without the five to ten cuticle cells arranged in overlapping stacks to form the cuticle sheath, the cortical cells would rapidly collapse. Moreover, the surface of the cuticle cells not only has a high degree of hardness but also contains a lubricious fatty layer and is therefore very resistant to friction/abrasion. Hair fibers need this type of surface structure as they are constantly in motion, rubbing against each other.

Physical parameters relevant to these properties are the dynamic and static friction coefficients of the cuticle cells, the strength of the cuticle cell cement (CMC), and the Bending, Extension, and Compression Modulus of the cuticle cells. Unfortunately, data on the various mechanical modulus of the cuticle cells is scarce. Experimental studies carried out by various researchers have revealed, however, that the mechanical behavior of cuticle cells is not elastic but, as in the case of the cortical cells, their behavior is also viscoelastic (54, 55). This is not surprising since the proteins making the various components in hair are bio-polymers and, therefore, the overall behavior of each one of these components is also viscoelastic.

The phenomena of cuticle cell lifting and buckling produced by various environmental, mechanical, and thermal stresses, and the time it takes to recover from these deformations, are proof of cuticle cell viscoelasticity (56). Lifting and buckling of the cuticle cells occurs often in hair when subjected to continual elongation during combing, and also by thermal stresses after blow-drying or hot iron applications. Cuticle cell cement breakage and buckling are two of the most common manifestations of viscoelastic material mismatch between the various layers of the cuticle cells. When hair fibers are stressed, either thermally (by rapid compression due to water evaporation), or mechanically during excessive tensile elongation, the internal components of the single cuticle cells, i.e., the epicuticle, exocuticle, endocuticle, and cell membrane complex, do not respond in the same manner. This causes an excessive accumulation of shear stresses at their junctions and, consequently, the weakest link within the cuticle cell fails. Depending on moisture conditions, the endocuticle or the cell membrane complex fails, causing either cuticle cell buckling or breakage (52).

Cuticle cell damage in the form of cement breakage and buckling is commonplace in most people and it is significantly increased by various damaging hair treatments (54–60). This type of hair damage is almost absent in hair sections close to the fiber root and it is commonplace at its tips. Thus, a strong possibility exists that the "cement" becomes weaker by various environmental oxidative stresses during the life of a hair fiber. Gradual oxidation of the various cuticle cell layer components and their junctions will make them more prone to breakage by mechanical extensions during grooming.

Figure 14a shows a typical image of hair near its tip taken from a female subject with long hair (60). The same type of cuticle cell damage can be produced in virgin hair in the laboratory after subjecting it to large elongations and to thermal stresses (see Figure 14b). A very interesting aspect of cuticle cell buckling is that the deformations causing it can be either viscoelastically reversible or irreversible. For instance, it has been found that most of the buckling deformations produced during a hair-damaging process are reversible, i.e., the buckled cuticle cells can actually recover their original shape if enough time is allowed for recovery. There is, however, depending on the damaging process, a fraction of cuticle cells that cannot recover their shape and remain permanently and irreversibly deformed (61).

It should be pointed out here that cuticle cell buckling always entails breakage of the "cement" or cell membrane complex (CMC). This is true regardless of whether the deformations in them are reversible or irreversible. In most cases, once the cuticle cells have undergone buckling their mechanical integrity is compromised. For instance, simple hair-strand swelling by water absorption and the resulting stresses are not capable of inducing cuticle cell lifting and buckling in virgin cuticle cells. Yet, after they undergo buckling, and after the cells have recovered from their deformations, they can be easily lifted and buckled again by simple water imbibition and resulting swelling. Studies have shown, however, that in certain cases the cell membrane complex by itself may have the ability to partially re-cement and re-glue the cuticle cells (61, 62). For instance, experiments have shown that, if deformed and lifted cuticle cells whose cement is broken are allowed to recover closing their gap, they will not lift again when immersed in water. In many cases the previously buckled and recovered cells will only buckle again when the levels of mechanical stresses are similar to the ones that initially produced cell lifting. This observation seems to indicate that, under certain conditions, the "cement" is able to partially re-cement the cuticle cells.

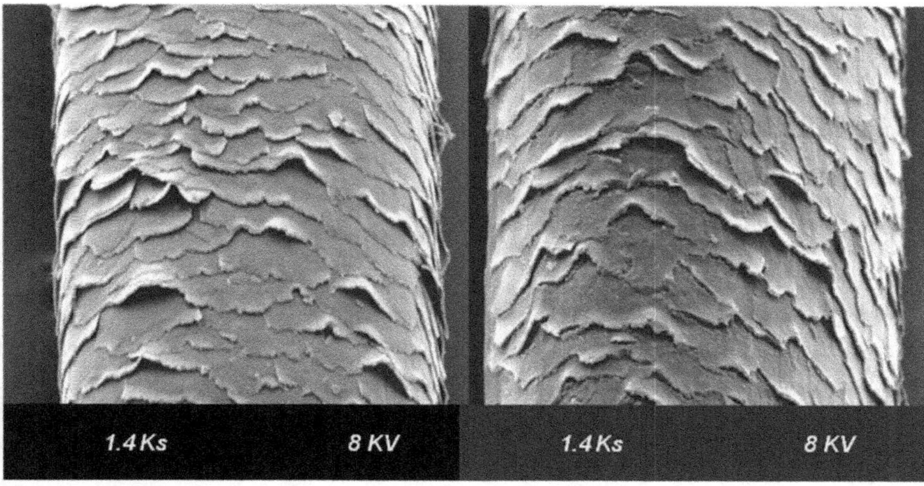

Figures 14a and 14b: SEM pictographs of cuticle cell buckling in hair as follows: (14a) as it appeared in a long hair of a female subject, and (14b) produced in the laboratory by mechanical stresses in an undamaged hair fiber (60).

c. Water and moisture absorption/desorption by cuticle cells

In the previous paragraphs we have pointed out that moisture absorption by the cortical cells has beneficial effects for the function of hair; among these benefits are scalp/skin temperature buffering, moisture transport, and a large contribution to softness/plasticization of hair fibers. We also pointed out that water is the main protein plasticizer, and we came to the conclusion that moisture makes hair softer because it plasticizes the amorphous protein in the cortex. An observation that is often ignored by many researchers studying keratin fibers is that the cuticle cells also absorb moisture and, most importantly, that their mechanical behavior is very sensitive to moisture. The strongest evidence of this sensitivity is the effect that moisture has on cuticle cell recovery from deformations that were caused by stress buckling. Figure 15a shows an SEM picture of a hair fiber whose cuticle cells underwent buckling deformations after the fiber was subjected to a mechanical elongation of about 15%. The same hair fiber with its cuticle cells recovered is shown in Figure 15b, where recovery of the buckled cuticle cells took place after the fiber was immersed in water absorption (61, 64). Likewise, Figure 16a shows a micrograph of deformed and buckled cuticle cells produced in hair by blow-drying in the presence of water and low-molecular-weight oils (58); while in Figure 16b the same hair fiber can be viewed with its cuticle cells recovered after they were allowed to absorb moisture. The pictures were obtained by optical microscopy using the technique of patterns of light interference analysis described in more detail in the following paragraphs.

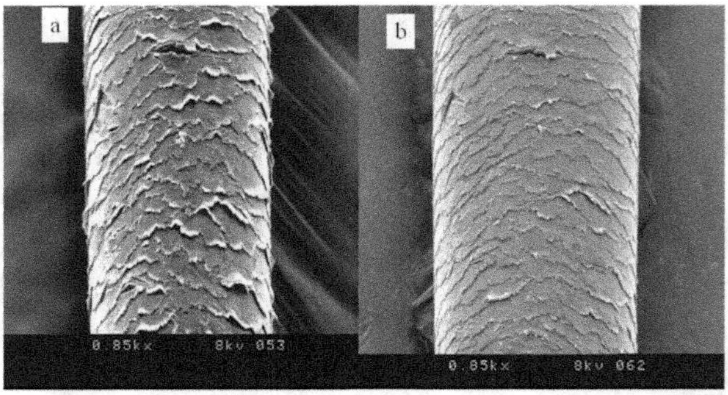

Figures 15a and 15b: SEM micrographs of cuticle cell buckling before (15a) and after water immersion (15b). Both micrographs correspond to the same spot in the hair fiber. As a point of reference, observe the elongated deep crack in the top section of the hair fiber (60).

Experimental observations made on those cuticle cells as depicted in Figures 16a show that their deformations do not recover if they are left alone for a good period of time at normal temperature (25°C) and under moisture conditions (53% RH). The experiments showed, rather, that the deformed and buckled cuticle cells recover only when moisture condenses on the cuticle cells, i.e., when the hair surface is above the dew point (65). These simple observations indicate the following: a) that cuticle cells need to absorb liquid water and not gaseous water molecules to recover by water plasticization and, b) that protein moisturization in the cuticle cells only occurs when multilayer adsorption occurs at protein chains by moisture condensation.

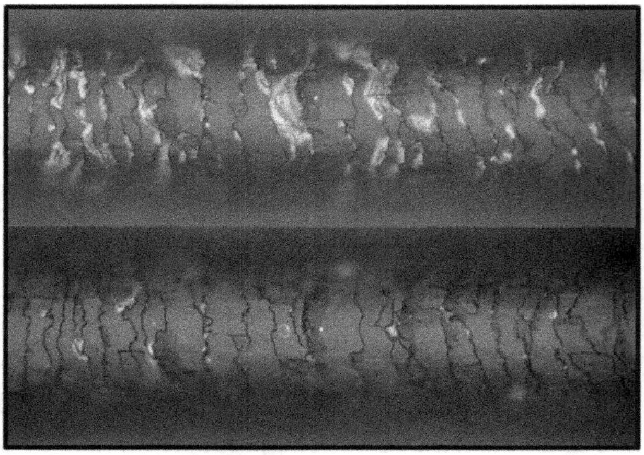

Figures 16a and 16b: Optical micrographs of buckled cuticle cells observed in a hair fiber blow-dried in the presence of low-molecular-weight oils by using the LIP technique (54). Figure 26a represents the state of the cuticles after the hair fiber was blow-dried, and Figure 16b shows the cuticle cells after the hair was immersed in water for a period of one minute (60).

Moisture absorption by the cuticle cells is thus crucial for the cells to recover from deformations and to comply mechanically with the deformation of the cortex and the whole hair fiber. Just as in the case of cortical cells, cuticle cells are also able to perform their beneficial function in hair if they are plasticized by water, i.e., "moisturized." It is important to mention here that the subjective perception of "hair dryness" is de facto associated to a lack of moisture in the cortical cells. However, studies have shown that this is an incorrect conception since hair swatches that were equilibrated at high relative humidities seemed to obtain higher "dryness perception" scores than those equilibrated at low relative humidities (66). An explanation of these contradictory facts has already been offered by some scientists. They have proposed that roughness on the hair surface, and not lack of moisture in the cortex, is what creates the perception of dryness in hair (66). Moisture content in the cuticle cells should, therefore, have a stronger correlation with the sensation of hair dryness.

d. Optical properties of the cuticle cells

Another important property of the cuticle cells is their optical set of properties. All the various layers composing the cuticle cells are transparent. When white light strikes a hair assembly the first component it encounters is the cuticle sheath. The main physical property that determines how a transparent material interacts with light is its index of refraction (IR). The IR of the cuticle sheath has been reported to be ~1.53 (67); the IR of each cuticle layer is not known, but because each one has a different composition and architecture, it is expected that its behavior will be somewhat different. The behavior of white light striking the cuticle cell—just as in the case of other transparent materials—thus, will be dependent on the IR of each layer. Its value will thus determine how much light is reflected, refracted, and absorbed by the cuticle cells. Reflected light can be of two types, specular or diffuse. If the reflected light is specular it will give rise to shine; if it is diffuse it will give a matt and dull appearance to hair. Light that is refracted passes through the cuticle cells and reaches the cortex, where it interacts with the pigments of melanin. There, a certain wavelength component of the light will be absorbed and the remainder of the light, which will not be white any more but colored, will be reflected back into the cuticle cells. The light will pass, then, throughout the cuticle cells and will appear to the eye as hair color (see Figure 17). If part of the light diffracts, penetrates into the cortex, and is absorbed by the melanin granules, the hair color will appear shiny and black, brown, or blond depending on the type of melanin. As it will be seen later, brown and blond colors are produced by different amounts of a brown melanin granule called eumelanin.

The condition of the cuticle cells thus determines the optical appearance of the hair assembly. If the cuticle cell cement is broken and the cuticle cells are lifted, light will not be properly transmitted to the cortex, and neither will it be specularly reflected. Rather, the light will be scattered and diffused and the hair will partially lose its shine and color, thereby, appearing dull and lifeless. Recently, it has been found that, either, when the cuticle cells are lifted, or whenever there are micro-pockets of air within the cuticle cell layers, the cuticle cells produce colorful microscopic light-interference patterns (LIPs) (see Figures 18a and 18b) (56). It is important to mention here that the vivid colors found in insects, butterflies, birds, and also in some mammals str created by such light-interference phenomena. These colors are usually very strong and they are not created by subtraction of colors from white light due to absorption by pigments. Rather they are created by the same mechanism used by soap bubbles to create color—a phenomenon based on the constructive and destructive interference of light (see Figure 19). This phenomenon is also known as iridescence, and the colors are called structural colors (68, 69). In the case of hair, if the interference colors produced by lifted cuticle cells could be made coherent at the macroscopic level, they would create strong and vivid colors.

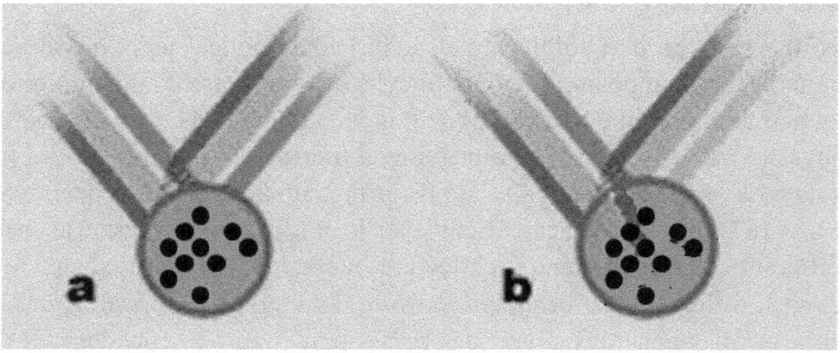

Figure 17: Diagrammatic representation of light interacting with hair showing (a) total reflection of colors, and (b) light reflection plus diffraction and absorption by melanin granules.

Unfortunately, the lifted cuticle cell areas containing air in their layers creating these strong LIPs are very small, and light-scattering edge effects dominate. In addition, because of the small size and discontinuity in the lifted cuticle cells, the strong interference colors are not coherent at the macroscopic level. Consequently, their final effect to hair appearance is rather deleterious. However, the weak patterns of iridescence produced by the layered structure of undamaged cuticle cells certainly will contribute to the final optical appearance of hair. Colored light coming from the melanin in the cortex will thus combine with colored light produced by the weak iridescent patterns of virgin cuticle cells, and both, just as in the case of cuticle cells of some mammals, should produce the final hair optical properties. Thus, the weak iridescence patterns of virgin cuticle cells contribute to the unique color properties of undamaged hair.

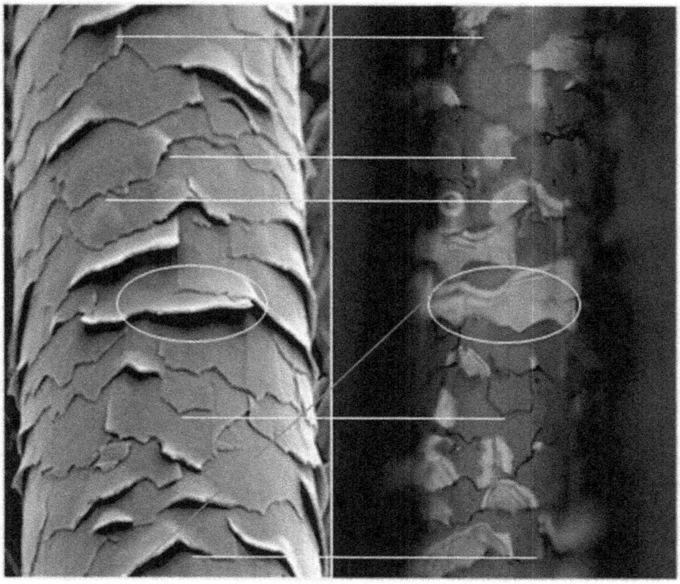

Figure 18: Micrographs showing lifted and buckled cuticle cells on the same fiber by SEM (left), and by optical microscopy (right) using the LIP technique. Lines and circles in the pictures identify same features (56).

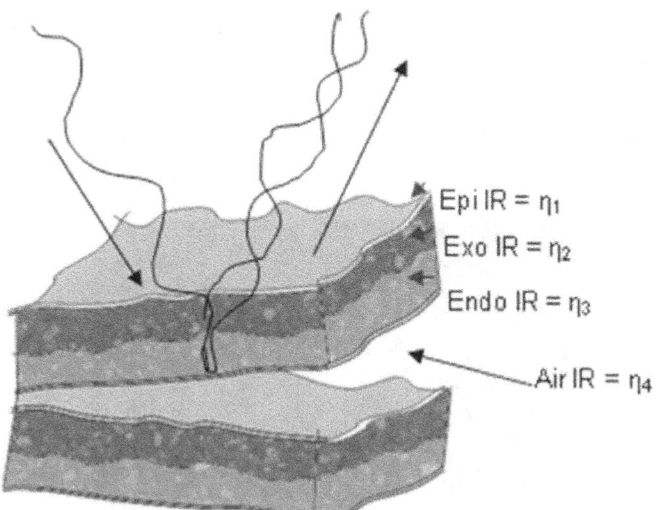

Figure 19: Diagram of lifted cuticle cells describing formation of light interference patterns by the phenomenon of thin-film light interference (56)

The color and shine enhancement often seen in hair when wet is a typical example of improved hair color perception due to changes in the IR of the cuticle sheath. Color enhancement in wet objects that absorb water can thus be explained by two mechanisms. The first is by the decrease in light scattering due to water filling of the otherwise empty pores containing air. The second is color and shine enhancement in hair by moisture absorption, also due to changes in the IR of the endocuticle, which enhances the phenomenon of iridescence. Polydimethylsiloxane polymers, oils, and some other high-molecular-weight polymers can also produce similar effects—as long as they are able either to penetrate into air gaps at the cuticle sheath or to smooth the cuticle cell surface to eliminate diffuse scattering.

e. The medulla cells

The medulla in hair refers to a region of very low density located at the center of a hair fiber (11). It is considered to be porous, irregular in shape; and, in human hair, in most cases, it is not continuous all along a single hair fiber. The regions of low density can be detected either by scanning electron microscopy or by optical microscopy (see Figure 20). In Figure 21, we can see a photograph showing the discontinuous presence of medulla along the hair fiber by which the hair was analyzed by transmission using optical microscopy (70). Not all hair fibers have medulla, but it is frequently found in thicker hair. Analyses have shown that, even in the case of thick hair, hair fibers from the same head may or may not have medulla cells. The medulla region is made of cells that are very different in structure to the cortical and cuticular cells; they are large and cuboidal in shape, and often, but not always, they are very porous. The structure, composition, and role of the medulla cells are not very well known. Because of their porous structure, the medulla cells are filled with air and it has been speculated that this cell-air system contributes to increase the hair's ability to provide thermal insulation. The medulla cells have also been reported to have a strong impact on hair optical properties (71).

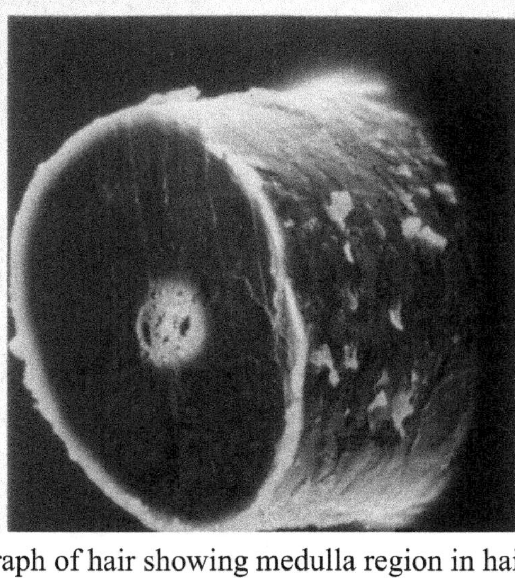

Figure 20: Micrograph of hair showing medulla region in hair (60).

3.3.1.7 MELANIN PIGMENTS IN HAIR

The melanin pigments in hair are made of very interesting molecules that play a crucial role in the function of hair. They act as free radical scavengers, antioxidants, UV light absorbers, heat radiation absorbers, and also as gamma rays absorbers (72–74). Melanin pigments not only protect the proteins in hair against oxidation and UV damage, but also help to protect the scalp from excessive harmful UV and heat radiation. They also provide color to hair for aesthetic and social communication. The protective action of melanin pigments is so important that nature does not use melanin only in hair, but also in the neurons of the brain as well as in the cells of eyes. Melanin has been found to provide important protection effects to the eyes; among these are the following: photoprotection, vision enhancement, decreases in the risk of cataract formation, and a lower risk of macular degeneration in the retina (73, 74).

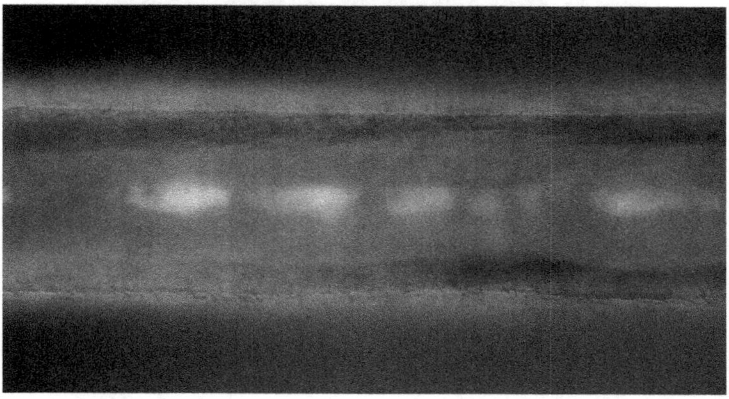

Figure 21: Micrograph showing discontinuity of medulla region along a hair fiber (60).

Melanin granules in hair are approximately 0.8 μm in diameter (see Figure 22). They are polymeric in nature and depending on their type they differ chemically. The various chemical moieties forming the melanin polymer are 5,6-dihydroxyindole (DHI) and 5,6-dihydroxyindole-2-carboxylic acid molecules (75, 76). A description of their composition is given in Figure 23. Melanin granules isolated from hair or skin display brown, black, green, and yellow colors.

There are many types of melanin and they can be grouped into two main types, namely, eumelanins and pheomelanins. Eumelanins can be further divided into brown and dark eumelanins. Brown eumelanin is common in people with lighter or brown color while dark melanin is typical of people with dark hair. Gray hair is caused by the absence of melanin in general while blond hair is produced by low amounts of brown eumelanin. Red hair contains mainly pheomelanin as pigment, which is also found in small amounts in skin together with eumelanin. The melanin granules are made in the follicle not by the cortical or cuticular cells, but rather, by specialized cells called melanocytes. Once the pigment granules are made, the melanocytes get instructions to excrete them and pass them into the cortical cells, where they are incorporated by phagocytosis (76, 77).

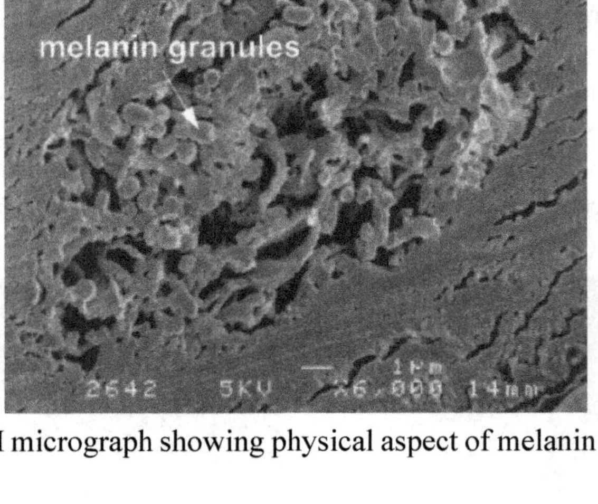

Figure 22: SEM micrograph showing physical aspect of melanin pigments in hair SEM (72–75).

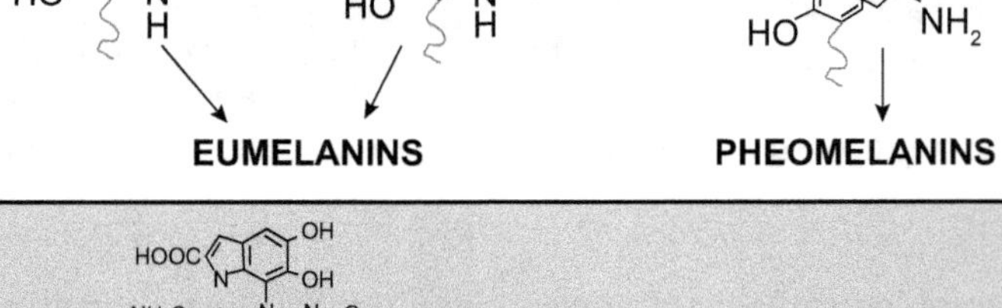

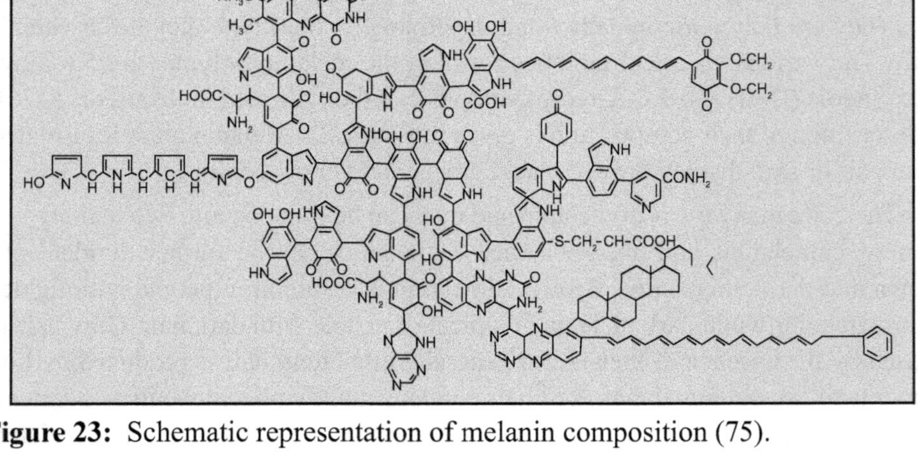

Figure 23: Schematic representation of melanin composition (75).

3.3.1.8 HAIR FUNCTION

As discussed in the previous paragraphs, the sequences of amino acids constituting the primary, secondary, tertiary, and quaternary structures in the proteins of hair are optimized so the fibers are capable of fulfilling their biological functions. Other biological substances in hair—such as lipids, polysaccharides, and complex polymeric molecules—are found in the cuticular cement and in the melanin pigments. These are also carefully structured in the hair cells to fulfill a specific function. This optimization of composition and structure in the cells occurs so that hair can, finally, serve its biological functions of temperature buffer by absorption/desorption of water, protection against harmful environmental radiation, thermal and mechanical insulation, and aesthetic agent in social communication. Hair with an undamaged structure is apt to perform its biological function, and it is not coincidental that undamaged hair is also aesthetically and cosmetically appealing.

3.3.1.9 THE FOLLICLE

As we have stated earlier, the follicle is the smallest organ in the body, and it is there where hair fibers are produced (see Figure 3). Also acknowledged previously, there is one single follicle for each hair fiber. This minute organ is essentially composed of various biological units, namely: bulb, dermal papilla, bulge, and external and internal root sheath (78). With these key basic units, follicles are able to produce and assemble hair cells to form hair fibers. There are between 100,000 and 150,000 follicles in a normal scalp, distributed on its surface in the form of clusters of three or four hair follicles (see Figure 24). Evidence suggests that the number of hair follicles is constant throughout one's life, so the number of hair fibers on a scalp will, at least, while one is alive, remain constant. The hair follicle, with all its basic internal units, regenerates itself approximately every four to six years. At each regeneration cycle, the hair fiber that has been produced falls out, and a new one starts to grow.

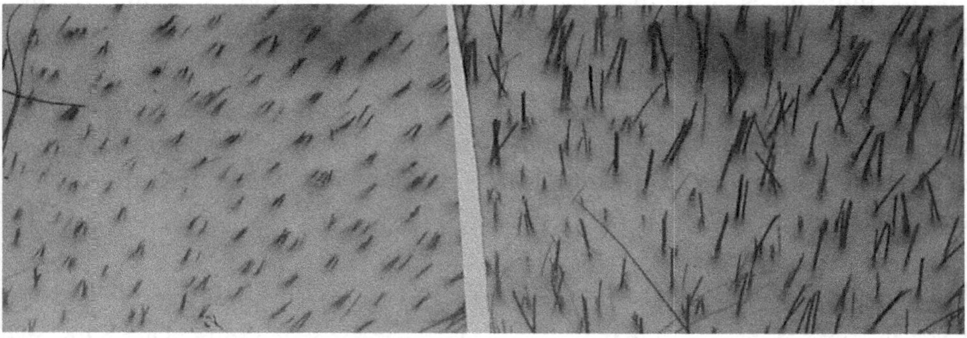

Figure 24: Clusters of various follicles in scalp (60).

a. Different zones in the follicle

All cells forming a hair fiber are made in the follicle from stem cells (79–81). The manufacture of hair cells involves a very well-organized process of stem cell preparation, shaping, and assembly in a way that is akin to a car assembly line. These various processes occur from bottom to top of the follicle in three main zones; namely: a zone of cell proliferation; a zone of gene expression and differentiation, and, finally, a zone of cell hardening or keratinization (see Figure 3) (11).

Each zone within the follicle has specific tasks crucial for hair production. At the bottom of the follicle is the first zone, and it is constituted by the dermal papilla and basal membrane. It is in this zone where epithelial stem cells that descend from the bulge are gathered to receive instructions from the dermal papilla to proliferate by mitosis. Moving towards the tip, in the next contiguous zone, the cells obtain instructions also from the dermal papilla to become differentiated into cuticle, cortical, and medulla cells. During this process they are packed and glued together, forming a cylindrical shape. Moving further towards the tip in the following third zone, located in the middle portion of the follicle, the hair cells are instructed to undergo apoptosis and become hard through a process of keratinization. In this zone, proteins in the cortical and cuticle cells become cross-linked to attain their final optimized, mechanical, thermal, and physical properties. In the zone of keratinization the hair reaches its final form and emerges from the scalp.

Just as in a car assembly line, where total production is controlled by external demands and internal constraints, there has to be a very well-coordinated process of communication within the follicle itself and with other body glands to successfully produce hair. For a period of approximately four to six years each hair follicle is instructed to keep its key components active making hair. The new portions of hair created in the follicle push out upper sections of the fibers and the hair grows. At the end of the sixth year of activity, the follicle gets instructions from the body's glands and genetic system to cease and stop the production of hair. The ancillary machinery in the various zones of the follicle is then shut down, and the three zones of the follicle become completely inactive. Subsequently, the key components of the follicle are dismantled and discarded as they are pushed out by new ones being formed underneath. In this way, the old grown hair fibers, together with their inactive follicle units, are pushed out from the scalp and the hair fibers fall out. The new components form a new follicle with new zones of cell proliferation, gene expression/differentiation, and cell keratinization, and a new hair fiber grows.

b. Life cycle of the follicle

From the time of its inception until it recedes, the regenerated follicle has a life cycle characterized by three different phases, namely: anagen, catagen, and telogen (see Figure 25) (82). In the anagen phase, the assembly line activity of the hair follicle is invigorated and has its maximum efficiency preparing and assembling cells into fibers. It is at this stage that the hair fibers in the three zones of cell creation, differentiation, and keratinization are continuously assembling and growing. An intensive production of cuticle and cortical cells via stem cell mitosis characterizes this stage. The produced cells are continuously shaped and assembled into hair fibers by instructions from the dermal papilla in coordination with other body glands. For instance, it is well known that the growth rate of hair is strongly dependent on certain hormones and that it is used by nature as a tool of social communication to assert gender differentiation. During the anagen phase most of the hair fibers thus acquire their main physical, mechanical, thermal, and optical properties. The overall characteristics of hair fibers are therefore dependent on nutritional and hormonal variations affecting this stage of follicle development. Then, in the catagen phase, which lasts only two to four weeks, the follicle lowers its cell production and a large part of its cells undergo apoptosis. In the telogen phase, which lasts only from two to three months, the inactive parts of the follicle are pushed out and the old hair falls out.

New research has actually shown that the activity of the follicle is even more complicated than described in the three stages mentioned above. Some researchers have already proposed the existence of various substages for each one of the three main phases (83). There are two main reasons behind these proposals:

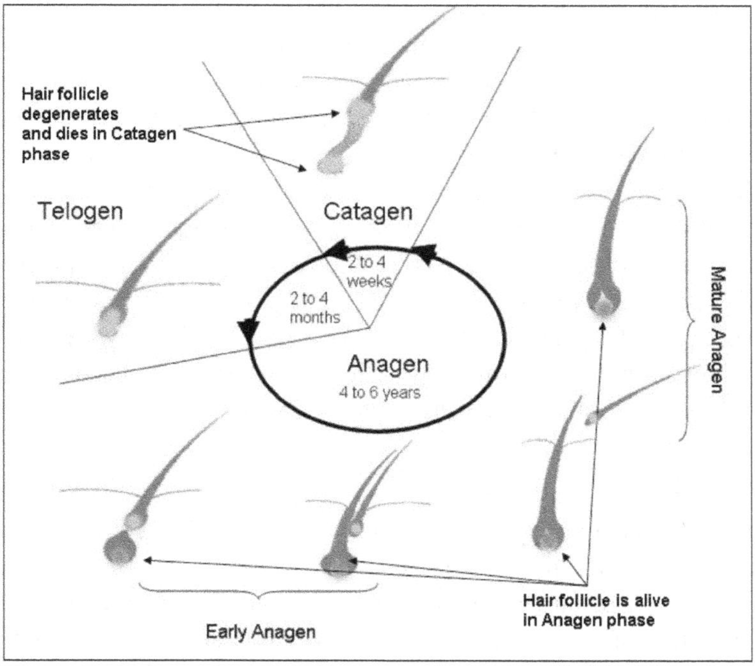

Figure 25: Life cycle of the follicle: anagen, catagen, and telogen (60).

namely, a) each stage has very well-differentiated activities that can be further divided, and b) it has been found that at the end of each stage there are already preparatory signals taking place for the next stage. In fact, the appearance of new follicle components producing a new hair fiber starts in the follicle even before the older fiber is pushed out; so the anagen phase of a new growing hair fiber in some cases overlaps with the telogen phase of a hair that is going to fall. Thus, some of the processes controlling the formation of new hair fibers and the shedding of old ones seem to overlap between phases. This process can easily be perceived in the picture of human scalp shown in Figure 24, where it can be seen that in certain areas there are two hair fibers emerging from the same follicle.

All processes taking place in the follicle, whether they occur in the anagen, catagen, or telogen phase, or in any of their substages, need to occur in synchrony. Their occurrence involves the timely interaction and participation of a large number of biopeptides, enzymes, and other biological factors that act as regulators, communicators, and controlling agents for the production of stem cells, cells division, cell apoptosis, keratinization, etc. Furthermore, the maintenance process of the hair shaft, after it has emerged from the scalp in all its length, is partially executed by the biological activity of the follicle. Sebum and enzymes are released from the sebaceous glands in concert with the follicle to maintain the integrity of the hair shaft.

Hair diseases, hair defects, or mechanical weaknesses in hair fibers are caused by internal or external factors that interfere, block, change, or damage the various biological processes involved in normal hair growth and hair maintenance. Traction alopecia, androgenetic alopecia, chemical alopecia, trichorrhexis nodosa, etc. are all hair ailments caused by some sort of internal or external interference. It has recently been discovered that the follicle is the target of major hormonal pathways, and that the follicle and sebum glands, both together, referred to as the pilosebaceous unit, can also act as a peripheral hormone-producing unit for a wide range of steroid hormones, neuropeptides, and neutrophins (84). Thus, proper growth of new hair fibers and shedding of old ones require no obstruction or interference with the biochemical substances involved within the follicle. Any internal or external factor interfering with the function of these biochemical substances will cause some sort of malfunctioning or disease in hair growth.

Acknowledgments

The author would like to thank Linda Foltis for her helpful discussions and support during the writing of the manuscript. Thanks also to Ashland, Inc. for providing the opportunity and resources to carry out this task. The editor-in-chief, Meyer R. Rosen, would like to thank Manuel Gamez-Garcia and Linda Foltis for an extraordinary, in-depth, diversely technical exploration of the physical and chemical nature of hair. We believe that knowledge at this depth will generate new ideas for ingredients and mechanistic approaches that address consumer needs in an aging society, which are strongly needed as hair and its appearance, both in women and men, is a major factor in the look-good, feel-good search occurring during the inevitable(?) aging process.

REFERENCES

1) F. Alan, Structure and mechanism in protein science: a guide to enzyme catalysis and protein folding. San Francisco: W.H. Freeman. (1999), ISBN 0-7167-3268-8.

2) F.J. Wortmann, G. Sendelbach, and C. Popescu, "Fundamental DSC Investigations of Alpha-Keratinous Materials as Basis for the Interpretation of Specific Effects of Chemical, Cosmetic Treatments on Human Hair," J. Cosmet. Scie, Vol. 58.

3) M. Lewin, Handbook of Fiber Chemistry 3th edition by CRC Press Taylor and Lewis Group, Boca Raton, Florida.

4) I.D. Kuntz, W. Kaufmann. Hydration of Proteins & Polypeptides. Adv Prot Chem (1974) 28:239-345.311-317, July/August.

5) L. Kubisz, The influence of storage time on the temperature dependence of the dc electrical conductivity of horn keratin, Bioelectrochemistry 53, 2001, 161–164.

6) R. Moll, M. Divo, and L. Langbein, The human keratins: biology and pathology, Histochem Cell Biol. 2008 June; 129(6): 705–733;

7) N.O. Ku, P. Strnad, BH Zhong, GZ Tao, and M.B. Omary, Keratins let liver live: Mutations predispose to liver disease and crosslinking generates Mallory-Denk bodies, Hepatology. 2007 Nov;46(5):1639–49.

8) M. Toni , L.D. Valle , and L. Alibardi, Hard (Beta-) Keratins in the Epidermis of Reptiles: Composition, Sequence, and Molecular Organization, Proteome Res., 2007, 6 (9), pp 3377–3392

9) P.A. Coulombe, X. Tong, S. Mazzalupo, Z. Wang, P Wong, Great promises yet to be fulfilled: defining keratin intermediate filament function in vivo, Eur J Cell Biol. 2004 Dec;83(11–12):735–46.

10) E. Fuchs E, Keratins and the skin, Annu Rev Cell Dev Biol. 1995;11:123–53.

11) C. Robbins, "Chemical and Physical Behavior of Human Hair" 3th. Ed. Springer-Verlag, New York, 1994, pp. 211–206

12) R.C. Marshall, D.F. Orwin, J.M. Gillespie, Structure and biochemistry of mammalian hard keratin, Electron Microsc Rev. 1991;4(1):47–83.

13) D.A. Parry, Hard alpha-keratin intermediate filaments: an alternative interpretation of the low-angle equatorial X-ray diffraction pattern, and the axial disposition of putative disulphide bonds in the intra- and inter-protofilamentous networks, Int J Biol Macromol. 1996 Jul;19(1):45–50.

14) L.N. Jones, F.M. Pope, Isolation of intermediate filament assemblies from human hair follicles, J Cell Biol. 1985 Oct;101(4):1569–77.

15) M. Feughelman, A Two Phase Structure for Keratin Fibers, Text., Res., J. 29: 223–228.

16) N.G. Jabloski, Skin; A Natural History, University of California Press LTD (2008).

17) J. A. Kushlan, The Evolution of Hairlessness in Man, The American Naturalist, Vol. 116, No. 5 (Nov., 1980), pp. 727–729, Published by: The University of Chicago Press

18) W.S. Simpson and G.H Crawshaw, Wool Science and Technology, CRC Press LLC, Boca Raton Florida, 2002

19) FJ Wortmann, A Hullmann, C Popescu, Water sorption performance of human hair and the influences of cosmetic products and processes, 15th International Hair-Science Symposium HairS'07; 12 Sep 2007–14 Sep 2007; Kloster Banz, Bad Staffelstein, Germany. 2007.

20) M. Feughelman, "Mechanical Properties and Structure of alpha-Keratin Fibres; Wool, Human Hair, and Related Fibers," Published by University of New South Wales Press, 1997

21) L. Kreplak et-al, A New Deformation Model of Hard-Keratin Fibers at the Nanometer Scale: Implications for Hard-Keratin Intermediate Filament Mechanical Properties, Biophysical Journal Volume 82 April 2002 2265–2274

22) D. V. Istrate, M. Heat induced denaturation of fibrous hard α-keratins and their reaction with various chemical reagents, PhD Dissertation Thesis, Aachen University, June 2011.

23) E.G. Bendit, A quantitative X-ray diffraction study of the alpha-beta transformation in wool keratin. Textile Res J 1960 30: 547.

24) I. M. Ward, J. Sweeney, Mechanical Properties of Solid Polymers, Publisher: John Wiley & Sons Inc, December, 2012

25) A. Lendlein, S. Kelch, "Shape-memory polymers." Angew. Chem. Int. Ed. 41: 2034–2057, (2002).

26) H. H. Winter, Viscous Dissipation in Shear Flows of Molten Polymers, Advances in Heat Transfer, Vol. 13, 1977

27) J. J. Aklonis, Introduction to Polymer Viscoelasticity, Wiley , 1995

28) M. L. Tate, Y. K. Kamath, S. B. Reutsch, and H.D. Weigmann, Quantification and prevention of hair damage, J. Soc. Cosmet. Chem., 44, 347–371, (November/December 1993);

29) F.J. Wortmann, C. Springob, G. Sendelbach, Investigations of cosmetically treated human hair by differential scanning calorimetry in water, J Cosmet Sci. 2002 Jul-Aug;53 (4): 219–28.

30) A.B. Hughes, Amino Acids, Peptides, and Proteins in Organic Chemistry, Vol-5 Analysis and Function of Amino Acids and Peptides, pp. 317–318, Wiley-VCH, Verlag and Co., Weinheim, Germany, 2012.

31) P. Milczarek, M. Zielinski, and M.L. Garcia, "The Mechanism and Stability of thermal Transition in Hair Keratin," Colloid & Polymer Science, Vol. 270, Num. 11, pp. 1106–1115.

32) E. Menefee, G. Yee, Thermally-Induced Structural Changes in Wool, Textile Research Journal September 1965 vol. 35 no. 9 801–812

33) P. Zuidema, L.E. Govaert, F.P.T. Baaijens, P.A.J. Ackermans, and S. Asvadi, The influence of humidity on the viscoelastic behaviour of human hair, Biorheology 40 (2003) 431–439

34) D.H. Johnson, Hair and Hair Care, Cosmetic Science and Technology Series, Vol 17, Marcel Dekker 1997, Phoenix Arizona;

35) Y.H. Roos, Phase Transitions in Food Engineering Vol-1, Academic Press, San Diego California, 1995;

36) H Maeda, Water in keratin. Piezoelectric, dielectric, and elastic experiments, Biophys J. 1989 November; 56(5): 861–868.

37) H.J. White, An Experimental and Theoretical Study of the Adsorption and Swelling Isotherms of Human Hair in Water Vapor, Textile Research Journal March 1949 vol. 19 no. 3 136–151

38) Y. K. Kamath, Effect of oil films on moisture vapor absorption on human hair, J. Cosmet. Sci., 58, 135–145 (March/April 2007)

39) A. B. D. Cassie, Absorption of water by wool, Trans. Faraday Soc., 1945,41, 458–464;

40) J. D. Leeder , I. C. Watt, The Role of Amino Groups in Water Absorption by Keratin, J. Phys. Chem., 1965, 69 (10), pp 3280–3284

41) I. C. Watt and J. D. Leeder, Role of Carboxyl Groups in Water Absorption by Keratin, J. appl. Chem., Vol. 18, January 1968

42) Y. Kajiura, S. Watanabe, T. Itou, K. Nakamura, A. Iida, K. Inoue, N. Yagi, Y. Shinohara, Y. Amemiya, Structural analysis of human hair single fibres by scanning microbeam SAXS, J Struct . Biol. 2006 Sep; 155(3):438–44.

43) S. Thibaut, P. Barbarat, F. Leroy, B.A. Bernard, Human hair keratin network and curvature, Int. J. Dermatol. 2007 Oct; 46 Suppl 1:7–10

44) B.A. Bernard, Hair shape of curly hair, J. Am. Acad. Dermatol. 2003 Jun; 48 (6 Suppl) S 120–6

45) L. N. Jones and D. E. Rivett, Role of 18-methyleicosanoic acid in the structure and formation of mammalian hair fibers, Micron, 28, 469 (1997).

46) U. Natarajan and C. Robbins, The thickness of 18-MEA on an ultra-high-sulfur protein surface by molecular modeling, J. Cosmet. Sci., 61, 467–477 (November/December 2010)

47) S. Breakspear, J.R. Smith, G. Luengo, Effect of the covalently linked fatty acid 18-MEA on the nanotribology of hair's outermost surface, Journal of Structural Biology, 149, (2005), pp 235–242

48) N.H. Leon, Structural aspects of keratin fibres, J. Soc.Cosmet. Chem. 23, pp. 427–445 (1972)

49) C. Robbins, H.D. Weigmann, S. Ruetsch, Y. Kamath, Failure of intercellular adhesion in hair fibers with regard to hair condition and strain conditions, J Cosmet Sci. 2004 Jul-Aug; 55 (4): pp. 351–71.

50) J.R. Smith and J.A. Swift, Lamellar subcomponents of the cuticular cell membrane complex of mammalian keratin fibers show friction and hardness contrast by AFM, J Microsc. 2002 Jun; 206 (Pt 3): pp. 182–93

51) A. Swift, The Hair Surface, in Hair Research, ed. By Orfanos Montagna, Stuttgen-Springer-Verlag, New York, 1994, pp. 211–226

52) S. B. Reutsch, H. D. Weigmann, "Mechanism of Tensile Stress Release in the Keratin Fiber Cuticle I," J. Soc. Cosmet. Chem., Vol. 47, pp. 13–26, (1996)

53) C. Robbins, The cell membrane complex: three related but different cellular cohesion components of mammalian hair fibers, J Cosmet Sci. 2009 Jul-Aug; 60 (4): 437–65

54) M. Gamez-Garcia, "The Cracking of Human Hair Cuticles by Cyclical Thermal Stresses," J. Soc. Cosmet. Chem., 49, 141–153 (1998)

55) M. Gamez-Garcia, "Cuticle De-cementation and Cuticle Buckling Produced by Poisson Contraction on the Cuticular Envelope of Human Hair," J. Soc.Cosmet. Chem., Vol 49, pp. 213–222, (1998).

56) M. Gamez-Garcia, Patterns of Light Interference Produced by Damaged Cuticle Cells in Human hair," J.Cosmet. Sci., Vol 58, No. 4, pp. 269–282, (July/August 2007)

57) R. McMullen and J. Jachowicz, "Thermal Degradation of Hair I. Effect of Curling Irons," J. Cosmet. Sci. 49, pp. 223–244 (July/August 1998).

58) Y. Zhou, etal, "Investigation of thermal Damage of Hair from Hot Flat Ironing and the Thermal Protective Effects of Cosmetic Pretreatments," presented at 26 th Congress of the IFSCC in Argentina, September 20–23, 2010.

59) S.B. Ruetsch and Y.K. Kamath, "Effect of Thermal Treatment with a Curling Iron on Hair

60) M Gamez unpublished results

61) M.Gamez-Garcia, The effects of lipid penetration and removal from subsurface microcavities and cracks at the human cuticle sheath, J. Cosm. Sci.Vol. 60, Issue 2

62) M Gamez unpublished results

63) M. Gamez-Garcia, Light interference phenomena produced by cuticle cells of human hair, www.skin-care-forum.basf.com 2012/light September 2012

64) M. Gamez-Garcia, "Plastic Yielding in Hair Cuticles," J Soc. Cosmet. Sci., 50, 69–77, (1999)

65) M. Gamez-Garcia, "The effects of oil sorption and desorption on the emolliency of hair," TRI Hair Conference on Hair Science, Princeton, NJ, September, 2012.

66) T. Evans. Adsorption Properties of Hair, in Practical Modern Hair Science, Eds., T. Evans and R. Wickett, Allured Books, Specialty Science Books, 2012.

67) S. Watanabe, H. Sato, S. Shibuichi, M. Okamoto, S. Inoue, and N. Satoh, Formation of nanostructure on hair surface: Its characteristic optical properties and application to hair care products, J. Cosmet, Sci., 58, 283–294 (July/August 2007)

68) R.O. Prum, T. Quinn, R.H. Torres, "Anatomically diverse butterfly scales all produce structural colours by coherent scattering," J. Exp. Biology, Vol. 209, pp., 748–765 (2006)

69) R.O. Prum, "Anatomy, physics, and evolution of certain avian structural colors," In Brod Coloration, Vol. 1, Mechanisms and Measurements, Ed. G.E. Hill and K.J. McGraw, pp. 295–353, Cambridge, Harvard University Press (2006)

70) M Gamez unpublished results

71) A. Kharin, B. Varghese, R. Verhagen, N. Uzunbajakava, Optical properties of the medulla and the cortex of human scalp hair, J Biomed Opt. 2009 Mar-Apr; 14(2):024035. doi: 10.1117/1.3116712.

72) P. Hallegot, R. Peteranderl, and C.Lechene, In-Situ Imaging Mass Spectrometry Analysis of Melanin Granules in the Human Hair Shaft, J Invest Dermatol 122:381 –386, 2004

73) L. Zeise, Melanin: Its Role in Human Photoprotection, Proceedings of the symposium held in Washington, D.C., March 11–12, 1994.

74) P. Proctor, Free Radicals and Human Disease, in CRC Handbook of Free Radicals and Antioxidants, vol 1 (1989), p209–221.)

75) Miyake, Y., Izumi, Y., Isutsumi, A., Jimbow, K (1986). "Chemico-physical properties of melanin." IV. In Structure and Functions of Melanins (K. Jimbow, ed.), Vol. 2, pp. 3–18, Fuji. Shoin Co. Ltd., Sapporo, Japan

76) Suman K. Singh*, Robin Kurfurst†, Carine Nizard†, Sylvianne Schnebert†, Eric Perrier† and Desmond J. Tobin*, Melanin transfer in human skin cells is mediated by filopodia—a model for homotypic and heterotypic lysosome-related organelle transfer, The FASEB Journal Vol. 24 no. 10 3756–3769, October 2010

77) J. H. Mottaz and A. S. Zelickson, Melanin Transfer: A Possible Phagocytic Process, The Journal of Investigative Dermatology, (1967) 49, 605–610

78) M.H. Hardy, The secret life of the hair follicle, Trends. Genet. (1992) 8: 55–61.

79) G. Cotsarelis, Epithelial Stem Cells: A Folliculocentric View, Journal of Investigative Dermatology (2006) 126, 1459–1468.

80) R.J. Morris, Y. Liu, L. Malres, Z. Yang, C. Trempus, S. Li, J.S. Lin, J.A. Sawicki, and G. Cotsarelis, Capturing and Profiling Adult Hair Follicle Stem Cells, Nature Biotechnology, Vol. 22, Number 4, April 2004.

81) M. Ohyama, Hair follicle bulge: A fascinating reservoir of epithelial stem cells, Journal of Dermatological Science (2007) 46, 81–89

82) K. S. Stenn and R. Paus, "Controls of Hair Follicle Cycling," Physiological Reviews, Vol. 81, No. 1, January 2001

83) A. Panteleyev, C. Jahoda, A. Christiano, Growth Characteristics of Hair Follicle are Predetermined by the Previous Anagen-Telogen Hair Cycle, Presentations on Hair Follicle Stem Cells Research 3rd Intercontinental Hair Research Societies

84) I. Borbiro, New Mechanisms in the Biological Process of Human Hair Growth Regulation, PhD Thesis, University of Debrecen, Doctoral School of Molecular Medicine, Debrecen, Hungary, 2011

PART 3.3.2

AN OVERVIEW OF HAIR FOLLICLE ANATOMY AND BIOLOGY

By

Paul Mouser Ph.D.
Ashland, Inc.,
Ashland Specialty Ingredients,
Bridgewater, NJ, United States

ABSTRACT

Since ancient times, the human hair has been an attribute for health, youth, and attractiveness as it plays a vital role in people's self-perception [1]. As a result, changes in the appearance of hair such as hair loss, hair thinning, and premature graying often cause psychological distress to the affected individuals.

Hair is produced by a multicellular entity; the **hair follicle**. The hair follicle is one of the most fascinating and dynamic organs of the human body and, unlike the hair itself, which is composed of dead keratinocytes, hair follicles undergo a process of regeneration that controls the production of the hair fiber. One can distinguish between three main types of hair follicles: the **lanugo**, the **vellus**, and the **terminal hair follicle**:

- **Lanugo hair** is very fine and normally shed *in utero*, or during the first weeks of life.
- **Vellus hairs** are very short, nonpigmented, nonmedullated hairs found all over the body surface.

Terminal hair is the large, and usually pigmented and medullated hair that is predominantly found on the scalp. It is estimated that humans have around 5 million hair follicles, of which 80,000 to 150,000 are located on the scalp. Scalp hairs grow at a rate of 0.3 to 0.4 mm per day [2]. **No additional follicles are produced after birth**, although the size of the follicles and hairs can alter with time, primarily under the influence of androgens. In pubic, axillary, and beard regions, androgens stimulate the conversion of vellus to terminal hairs, whereas in frontal scalp regions of genetically predisposed individuals, androgens trigger miniaturization of hair follicles via conversion of terminal to vellus hair follicles [3].

The most unique feature of hair growth is its cycle. Hair follicles undergo repeated cycles of anagen (growth), catagen (degeneration), and telogen (quiescence). During anagen, hair follicle stem cells sustain the steady production of matrix cells in the hair bulb. These proliferate several times and terminally differentiate into the companion layer, the inner root sheath, and the hair shaft.

Unwanted hair loss is a common problem and is suffered by much of the world's population in both women and men. The condition is characterized by premature hair loss and excessive hair shedding. The process is caused by an interruption in the normal hair growth cycle, which can lead to the development of baldness with insufficient replacement of hairs in human scalp. This can have negative effects on an individual's self-esteem and thus products that claim to be useful for treating hair loss target a steadily growing, multibillion-dollar market worldwide.

The field of human follicle biology is progressing rapidly largely because of technical advances in molecular and cellular biology as well as sophisticated cell culture techniques. This chapter reviews the structure of hair, the biological processes occurring during the hair growth cycle, and the changes that occur with hair aging.

TABLE OF CONTENTS

3.3.2.1 HAIR FOLLICLE STRUCTURE

The hair follicle is a three-dimensional tube, composed mainly of epithelial cells, which protrude down through the epidermis and dermis of the skin (Figure 1).

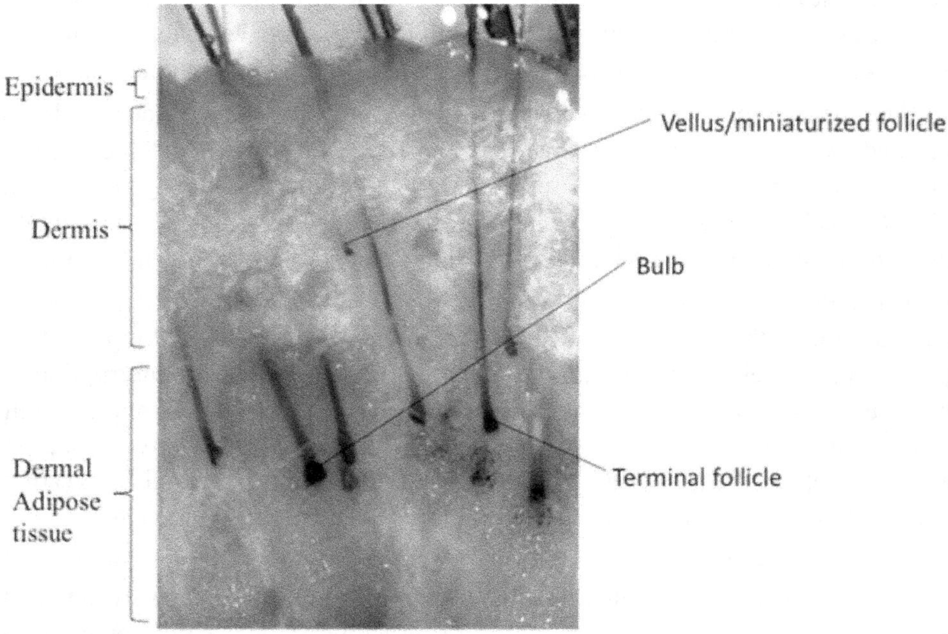

Figure 1. Human scalp tissue isolated from the scalp. Hair follicles protrude down through the epidermis and dermis of the skin (photo kindly provided by Dr Claire Higgins)

Hair follicles vary considerably in shape and size, depending on their location, but they all have common architecture. Anatomically, the hair follicle is most commonly described when it is in the mature anagen stage (Figure 2A). The mature anagen follicle can be divided into an upper permanent portion (infundibulum and isthmus), which does not cycle, and a lower part (bulb and suprabulbar), which is remodeled in each hair cycle. The infundibulum is the opening of the hair canal to the skin surface, and the isthmus is the permanent middle section extending from the sebaceous duct opening to the point of arrector pili insertion. The lower isthmus also contains the bulge region (Figure 2B), which is a region of functional importance as it is in this location that a reservoir of stem cells reside. Stem cells are unique, as they have the capacity to generate all the differentiated cell types within tissue and to self-renew in order to replenish their pool. Earlier studies have demonstrated that all epithelial layers within the hair follicle and hair originated from bulge cells [4, 5]. Hair follicle stem cells therefore appear to be responsible for regenerating the hair follicle in each cycle. Up until recently the location of the bulge in human follicles was unclear. By contrast with the bulge in rodent follicles, human follicles are not morphologically distinct. However, identification of unique bulge markers in the human follicle has enabled the human anagen bulge to be defined as a distinct region [6, 7].

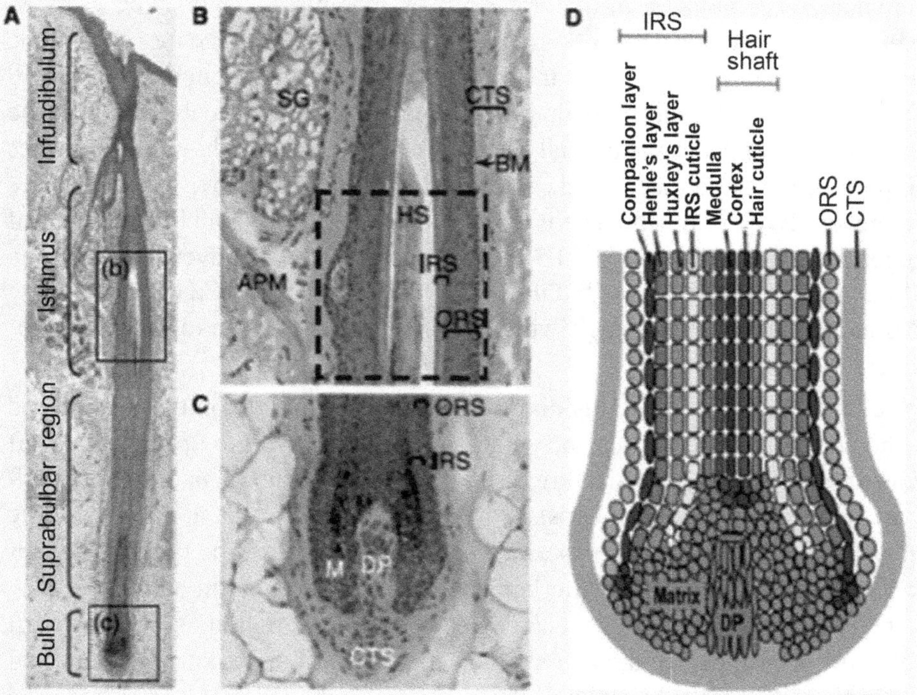

Figure 2. Structure of human anagen hair follicle. (A) Longitudinal section of a human scalp hair follicle showing the permanent (infundibulum and isthmus) and cycling (suprabulbar region and bulb) components of the hair follicle. (B) High magnification image of the isthmus. The dashed square indicates the approximate location of the bulge. (C) High magnification image of the bulb showing the outer root sheath (ORS), inner root sheath (IRS), matrix zone (M), dermal papilla (DP) and connective tissue sheath (CTS). (D) Schematic drawing illustrating the concentric layers of the ORS, IRS and shaft in the bulb. Current Biology 19, R132-R142 2009 ©2009 Elsevier

The anagen bulb (Figure 2C) is one of the most rapidly dividing tissues in the body. The bulb represents the hair shaft factory; it contains the proliferating matrix keratinocytes and pigment-producing melanocytes (matrix zone). The hair matrix keratinocytes move upwards and differentiate into the hair shaft, as well as into the inner root sheath; the melanocytes transfer pigment into the developing hair keratinocytes to give hair its color [8]. These cells are supplied by the pluripotent stem cells existing in the bulge. The hair bulb surrounds the dermal papilla, which comprises a group of specialized cells (dermal papilla cells) with important inductive properties. The dermal papilla is believed to be one of the most important drivers that instruct the hair follicle to grow, and dictates hair bulb size, hair shaft diameter, length, and anagen duration.[9] The dermal papilla is known as the "conductor of the orchestra" or "command center," and is an essential source of growth factors (keratinocyte growth factor, bone morphogenetic protein, hepatocyte growth factor, insulin-like growth factor, stem cell factor), all of which are critical for hair growth and melanogenesis [8]. Surgical removal of the dermal papilla and the lower dermal sheath prevents hair growth, which indicates the importance of these specialized cells as the key signaling center in hair follicles [10]. Interestingly, dermal papilla cells from balding scalp have both higher levels of androgen receptor (AR) and type II 5-alpha reductase, which converts testosterone to dihydrotestosterone (DHT) [11]. DHT can induce dermal papilla cells to secrete factors including transforming growth factor beta 1 (TGFb1) and DKK-1 that inhibit keratinocyte growth [12, 13].

The hair shaft (Figure 2D) is divided into the hair cuticle on the outside and both the cortex and medulla in the center. The cells that make up the hair shaft are known as trichocytes, which are terminally differentiated hair follicle keratinocytes. The hair shaft cuticle consists of overlapping cells that are arranged like shingles pointing outward and upward. The hair shaft cortex, the bulk of the hair shaft, is composed of hair-specific keratin filaments and keratin-associated proteins with melanin produced by melanocytes in the matrix region [2]. The hair shaft medulla, the central part of the hair shaft, is composed of large, loosely connected keratinized cells with large intercellular air spaces. The hair shaft is surrounded and supported by the inner root sheath (IRS), the companion layer, and the outer root sheath (ORS).

The IRS consists of three distinct layers: the cuticle, Huxley's layer, and the Henle's layer (Figure 2D). The IRS cuticle layer adjoins the cuticle of the hair shaft and anchors the hair shaft to the follicle. IRS keratinocytes produce keratins and trichohyalin that serve as an intracellular "cement" giving strength to the IRS to support and mold the growing hair shaft, as well as guide its upward movement [8].

The ORS surrounds the IRS and is continuous with the basal layer of the epidermis. Distinct from the other epithelial components, the ORS does not generate by upwards growth from the matrix zone, but rather directly from the stem cell bulge. The bulge region of the ORS is located just below the sebaceous gland and at the insertion site of the arrector pili muscle. Stem cells leave the bulge in the ORS and migrate toward the matrix zone, where they begin to proliferate and subsequently differentiate into new hair shafts [14].

Hair follicles grow in an oblique angle towards the epidermal surface. This angle can be varied by the contraction of a bundle of muscle, collectively called the arrector pili muscle (APM). The APM is under adrenergic control and thus, in situations of cold temperature and emotional stressors, it gives rise to the interesting phenomenon of involuntary contraction resulting in the hair standing up!

3.3.2.2 HAIR FOLLICLE CYCLING

Hair growth and loss in humans is controlled by a specific follicular cell cycle (Figure 3) that includes three major stages [9]:

- growth and differentiation (**anagen**)
- regression and apoptosis (**catagen**) and
- rest (**teleogen**)

Additional phases recently discovered include exogen, in which the fiber is actively shed [15], and kenogen, when the follicle is empty [16].

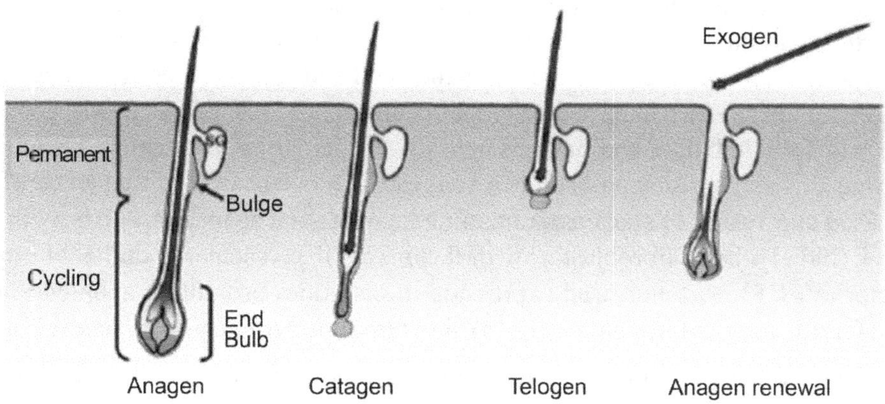

Figure 3. Hair Follicle Cycle. The different stages of the adult hair follicle are divided into three main categories known as anagen, catagen, telogen, which continually cycle throughout the life of the follicle. During anagen the matrix cells of the bulb (red) rapidly proliferate and differentiate to produce the hair fibre and layers of the inner root sheath. The hair follicle enters catagen which is characterized by apoptosis of the epithelial cells, and the formation of the club fiber. The dermal papilla (blue) moves up to the base of the permanent section of the follicle, in close proximity to the bulge (green). A resting phase known as telogen then occurs before the renewal of a subsequent anagen phase. Exogen describes the removal of the remaining club fiber which typically occurs close to the time of renewed anagen onset. Seminars in Cell & Developmental Biology 18 245-254 2007 ©2007 Elsevier

Hair follicle cycling is driven in response to continuing molecular interactions between the dermal papilla and the epithelial components of the follicle [17, 18].

The duration of the different growth phases depends on the type and localization of the hair follicle. Scalp follicles stay in the anagen stage for two to six years and produce long hairs, whereas eyebrow or eyelash hair follicles do so for only one to three months and produce short hairs. An in-depth description of eyelash hair follicles may be found elsewhere in this book. What determines the clock mechanism and the duration of anagen in individual hair follicles is not known, although one candidate for consideration is the circadian clock, a molecular oscillatory system [19, 20].

Following morphogenesis, the hair follicle enters the regression phase (catagen). The catagen stage lasts approximately two weeks, during which time the hair fiber ceases to grow. During the catagen stage, cells located in the lower portion of the hair follicle undergo programmed cell death (apoptosis). The hair follicle shortens and the hair bulb loses its internal and external sheaths. During this process the hair follicle acquires a club-shaped end and is subsequently referred to as the "club fiber." Additionally the dermal papilla condenses, moves upward beneath the hair follicle bulge, and halts its activity. Follicular melanogenesis also ceases during this stage. Catagen has been suggested to occur as a consequence of decreased expression of anagen maintaining factors, such as insulin-like growth factor 1 (IGF-1), basic fibroblast growth factor (bFGF), vascular endothelial growth factor (VEGF), and increased expression of cytokines promoting apoptosis, such as TGFb 1, interleukin-1alpha (IL-1a), and tumor necrosis factor alpha (TNFa) [21].

Upon catagen completion, hair follicles enter a resting stage (telogen) for an average of three months. In the telogen stage, the hair follicle has decreased to about half of its previous size and the stem cells are thought to be quiescent. However, by the end of the telogen stage, hair follicle stem cells become activated by Wnt and TGFb signals from the dermal papilla and form a new hair follicle [22–24]. Anagen involves the complete regrowth or regeneration of the lower, cycling portion of the follicle, i.e., the hair shaft factory. The cross-talk of dermal papilla with neighboring matrix cells results in the maintenance of hair fiber production (i.e., the hair continues to grow). Two secreted molecules that have important roles in hair follicle cycling are IGF-1 and bFGF. Both are produced by the dermal papilla, and their receptors are found predominantly in the overlying matrix cells [25].

Sometime after new shaft production begins, the club fiber is shed [26]. The term 'exogen' has been introduced to identify the hair fiber shedding event as a separate process during hair follicle cycling [15]. Shedding of 100–150 hairs per day is normal [2]. Previously, hair fiber shedding was believed to be passive, but recent research suggests that shedding is an active and highly controlled process [15, 27, 28]. Empty hair follicles, after shedding of the club fiber, but before the onset of renewed anagen, are in a stage called "kenogen." Kenogen can be observed in healthly skin, but the frequency and duration are significantly greater in individuals with androgenetic alopecia [16].

In addition to hair follicle tissue modeling, skin innervations and vascular networks also undergo substantial changes with the progression of the anagen stage [17, 29]. Perifolicular vascularization is significantly increased during anagen. It correlates with the up-regulation of the expression of vascular endothelial growth factor (VEGF) mRNA, a potent angiogenic growth factor, produced by keratinocytes of the outer root sheath [8].

Each follicle can undergo repeated cycles until it eventually dies or miniaturizes to give rise to a vellus hair [30, 31]. **Disturbances of hair follicle cycling lie at the heart of most hair growth disorders, and have dramatic effects on visible hair growth and shedding**. For instance the most common alopecia, *androgenetic alopecia*, produces a patterned baldness involving a reduction in the percentage of scalp hair follicles in anagen, a reduction in the anagen growth phase duration, and a corresponding increase in the percentage of hair follicles in telogen and an increase in the duration of telogen. These alterations (in combination with a shift in the exogen phase from primarily occurring in early anagen to initiation primarily during telogen) result in thinning hair coverage [32, 33]. The most effective therapeutic strategies for hair loss therapy inhibit catagen development so as to prolong anagen, to induce anagen in telogen follicles, and/or to inhibit exogen [34].

3.3.2.3 AGING OF THE HAIR FOLLICLE

While consumers are increasingly concerned with diminishing the signs of aging, especially the aesthetic of hair, addressing the cellular mechanisms behind them represents a decisively new direction in hair care strategies. Like all biological systems, the hair follicle also undergoes an aging process. This process is not only characterized by loss of pigmentation, but changes in growth characteristics that include decreased hair follicle density, increased number of telogen hairs, a decrease in the diameter of hair shafts, and slower hair growth rates [35–38].

The color of hair mainly relies on the presence or absence of melanin pigment. Two types of pigment can be produced by the hair follicle. The first type is eumelanin, which is the pigment in brown-black hairs, while the second type is pheomelanin, the pigment in red-blond hairs. Melanin is produced by the melanocytes, and is the result of a complex biochemical pathway (melanogenesis) with tyrosinase being the rate-limiting enzyme. Hair melanins are formed in cytoplasmic organelles called melanosomes. The melanosomes travel out to the tips of the melanocyte's dendrites where they are transferred to the hair follicle keratinocytes of the hair cortex and medulla. Each hair cycle can produce a long pigmented terminal hair because the follicle is able to replace these melanocytes from a reserve found in the bulge region of the ORS (39). As individuals age, the melanin content of the hair follicle decreases, causing graying and eventual whitening of the hair. Although poorly understood, numerous mechanisms have been suggested for this loss of hair follicle pigment, including pigmentary machinery malfunction or loss, melanocyte apoptosis, anagen defects, the loss of melanocyte stem cells or their failure to differentiate, and melanocyte migration defects (40).

Hair graying, sometimes referred to as canities, is one of the most prominent signs of human aging. A recent worldwide survey showed that 74% of people between the ages of 45 and 65 have gray hair, and that it occurs earliest in people of Caucasian descent, followed by lesser occurrence in Asians and Africans (41). The age of graying onset is genetically controlled and inheritable. Hair is considered to gray prematurely only if it occurs before the age of 20 years in Caucasians, before 25 years in Asians, and before 30 years in Africans (42). As hair color is socially important, premature graying imposes a psychosocial distress and is often perceived as a sign of stress, old age, ill health, and bodily decline (42, 43).

Both the hair and scalp are constantly exposed to various environmental stressors. These include UV irradiation as well as oxidative and chemical stressors. The effect of external stressors on the hair fiber is quite well documented. In particular, repeated sun exposure impairs the structure of the hair shaft keratin fiber, while UV radiations induce hair protein loss and color changes (44). Recent *in vitro* and *ex vivo* studies have investigated the damage caused by UV radiation and oxidative stress on the hair follicle (45, 46). Upon exposure to repetitive UVB irradiation isolated hair follicles in culture demonstrated reduced hair shaft elongation and premature entry into the catagen phase. Moreover, oxidative DNA damage was observed in hair follicle submitted to low UVB doses (45). Gondran et al. examined the effects of UV radiation and oxidative stress generated by H_2O_2 on human scalp skin grafts containing hair follicles (46, 47). *Oxidative stress impaired hair follicle structure as indicated by increased number of vacuoles and edema mainly observed in the outer root sheath.* Emerging evidence shows that reactive oxygen species (ROS) accumulate in human gray/white scalp follicles up to millimolar concentrations. The presence of ROS is believed to cause oxidative damage (free radical-induced aging) to the hair follicle melanocytes (48, 49). In addition catalase (the enzyme involved in cell response to oxidative stress), expression is reduced in unpigmented and older follicles (48, 50, 51). Altogether, the data strongly suggest that the hair follicle itself is a direct target of oxidative stress and underline the interest of applying a specifically developed cosmetic follicle ingredient to protect the hair follicle from endogenous or environmental stressful processes (46, 47).

CONCLUSION

Hair care formulations have traditionally relied on ingredients that treat the hair fiber to improve appearance. However, vibrant and healthy-looking hair starts at the roots and, therefore, cosmetic biofunctionals that target the hair follicle provide product manufacturers with new innovative ways to bring back beauty to the hair.

REFERENCES

1. Trueb RM. Aging of hair. J Cosmet Dermatol 2005;4:60–72.
2. Paus R, Cotsarelis G. The biology of hair follicles. N Engl J Med 1999;341:491–7.
3. Hamilton J. Patterned loss of hair in man; types and incidence. Ann N Y Acad Sci 1951;53:708–28.
4. Cotsarelis G. Epithelial stem cells: a folliculocentric view. J Invest Dermatol 2006;126:1459–68.
5. Cotsarelis G, Sun TT, Lavker RM. Label-retaining cells reside in the bulge area of pilosebaceous unit: implications for follicular stem cells, hair cycle, and skin carcinogenesis. Cell 1990;61:1329–37.
6. Lyle S, Christofidou-Solomidou M, Liu Y, et al. Human hair follicle bulge cells are biochemically distinct and possess an epithelial stem cell phenotype. J Investig Dermatol Symp Proc 1999;4:296–301.
7. Ohyama M, Terunuma A, Tock CL, et al. Characterization and isolation of stem cell-enriched human hair follicle bulge cells. J Clin Invest 2006;116:249–60.
8. Randall VA. The biology of hair growth. In: Cosmetic applications of laser and light based systems. William Andrew Inc; 2009. p.3–35.
9. Schneider MR, Schmidt-Ullrich R, Paus R. The hair follicle as a dynamic miniorgan. Curr Biol 2009;19:R132-R142.
10. Oliver RF. Whisker growth after removal of the dermal papilla and lengths of follicle in the hooded rat. J Embryol Exp Morphol 1966;15:331–47.
11. Hibberts NA, Howell AE, Randall VA. Balding hair follicle dermal papilla cells contain higher levels of androgen receptors than those from non-balding scalp. J Endocrinol 1998;156:59–65.
12. Inui S, Fukuzato Y, Nakajima T, Yoshikawa K, Itami S. Androgen-inducible TGF-beta1 from balding dermal papilla cells inhibits epithelial cell growth: a clue to understand paradoxical effects of androgen on human hair growth. FASEB J 2002;16:1967–9.

13. Kwack MH, Sung YK, Chung EJ, et al. Dihydrotestosterone-inducible dickkopf 1 from balding dermal papilla cells causes apoptosis in follicular keratinocytes. J Invest Dermatol 2008;128:262–9.
14. Oshima H, Rochat A, Kedzia C, Kobayashi K, Barrandon Y. Morphogenesis and renewal of hair follicles from adult multipotent stem cells. Cell 2001;104:233–45.
15. Stenn K. Exogen is an active, separately controlled phase of the hair growth cycle. J Am Acad Dermatol 2005;52:374–5.
16. Rebora A, Guarrera M. Kenogen. A new phase of the hair cycle? Dermatology 2002;205:108–10.
17. Botchkarev VA, Kishimoto J. Molecular control of epithelial-mesenchymal interactions during hair follicle cycling. J Investig Dermatol Symp Proc 2003;8:46–55.
18. Rendl M, Lewis L, Fuchs E. Molecular dissection of mesenchymal-epithelial interactions in the hair follicle. PLoS Biol 2005;3:e331.
19. Lin KK, Kumar V, Geyfman M, et al. Circadian clock genes contribute to the regulation of hair follicle cycling. PLoS Genet 2009;5.
20. Al Nuaimi Y, Hardman JA, Biro T, et al. A meeting of two chronobiological systems: circadian proteins Period1 and BMAL1 modulate the human hair cycle clock. J Invest Dermatol 2014;134:610–9.
21. Trueb RM. Molecular mechanisms of androgenetic alopecia. Exp Gerontol 2002;37:981–90.
22. Enshell-Seijffers D, Lindon C, Kashiwagi M, Morgan BA. beta-catenin activity in the dermal papilla regulates morphogenesis and regeneration of hair. Dev Cell 2010;18:633–42.
23. Greco V, Chen T, Rendl M, et al. A two-step mechanism for stem cell activation during hair regeneration. Cell Stem Cell 2009;4:155–69.
24. Oshimori N, Fuchs E. Paracrine TGF-beta signaling counterbalances BMP-mediated repression in hair follicle stem cell activation. Cell Stem Cell 2012;10:63–75.
25. Danilenko DM, Ring BD, Pierce GF. Growth factors and cytokines in hair follicle development and cycling: recent insights from animal models and the potentials for clinical therapy. Mol Med Today 1996;2:460–7.
26. Milner Y, Sudnik J, Filippi M, et al. Exogen, shedding phase of the hair growth cycle: characterization of a mouse model. J Invest Dermatol 2002;119:639–44.

27. Higgins CA, Westgate GE, Jahoda CA. Modulation in proteolytic activity is identified as a hallmark of exogen by transcriptional profiling of hair follicles. J Invest Dermatol 2011;131:2349–57.

28. Bhogal RK, Mouser PE, Higgins CA, Turner GA. Protease activity, localization and inhibition in the human hair follicle. Int J Cosmet Sci 2013.

29. Mecklenburg L, Tobin DJ, Muller-Rover S, et al. Active hair growth (anagen) is associated with angiogenesis. J Invest Dermatol 2000;114:909–16.

30. Whiting DA. Male pattern hair loss: current understanding. Int J Dermatol 1998;37:561–6.

31. Ishino A, Uzuka M, Tsuji Y, et al. Progressive decrease in hair diameter in Japanese with male pattern baldness. J Dermatol 1997;24:758–64.

32. Mei Yu. Hair follicles and their role in skin health. Expert Review of Dermatology 2006;1:855–71.

33. K J McElwee. Hair physiology and its disorders. Drug Discovery Today Disease Mechanisms 2008;5:e163–e171.

34. Paus R. Therapeutic strategies for treating hair loss. Drug Discovery Today: Therapeutic Strategies 2014;3:101–10.

35. Barman J. The Normal Trichogram of the Adult. J Invest Dermatol 1965;44:233–6.

36. Paradi Mirmirani. Hair Growth Parameters in Pre- and Postmenopausal Women. In: Aging Hair. Springer; 2010. p.49–60.

37. Van Neste D. Thickness, medullation and growth rate of female scalp hair are subject to significant variation according to pigmentation and scalp location during ageing. Eur J Dermatol 2004;14:28–32.

38. Tobin DJ. Aging of the hair follicle pigmentation system. Int J Trichology 2009;1:83–93.

39. Nishimura EK, Granter SR, Fisher DE. Mechanisms of hair graying: incomplete melanocyte stem cell maintenance in the niche. Science 2005;307:720–4.

40. Seiberg M. Age-induced hair greying - the multiple effects of oxidative stress. Int J Cosmet Sci 2013;35:532–8.

41. Panhard S, Lozano I, Loussouarn G. Greying of the human hair: a worldwide survey, revisiting the '50' rule of thumb. Br J Dermatol 2012;167:865–73.

42. Tobin DJ. Human hair pigmentation--biological aspects. Int J Cosmet Sci 2008;30:233–57.

43. Commo S, Gaillard O, Bernard BA. Human hair greying is linked to a specific depletion of hair follicle melanocytes affecting both the bulb and the outer root sheath. Br J Dermatol 2004;150:435–43.
44. Lee WS. Photoaggravation of hair aging. Int J Trichology 2009;1:94–9.
45. Lu Z, Fischer TW, Hasse S, et al. Profiling the response of human hair follicles to ultraviolet radiation. J Invest Dermatol 2009;129:1790–804.
46. Gondran C. Hair follicle protection from oxidative damage. Personal Care 2012;February:89–92.
47. Gondran C. Hair Follicle Protection. SOFW Journal 2012;138:38–42.
48. Wood JM, Decker H, Hartmann H, et al. Senile hair graying: H2O2-mediated oxidative stress affects human hair color by blunting methionine sulfoxide repair. FASEB J 2009;23:2065–75.
49. Arck PC, Overall R, Spatz K, et al. Towards a "free radical theory of graying": melanocyte apoptosis in the aging human hair follicle is an indicator of oxidative stress induced tissue damage. FASEB J 2006;20:1567–9.
50. Shi Y, Luo LF, Liu XM, et al. Premature graying as a consequence of compromised antioxidant activity in hair bulb melanocytes and their precursors. PLoS One 2014;9:e93589.
51. Kauser S, Westgate GE, Green MR, Tobin DJ. Human hair follicle and epidermal melanocytes exhibit striking differences in their aging profile which involves catalase. J Invest Dermatol 2011;131:979–82.

GLOSSARY

Alopecia: Abnormal hair loss.

Androgenetic alopecia: Loss of hair caused by miniaturization of genetically predisposed follicles

Anagen: Growing stage of the hair follicle cycle.

Bulb: Lowermost portion of the anagen follicle containing rapidly proliferating cells that generate the hair fiber

Bulge: Site of stem cells within the follicle outer root sheath, located at the insertion site of the arrector pili muscle just below the sebaceous gland.

Catagen: Regression stage of the hair follicle cycle.

Club hair: Fully keratinized, dead hair formed during catagen.

Dermal papilla: Signaling control center of the hair follicle consisting of dermal papilla cells.

Exogen: Stage of the hair follicle cycle when hair is shed from the follicle.

Hair shaft: The hair *per se,* composed of trichocytes, which are terminally differentiated hair follicle keratinocytes. It is composed of the medulla and the cortex.

Infundibulum: Most proximal part of the hair follicle relative to the epidermis, extending from the sebaceous duct to the epidermal surface.

Inner root sheath: Surrounds and protects the growing hair.

Isthmus: Permanent middle section of hair follicle extending from the sebaceous duct to the point of arrector pili insertion

Kenogen: Stage of the hair follicle characterized by empty hair follicles after the hair fiber is shed before a new anagen hair emerges.

Outer root sheath: The outermost layer of the hair follicle. Merges proximally with the basal layer of the epidermis and distally with the hair bulb.

Telogen: Resting stage of the hair follicle cycle.

Terminal hair: Large, usually pigmented hairs (e.g., those found on the scalp).

Vellus hair: Very short, nonpigmented hairs (e.g., those found diffusely over nonbeard area of the face and bald scalp as a result of miniaturization of terminal hairs).

HAIR AGING: FUNDAMENTALS, PROTECTION AND REPAIR

Padmaja Prem, Ph.D

Vice President, Research & Development

Combe Incorporated, 1101 Westchester Avenue
White Plains, NY 10604

ABSTRACT

Aging skin is a concept easily grasped; aging hair is not. However, changes in hair with aging are consumer perceivable and measurable. This chapter describes the structure of hair, fundamentals of aging hair, signs of aging hair, and causes of the visible signs of aging hair. Further, it also covers remedies for protection of hair fibers, the scalp from which it grows, as well as hair products and ingredients formulated to maintain and restore youthful hair. Beyond these approaches, the author has also provided a unique cosmeticological look at selected products and ingredients on the market with commentary on their performance.

While considerable attention has been paid to the many factors affecting aging skin, it is only recently that a shift in the perception that hair is "dead" has begun to accelerate. Actually, while this is true, in part, it is also true that the core of the hair fibers is alive as well as the skin from which it grows, and much has been done and needs doing to bring it to life again.

The understanding of the hair-scalp system described in this chapter provides important leads to ingredient-seekers and product formulators and presents an opportunity for a myriad of novel products that consumers long for. The chapter is also unique in that it provides thoughtful, practical recommendations for hair care and protection. This wisdom goes beyond the traditional approach of finding new ingredients or formulations to achieve the goals of beautiful hair. It is recommended that these approaches be incorporated in recommendations by product manufacturers as important information to consumers.

TABLE OF CONTENTS

3.3.3.1 INTRODUCTION

Similar to skin, with aging, the scalp and hair are subject to intrinsic or chronological aging, and extrinsic aging due to environmental factors. The changes associated with aging skin and the mechanism of skin aging has been well researched and published extensively over the past decades. According to Mintel's global product database, nearly half of the skin care products in the market are anti-aging products.

While the aging of hair has not been studied extensively like skin aging, there are numerous studies published on hair aging[1–3], and the number of anti-aging hair care products continues to increase year by year[4]. The most obvious sign of hair aging is the appearance of gray hair that correlates closely with intrinsic aging. Melanin pigment is responsible for the natural color of hair and it is produced by melanocytes in the hair follicles. With aging, melanocytes stop producing melanin pigment, resulting in gray hair. The loss of melanin has been linked to a decrease in the number of melanocytes in the hair follicle as well as a possible decrease in the activity of the enzymes involved in melanogenesis[5]. A recent publication by Wood et al.[6] showed for the first time high accumulation of hydrogen peroxide in human gray scalp hair shaft, thus supporting the theory of oxidative stress in gray hair formation. These researchers also demonstrated that H_2O_2-mediated oxidation of methionine in tyrosinase enzyme limits its functionality, which leads to gradual loss of hair color.

In addition to graying of hair, with aging, your hair will become deficient in essential nutrients and the hair follicles shrink, it loses its elasticity, lipid and keratin production diminish, and many hair follicles stop producing new hairs altogether. These internal changes cause hair to become thin, dry, less manageable, brittle and less shiny, and ultimately lead to hair fall.

Externally, the hair shaft is exposed to sunlight, environmental pollutants, chemical and heat treatments, and subjected to daily grooming and mechanical aggression-in-search-of- "beauty." These environmental insults and daily aggressors alter the chemical and physical properties of the hair fiber. When hair is exposed to sunlight, severe damage occurs due to lipid, protein, and melanin oxidation. This results in loss of mechanical strength, loss of color, an increase in porosity, as well as an increase in surface roughness. Other environmental pollutants such as cigarette smoke, car exhaust fumes, and smog also impart hair damage, resulting in dull and brittle hair. These physicochemical changes in hair structure and damage caused by aging are measurable and also perceivable to the consumer.

Several methods involving microscopic techniques, differential scanning calorimetric, wet and dry combing measurements, protein loss, and assessment of tensile properties of the hair are generally used to evaluate the various physicochemical changes to hair[7]. These approaches are useful in characterizing aging changes as well as the effect of "treatments" that may improve the detrimental effects of the various stressors.

Hair loss is another significant aspect of aging that occurs gradually with a progressive thinning of hair. With aging, less protein is produced in the hair follicle that can cause hair to fall out and not to be replaced as quickly as desirable. This causes baldness, as well as thinning of hair. Unlike the long term, initial focus on the skin of women, the baldness phenomenon is also a men's "condition" and any impact of novel approaches to reduce hair loss and hair thinning represents an area of potential product growth for both men and women.

Experimental evidence supports the hypothesis that oxidative stress also plays a role in hair aging. The damaging effects of these reactive oxygen species are induced internally during normal metabolism and externally through exposure to various oxidative stresses from the environment. The body possesses endogenous defense mechanisms, such as antioxidant enzymes (superoxide dismutase, catalase, glutathione peroxidase) and non-enzymatic antioxidative molecules (e.g., vitamin E, vitamin C, glutathione, ubiquinone), protecting it from free radicals by reducing and neutralizing them.[9] With age, the production of free radicals increases, while the endogenous defense mechanisms decrease. This imbalance leads to the progressive damage of cellular structures, presumably resulting in the aging phenotype.

Nourishment and proper grooming are very important to maintain the beauty of hair as perceived by: good hair texture, healthy growth, shine, and luster. Eating foods rich in vitamin A, B, minerals, and proteins is necessary for promoting a healthy scalp and hence healthy hair growth. Eating a diet rich in dark green vegetables, orange and yellow fruits, sprouted whole grains, cereals, meat, and soy helps maintain a healthy follicle. It is equally important to use good scalp care and hair care products to protect the hair shaft from damage due to sunlight, pollution, and other daily aggressors. For daily washes, use a shampoo that is mild, gentle, and moisturizing. Anti-aging hair care topical and ingestible products enriched with vitamins, lipids, proteins, vegetable oils, and antioxidant rejuvenate the scalp and follicle, and encourage new, more resilient growth from the root.

This chapter describes the fundamentals of aging hair, signs of aging hair, and the causes of visible signs of aging. Further, it also surveys current remedies for protection of the hair fiber, along with hair products formulated to maintain and restore youthful hair.

3.3.3.2 STRUCTURE, COMPOSITION, AND NATURAL COLOR OF HAIR

Hair is composed of two parts, the hair follicle and the hair shaft. The hair follicle is a tiny cup-shaped point located in the dermis from which the hair grows. The hair follicle consists of the hair bulb, the inner root sheath, and the hair shaft (see Figure 1).

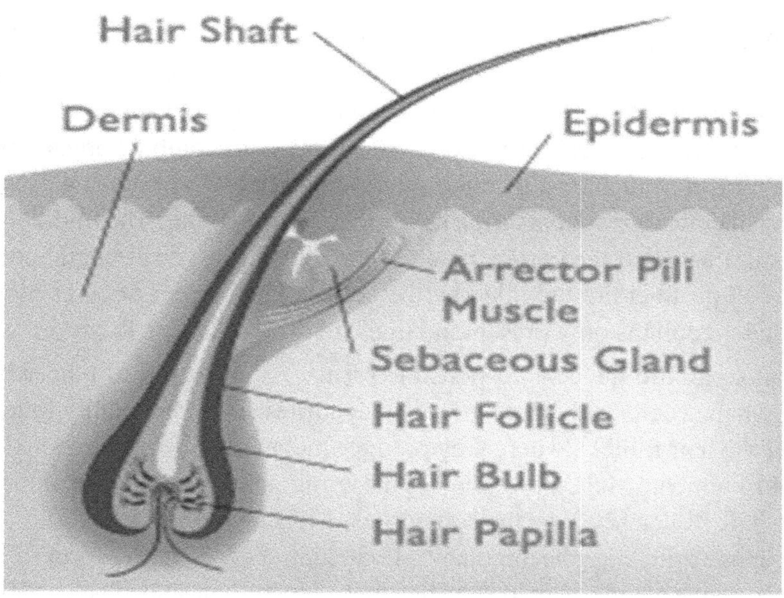

Figure 1. Cross-Sectional Image of Hair Bulb Structure

New hair is made inside the onion-shaped hair bulb that lies within the hair follicle. The hair bulb also contains some special cells called melanocytes that produce melanin, the pigment responsible for the natural color of hair. The part of the hair seen above the scalp is called the hair shaft. It consists of three layers; cuticle, cortex, and medulla (see Figure 2).

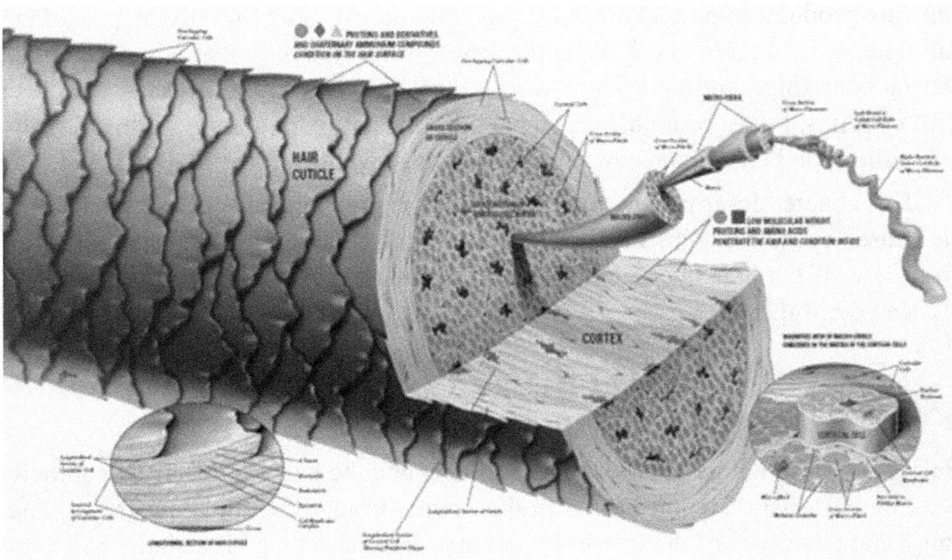

Figure 2. Structure of Human Hair Fiber

The outermost layer called cuticle is a thin and colorless layer made of several overlapping scale-type structures. It is responsible for the visual attributes of hair such as shine and smoothness. It is also responsible for the friction effect of hair, which determines manageability (i.e., how easy it is to comb or brush hair). The cuticle layer can be damaged by daily grooming such as combing and brushing as well as by chemical treatments such as bleaching or relaxing. The middle layer of the hair shaft is called the cortex, made of keratin fibers. The strength, color, and texture of a hair fiber are provided by the cortex. The innermost layer of the hair shaft called medulla is only present in large and thick hairs.

Melanocytes are the cells responsible for the natural color of hair, which are large star-shaped cells with branches called dendrites. They are mainly found at the bottom of the hair follicle, where they produce melanin in the form of small grains of colored pigment. Melanocytes inject these pigments into the keratinocytes of the hair shaft by lengthening their dendrites. Melanocyte produces two types of melanin: eumelanin and phaeomelanin. Eumelanin occurs in the form of a small rice-like granule having a color varying between brown and black. Melanin is formed by the oxidation of an amino acid, tyrosine by the enzyme tyrosinase. The higher the concentration of eumelanin, the darker the color of hair.

The actual appearance of hair, and its overall reflective quality, is determined primarily by the pigment type, but also by the density and distribution of the pigment granules. Phaeomelanin has a less precise shape and can be seen in the form of diffuse spots. Its color varies from yellow to red. Phaeomelanin differs from eumelanin because, in addition to tyrosine, another amino acid, rich in sulfur (cysteine), is involved in its production. There are two different types of eumelanin (brown eumelanin and black eumelanin). A small amount of brown eumelanin in the absence of other pigments apparently causes blond hair.

Although people with dark hair may still produce the yellow-orange pheomelanin, it is largely masked by the dark eumelanin pigment and cannot easily be seen. However, the red-yellow pheomelanin is believed to cause the warm, golden, or auburn tones found in some types of brown hair. The range of colors produced by melanins is limited to shades of yellow, brown, red, and black. Gray hairs contain only a few melanin granules, spread throughout the hair. White hairs contain no melanin at all: their whiteness is an optical effect, due to the way they reflect the light.

3.3.3.3 FUNDAMENTALS AND SIGNS OF AGING HAIR

When considering the phenomenon of hair aging, genetic, hormonal, and environmental factors need to be taken into account. Similar to skin, the scalp and hair are subject to intrinsic aging depending on individual genetics and hormonal factors and extrinsic aging due to environmental factors. Intrinsic aging or chronological aging results in graying of hair due to a decrease in melanin production and loss of hair due to androgenic alopecia. Extrinsic factors include ultraviolet radiation, pollution, smoking, diet, and lifestyle. All these extrinsic factors progressively degrade the hair fiber through oxidation of lipids, cleavage of disulfide bond, degradation of amino acids, and oxidation/bleaching of melanin pigment.

The effects of age-related changes in hair density, hair diameter, hair lipids, and hair color (graying) produce changes in hair fiber properties. These changes in properties impact important consumer hair assembly properties such as ease of combing, hair body, hair coverage, frizziness, shine, manageability, and style retention. There are many visible signs of aging hair that are measurable and consumer perceivable. *The most critical aging attributes are thinning of hair, loss of color, moisture, shine, and manageability.*

Thinning of Hair

Both men and women tend to lose hair thickness and amount as they age. Baldness is not usually caused by a disease. It has been found that poor diet, stress, aging, and pollution are the most common factors that damage hairs and cause hair loss. Scientifically, health experts have found that the growth of dihydrotestosterone (DHT) hormone on the scalp is responsible for hair loss. With aging, hair loss is experienced more rapidly because the amount of DHT increases with increase in age. This hormone makes hair follicles weaker and weaker by blocking the nutrients and water to the hairs. Over time, the follicle can shrink, causing the hair to become shorter and finer and finally the hairs fall from the scalp. Figure 3 shows the picture of a normal hair follicle compared to a finer follicle and a very small hair follicle, which results in baldness.

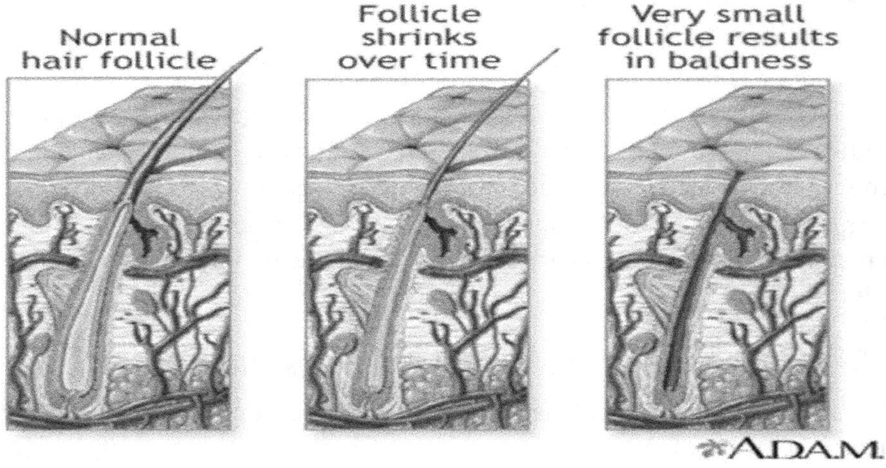

Figure 3. Picture of a hair follicle showing shrinkage over time

According to the American Hair Loss Association, around two-thirds of U.S. men will have experienced some degree of hair loss by the age of 35, and about 85% of men will have significantly thinning hair by the age of 50. Although hair loss is typically associated with men, figures state that women make up 40% of all hair loss sufferers in the U.S., showing that hair loss is a condition that can affect us all. Recent studies claim that 16% of women under age 50 are affected, which increases to 30–40% of women aged 70 years and over[10]. The thinning of hair in women may become rather more pronounced after menopause when there are fewer estrogen hormones to counteract the androgens. Men tend to have baldness while women have thinning of hair and preservation of the frontal area.

Hair loss treatment products are mostly designed to act as DHT blockers. In recent years, two pharmacological agents have become available to treat male pattern baldness. Neither is fully effective in all cases. Both need long-term administration or there will be recurrence. Both must be prescribed on private prescription. Minoxidil is provided in 2% and 5% solutions that are applied to the scalp twice daily. The 5% solution is for men only. One study found that the 5% solution was 45% more effective than the weaker strength after a 48-week trial and was the preferred treatment for men[11]. It may well be months before any improvement is seen and it should be discontinued if there is none after a year. A solution of 5% minoxidil in cutaneous foam is now available, which is developed for ease of use. The product instruction requires application of half a capful to the scalp twice a day but the treatment should be stopped if there is no improvement after four months.

Recently, the natural hair loss treatment, **Provillus™**, has gained significant popularity for its effective dual-step formula to treat the hairs of men and women accordingly as it offers different formulations for both. The treatment, clinically proven to regrow hair, consists of a powerful blend of natural herbs and has been approved as safe and beneficial formula by health experts and FDA. The two-step formula consists of a hair regrowth supplement and a hair regrowth spray with 5% minoxidil for men and 2% minoxidil for women, which performs dual action of preventing hair loss first and then promoting hair regrowth. The consumption of this supplement twice a day makes the hairs strong enough to fight against DHT hormone and to survive. The hair regrowth spray is a liquid to be applied over the scalp. The use of that spray twice a day promotes a thicker, stronger, and healthier hair regrowth. The product nourishes the overall health of hairs and makes them healthy, shiny, and beautiful, without any negative side effects.

Change in hair fiber diameter (fine-coarseness) is another parameter that is influenced by age. Large increases in hair fiber diameter occur during the first year in life and during the teenage years. Diameter tends to peak at about age 20 for men and in the mid-40s for women (see Figure 4). Figure 4 shows a steeper drop for the scalp hair fiber diameter of Japanese males versus Caucasian males. A decrease in hair fiber diameter results in thin hair.

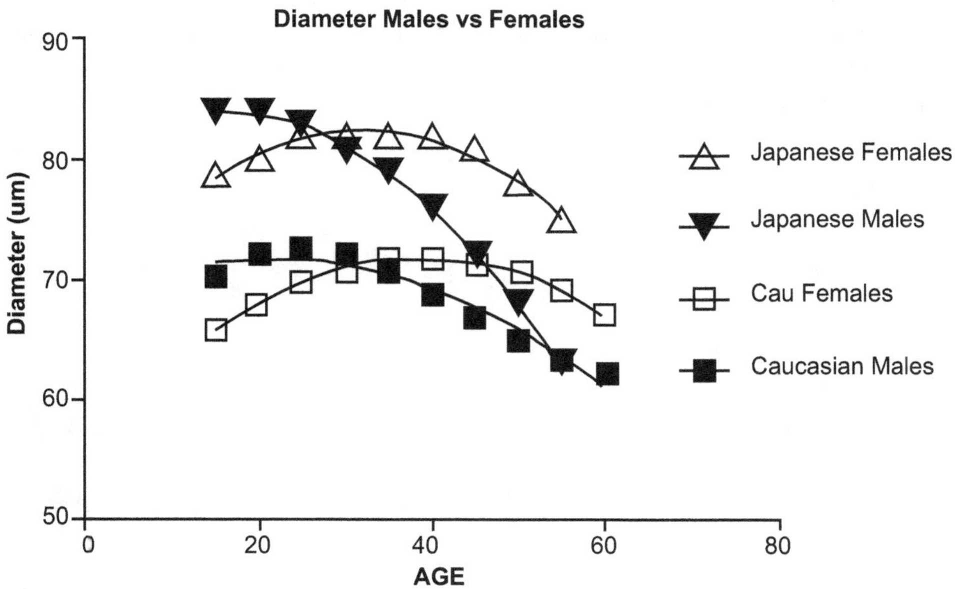

Figure 4. Hair fiber diameter of Japanese males vs. Caucasian males as a function of age (C.R Robbins pp 120)

Loss of Hair Color (Graying of Hair)

Graying of hair is a natural age-related phenomenon that varies between individuals and between different ethnicities. The biological process of hair aging has been attributed to the loss of pigment-forming melanocytes from the aging hair follicle[12]. There are many theories that explain the gradual loss of pigmentation with aging, including inactivation of tyrosinase enzyme[5] and decrease in stem cell factor[13]. Recently, a free radical theory of graying has been proposed by Arck et al.[14]. These authors found evidence of melanocyte apoptosis and increased oxidative stress in the pigmentary unit of graying hair follicles. Recently Wood et al.[6] have shown for the first time accumulation of high levels, millimolar concentration, of H_2O_2 *in vivo* in human gray/white scalp hair shaft by FT-Raman Spectroscopy. These authors further demonstrated absence of catalase and methionine sulfoxide reductase A and B enzymes. In younger people, catalase enzyme breaks down hydrogen peroxide into water and oxygen, thereby protecting melanocytes from oxidative damage by hydrogen peroxide. As we age, the decrease in the levels of catalase, combined with lower levels of methionine sulfoxide reductase enzymes, MSR A and B, which repair hydrogen peroxide damage, cause hair to turn gray. A recent study by researchers at University of Bradford demonstrated repigmentation of eyelashes and skin after reduction of epidermal H_2O_2 with topically applied narrow-band UV activated pseudo-catalase PC-KUS.[15] This further supports that accumulation of hydrogen peroxide due to decrease in catalase enzyme causes hair graying and reversal of pigment formation is possible through introduction of pseudo-catalase type molecules through topically applied products.

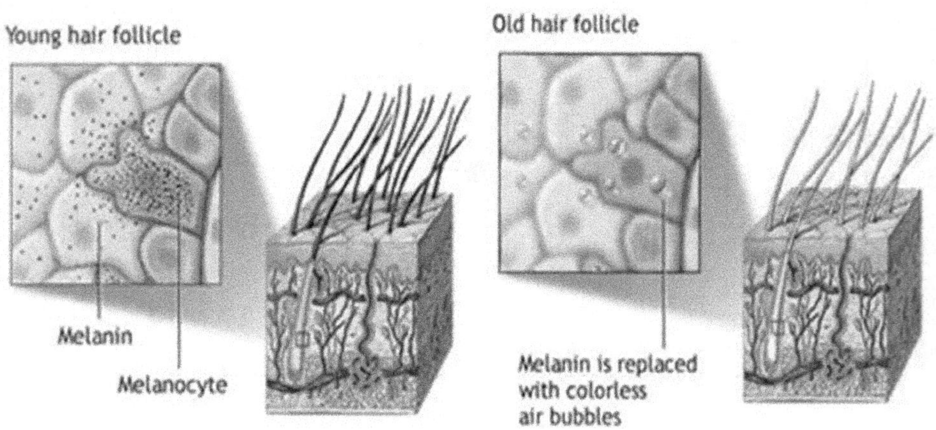

Figure 5. Picture of a young hair follicle vs. gray hair follicle showing melanin particles replaced with colorless air bubbles (www.nlm.nih.gov)

Hair Dryness, Shine, and Manageability

Hair dryness also results from both intrinsic and extrinsic aging. The sebaceous gland in the hair follicle produces sebum that normally hydrates the scalp and moisturizes the hair by surrounding it with a protecting microfilm. A deficiency or lack of sebum makes the scalp more fragile, resulting in irritation and itchiness. The loss of sebum also results in loss of hair elasticity and the hair becomes dry, dull, and prone to breakage. The intrinsic production of sebum from sebaceous glands in the follicle decreases with age, particularly in females as shown in Figure 6 below.

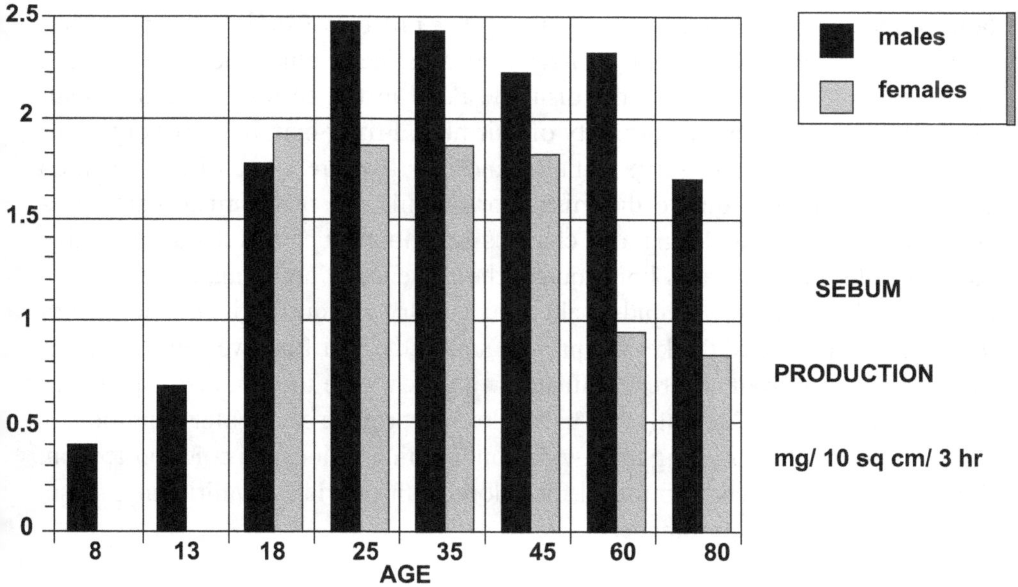

Figure 6. Variation of sebum production on foreheads with age. Data are from C.R. Robbins, *Chemical and Physical Behavior of Human Hair, 4th edition, p. 79*

Additionally, extrinsic parameters such as frequent washing of hair, use of alcohol-containing hair products, chemical treatments, exposure to sunlight, and frequent blow-drying also cause hair dryness. Each healthy hair strand has an outer protective layer (cuticle), which is composed of fatty acids, ceramides, and cholesterol. Together, these account for 0.7–1.3% of the total chemical content of hair. Integral hair lipids are located in the cell membrane complex (CMC) of hair cuticles, and are important in the maintenance of hair integrity due to hydrophobicity, moisturization, and stiffness.

Exposure to sunlight results in degradation of cuticle lipids by oxidative damage, and exposure to alcoholic cosmetic products solubilizes lipids and removes them from hair surface. Blow-drying and frequent washing with harsh surfactants also removes cuticle lipids. The appearance of your hair, and its reflective quality, depends heavily on the condition of the cuticle. Light reflection from a smooth and intact cuticle gives shine and glossiness, resulting in youthful appearance. Loss of cuticle also makes combing and brushing difficult. A flat and smooth cuticle structure reflects light, and it is important to keep healthy and shiny hair. It is reported that replacing the essential hair lipid, **18 MEA**, results in healthier-looking and -feeling hair through restoration of the hydrophobicity of hair fiber. Further, lipid replenishment protects the hair from further damage[16].

Chemical treatments such as hair relaxing and permanent hair coloring chemically modify the hair keratin structure by disrupting the disulfide bond, which is responsible for the strength of hair. Curly hair has a higher degree of disulfide bond in the cortex compared to straight hair. The process of straightening or relaxing changes curly hair into straight hair using alkaline or other chemical relaxers. The chemical modification of the disulfide bond in the cortex of the hair shaft affects the physicochemical property of hair fiber. Frizzy hair, hair breakage, hair thinning, scalp irritation, scalp damage, and hair loss are some of the common consumer complaints due to the misuse or chronic use of chemical hair relaxers[17]. Permanent hair coloring also changes hair fiber properties due to oxidative damage of hair proteins and lipids due to the presence of ammonia and hydrogen peroxide. The oxidation of lipids makes the hair dry and dull and the oxidation of the disulfide linkage of the keratin protein makes the hair fiber weaker. However, recent hair color products are formulated with great care to minimize damage as much as possible. Additionally, the hair color kits provide after-color conditioners to be used right after coloring to provide conditioning, shine, and color protection. Regular use of products formulated for colored hair provides conditioning, shine, and overall youthful appearance.

3.3.3.4 PHOTO-AGING OF HAIR

Photo-damaged hair shows dryness, an increase in fiber porosity, reduced strength and an increase in surface roughness. Long-term exposure to UV radiation causes severe chemical degradation to hair proteins and lipids. Photo-aging of hair results in lipid oxidation, disulfide bond cleavage, tryptophan degradation, and cysteic acid formation. Hair exposed to sunlight is claimed to be more brittle, stiffer, and drier than before irradiation and exhibits a reduced water-absorption capacity. Hair pigments provide photochemical protection to hair proteins by absorbing and filtering the impinging radiation and subsequently dissipating this energy as heat. However, in the process of protecting the hair proteins from light, the pigments are degraded or bleached. Dark hair is more resistant to photo-degradation than light hair. This is due to the higher photostability of eumelanin compared to pheomelanin[2].

The most obvious effect of the photo-aging of human hair is hair lightening, an effect that is accelerated by moisture. The extent of this photochemical-induced color change is dependent on the nature of the hair pigment and is understood to involve an oxidative attack on the eumelanin or pheomelanin melanosomes. Black hair is more photostable than blond hair. This color of hair seems well protected against UV light, and light brown hair is obviously damaged by a wide range of natural sunlight. The protective action of melanin granules is limited to the melanin-rich cortex of black hair, which shows only a slight modification of fiber proteins under irradiation[18].

3.3.3.5 PROTECTION OF HAIR FROM AGING

a. Scalp Care

Adequate care of scalp and shaft hair is critical to protect the hair from aging and to have healthy beautiful hair. Beautiful hair comes from a healthy scalp and hence taking care of the scalp is just as important as taking care of hair shaft. Hair problems such as thinning or falling of hair, premature graying or breakage, dandruff, and flaking could be symptoms that indicate an unhealthy scalp. Scalp care should be chosen based on the nature of your scalp, whether it is normal, oily, or dry. Normal scalp has the right balance of sebaceous glands, so it is generally not prone to problems like dandruff or excessive oil deposition. Shampooing three to four times a week with a normal shampoo and a light conditioner will be sufficient for this type of scalp. A warm oil treatment and massaging the scalp one to two times a month stimulates the oil gland and the massaging action improves blood circulation[i]. Coconut oil is great for all hair types. Avocado oil is one of the most emollient and moisturizing oils and is particularly good for really dry and frizzy hair.

If your scalp is oily, it is the most prone to dandruff and flaking. The excess oil that the sebaceous glands in the scalp produce tends to accumulate around the roots, clogging the pores. Such hair is usually limp and flat, making it almost impossible for volumizing or styling products to hold. Shampooing your hair every day with a deep cleansing shampoo is suitable for oily hair. If you suffer from dandruff, choose an anti-dandruff variety. Avoid using leave-in conditioners. A dry scalp causes constant itching and flaking, leaving the hair rough, dull and frizzy. As the oil secreted by the sebaceous glands is insufficient, apply oil externally and massage the scalp regularly to nourish the scalp. For dry hair, shampoo once or twice a week with a product that contains natural oils and moisturizing agents is sufficient. A thick cream-based conditioner and leave it on for about ten minutes before rinsing off makes hair smooth and soft. Get a warm oil treatment every week to stimulate the sebaceous glands. Massage your scalp thoroughly to stimulate oil secretion.

Unilever has recently launched Scalp and hair beauty therapy line of products formulated with Nutrium 10, an advanced moisturizing complex. A well-nourished scalp is the right foundation for strong, beautiful hair. For years women have been treating the wrong end of their hair. Clear Scalp & Hair Beauty Therapy made with Nutrium 10 nourishes the scalp, creating the right foundation for strong, beautiful hair. The regimen of shampoo and conditioner together is clinically proven to help restore scalp's natural moisture balance to create the right foundation for strong, beautiful hair from root to tip. There are various regimens of shampoo and conditioner to address the needs of different hair types.

b. Hair Care

Most women will see their hair become frizzier and less manageable due to chemical treatments such as coloring, straightening, perms, and frequent washing with harsh shampoos that strip the hair of natural oils. Everyday caring of hair starting with the right shampoo, conditioner, and styling product could cosmetically improve the appearance of shaft hair. Nourishment and proper grooming is very important to keep the hair texture, growth, shine, and luster in a good condition. For daily care, choose cleansing products that are gentle and moisturizing, preferably without harsh surfactants like sodium lauryl sulphate. Daily massaging of your hair with your fingertips helps proper blood circulation in the scalp. Apply heat-styling products to your hair before blow-drying and try to keep the setting on medium, not high. Use UV-protection hair products or wear a hat if your hair is brittle or color-treated. Choose a demi-permanent hair color product for covering gray; it doesn't contain ammonia and has less hydrogen peroxide. This type of product may not be an option if you have a lot of gray hair (more than 50%) and want to cover it, in which case you'll need permanent color.

3.3.3.6 ANTI-AGING HAIR CARE PRODUCTS

One of the latest trends in the global beauty industry is the proliferation of anti-aging hair products in the marketplace. Consequently, beauty product developers, ingredient suppliers, and brands large and small have been busy addressing the graying population in hopes of attracting the baby boomer marketplace[4].

Ingredients for hair care include the well-established ones such as: silicones for shine, quaternary ammonium compounds for ease of combing, thickening approaches such as proteins and high-molecular-weight polyquaternium polymers for conditioning[19] and polyvinylpyrrolidone for shaping and styling[20].

The hair shaft lacks biochemical processes, which gave the traditional concept that hair is dead and cannot be repaired and restored. As the root of the hair shaft is alive, hair treatments using anti-aging ingredients such as small-molecular-weight peptides, alpha hydroxyl acids, certain vegetable oils, amino acids, peptides, and ceramides can provide benefits to both the shaft and the hair root. In recent times, the hair care sector is being enlivened by entirely new ingredients as well as proprietary packages that combine the old standbys in novel ways. Anti-aging hair care specifically focuses on ingredients and products (applied both topically and in ingestible form) that can repair hair, providing more manageable and healthy looking hair.

Many ingredients are recently launched to address hair and scalp aging at the cellular level, improve follicle health, reduce hair loss, and offer antioxidant properties. These low-molecular-weight compounds penetrate the cuticle layers of the hair shaft, enhancing its softness, protection, and manageability. They can also penetrate the scalp, enhance scalp microcirculation, and improve follicle health, thereby promoting healthier new hair growth. Recently, researchers at DuPont have shown that hair care products with the well-known anti-aging ingredient, glycolic acid (marketed as DuPont™ Glypure), penetrates through the hair shaft and delivers enhanced protection and manageability to hair by conditioning, moisturizing, strengthening, and preventing breakage[8]. It also moisturizes and exfoliates the scalp, resulting in less flaking to give the scalp a healthy look and feel.

Natural vegetable oils provide nourishing conditioning and shine to hair. Coconut oil, being a triglyceride of lauric acid (principal fatty acid), has a high affinity for hair proteins and, because of its low molecular weight and straight linear chain, is able to penetrate inside the hair shaft[21]. It is an excellent conditioner and helps in the regrowth of damaged hair. It also provides the essential proteins required for nourishing damaged hair and it softens the hair and conditions the scalp. Avocado and Jojoba oil are other oils for nourishing, conditioning, and shine benefits.

Amino acid-like L-Arginine is a nitric oxide precursor found to stimulate hair regrowth by stimulating the production of hair follicles and also to strengthen hair by nourishing the hair roots. Sunscreens are another category of anti-aging ingredients now found in a variety of hair care products, including shampoos, conditioners, and hairsprays. They prevent breakdown of keratin due to sun exposure and also keep hair dye from fading in ultraviolet light. Ingredients like Crodasorb™ UV-HPP from Croda and PARSOL® SLX provide multiple benefits like prevention of color fading, strengthening hair body, and enhancing gloss when delivered through hair color, or hair care products, especially leave-on sprays. The table below lists some advanced functional hair care ingredients popular in today's hair care market.

Table 1. Advanced hair care ingredients popular in current hair care products[ii]

Hair Care Ingredients	Benefits	Supplier
Crodafos™ HCE	Increases color intensity & color uptake. Provides better color wash fastness. Reduces hair damage as shown by hydrophobicity and combing studies.	Croda Inc
Incroquat™ Behenyl TMS-50	Hair conditioning agent, suitable for cationic emulsions, provides soft touch.	Croda Inc
ChromAveil ®	Protects the hair from the damaging effects of sunlight. Gives color protection benefits to dyed hair from UVA and protects the mechanical properties of the hair from UVB.	Croda Inc
Crodasorb™ UV-HPP	Polyester polyquaternized ingredient that is substantive to hair and protects against the damaging effects of UV-B radiation.	Croda Inc
Lustreplex®	Creates lustrous, healthy-looking hair from anionic systems. Provides frizz control, shine, detangling, and conditioning benefits.	Croda Inc
Dow Corning® CE-8411 Smooth Plus Emulsion	Repairs colored, gray, and heat-damaged hair by restoring moisturized feel, shine, & alignment. Protects hair from further damage and color loss.	Dow Corning
Dow Corning® 5-7113 Silicone Quat Microemulsion	Restores smoothness, shine, and Alignment. Prolongs hair color. Protects hair from breakage.	Dow Corning
HYDROVANCE®	Improves water retention and helps to strengthen and even repair damaged hair, for benefits the consumer can clearly feel and see.	Akzo Nobel
STRUCTURE® PQ-37P	Cationic acrylic homopolymer multifunctional rheology modifier that provides thickening and conditioning.	Akzo Nobel
Procapil™	Reinforces hair anchoring. Reduces hair loss.	Sederma

Hair Care Ingredients	Benefits	Supplier
Glypure® glycolic acid	Glypure® penetrates the hair shaft to enhance the softness and manageability of hair.	DuPont
L-Arginine	Helps hair regrowth by stimulating the production of new hair follicles. It nourishes the hair root and strengthens hair.	Ajinomoto
PARSOL® SLX	PARSOL® SLX is a silicone-based UV-B absorber. Delivers multiple benefits including prevention of color fading, gloss enhancement, and conditioning.	DSM

Table 1. Shows ingredient information obtained from supplier websites

Anti-aging hair care products are designed to address the consumer needs such as thinning, coloring, breakage, and drying, with emphasis on particular ingredients that target specific hair issues. Such hair care formulations are designed to deliver conditioning, thickening, and color protection, strengthening, and nourishing properties through deposition of essential oils, cationic polymers, proteins, and other nutrients. For gray hair, so far, there are no solutions for reversing the color. Hair colorants are used for covering gray, to impart color and shine and hence youthful appearance. Therefore, hair colorants can also be classified as anti-aging hair color products.

Pantene has launched PRO-V Expert Age Defy shampoo, conditioner, and advanced thickening treatment designed to work together for thicker hair strands. These products are claimed to be gentle enough for daily use on color-treated hair. Formulated with a triple blend complex (mixture of amino acids), the shampoo and conditioner help fight seven signs of aging hair: reduces breakage, prevents split ends, reduces frizz, controls unruly grays, minimizes lackluster color, improves a thin look, and minimizes dryness.

There are several professional hair care products formulated with advanced technologies that restore oils vitamins and other essential nutrients. Nexxus has launched its first anti-aging range of products that combats eight signs of aging hair: volume loss, breakage, roughness, less shine, dryness, brittleness, unruliness, and loss of color vibrancy. It replenishes and revitalizes for more vibrant, youthful-looking hair.

Nexxus Youth Renewal™ Rejuvenating Shampoo gently cleanses hair to help rebuild volume, vibrancy, and vitality. Nexxus Youth Renewal™ Rejuvenating Conditioner provides lightweight nourishment to help preserve volume, vibrancy, and vitality. Youth Renewal™ Rejuvenating Elixir lightweight leave-in treatment helps rebuild hair's strength by reducing breakage while making hair look more youthful and vibrant in just seven days.

Alterna has launched CAVIAR Anti-Aging® Replenishing line of products comprising moisturizing shampoo and conditioner that transforms dry, brittle hair by sealing in a rich blend of lipids and essential ingredients to continually nourish and hydrate the hair. The shampoo is a luxurious, sulfate-free cleanser that restores moisture while protecting hair from color fade, daily stresses, and future damage. Both shampoo and conditioner are infused with Seasilk®, Age-Control Complex®, Enzymetherapy®, and Color Hold®. It not only helps maintain moisture, but also protects from daily stresses and delivers what your hair needs to become strong, healthy, and younger-looking. The anti-aging rapid repair spray helps add moisture and vibrancy to hair while combating natural, chemical, and environmental stresses. It may be used as a thermal protectant when applied pre-styling, or as a finishing shine spray.

Keranique® has launched a hair revitalization system developed for women to strengthen, fortify, and thicken each and every hair shaft. There are three key components to the Keranique® System. Step 1 includes a revitalizing shampoo and volumizing conditioner. Step 2 has the hair regrowth treatment with clinically proven FDA approved ingredient, Minoxidil, and Step 3 is an amplifying lift spray to provide fullness, volume, and body.

CONCLUSION

Hair, like skin, undergoes aging both intrinsically due to chronological aging and extrinsically as a result of exposure to environmental factors such as sun, pollution, and daily grooming habits. The aging of hair results in a series of visual and measurable changes both in the scalp and hair shaft. The most obvious sign of hair aging is graying of hair while the consumer also perceives a series of changes such as thinning of hair, dryness, brittleness, loss of shine, and manageability. Prevention of scalp and hair aging is not completely possible, but there are ways to protect scalp and hair fiber from damage due to external aggressors and to minimize damage from daily grooming by choosing the right products. The chapter provides an overview of the cause of hair aging, the factors that contribute to hair aging, the visual and perceptional signs of aging, and finally a compilation of some hair ingredients and anti-aging products currently available in the market.

REFERENCES

1. Trueb R.M. Pharmacological interventions in aging hair. *Clinical Interventions in Aging*. 2006: 1, 121–129.
2. Lee, W-S, Photoaggravation of hair aging. *Int. J. Trichology*. 2009: 1, 94–99.
3. Trueb R.M. Oxidative Stress in Aging of Hair. *Int. J. Trichology*. 2009: 1, 6–14.
4. Serviss N. The Rise of Anti-aging Hair Care. 2013. July Issue of GCI Magazine.
5. Commo S, Gaillard O, Bernard B.A. Human hair graying is linked to a specific depletion of hair follicle melanocytes affecting both the bulb and the outer root sheath. *Br. J. Dermatology*. 2004: 150, 434–443.
6. Wood J.M, Decker H, Hartmann H, Chavan, B, Rokos, H, Spencer, J-D, Hasse, S., Thornton, M-J, Shalbaf, M., Paus, R, and Schallreuter. Senile hair graying: H_20_2-mediated oxidative stress affects human hair color by blunting methionine sulfoxide repair. *FASEB J.*2009; 23:2065–2075.
7. Robins, C. R, Chemical and Physical Behavior of Human Hair, 4th Edition, 2002; pp 386–469.
8. Evans, TA, Altland JM, and Horsager J. Glycolic Acid-No longer just for Skin. Changing the Internal Properties of Hair. *Cosmetics and Toiletries*. 2013: 128, 816–820.
9. Shindo Y, Witt E, Han D, Epstein W, Packer L. Enzymatic and Non-enzymatic antioxidants in epidermis and dermis of human skin. *J. Invest Dermatol*. 1994: 102, 122–124.
10. Norwood OT, Incidence of Female Androgenic Alopecia (female pattern alopecia). *Dermatol Surg*. 2001: 27, 53–54.
11. Olsen EA, Dunlap FE, Funicella T, Koperski JA, Swinehart JM, Tschen EH and Trancik RJ. A randomized clinical trial of 5% topical minoxidil versus 2% topical minoxidil and placebo in the treatment of androgenetic alopecia in men. *J. Am. Acad. Dermatol*. 2002: 47, 377–385.\
12. Tobin D.J, Slominski, A, Botchkarev, V, and Paus, R. The fate of hair follicle melanocytes during the hair growth cycle. *J. Invest. Dermatol. Symp. Proc*. 1999: 4, 323–332.
13. Sarin, KY, and Artandi, S.E. Aging, graying and loss of melanocyte stem cells. *Stem Cell Rev*. 2007:3, 212–217.
14. Arck, PC, Overall, R, Spatz, K, Liezman C, Handjiski B, Klapp, BF and Peters EM. Towards a "free radical theory of graying": melanocyte apoptosis in the aging human hair follicle is an indicator of oxidative stress induced tissue damage. *FASEB J*. 2006: 20, 1567–1569.

15. Schallreuter, KU, Salem, AEL, Holtz, S and Panske, A. Basic evidence for epidermal H_2O_2/ONOO-mediated oxidation/nitration in segmented vitiligo is supported by re-pigmentation of skin and eyelashes after reduction of epidermal H_2O_2 with topical NB-UVB activated pseudo-catalse PC-KUS. *FASEB J.* 2013: 27, 1–10.
16. Tillou, R. Restoring Essential Hair Fiber Lipids with Quaternized 18-MEA. Cosmetics and Toiletries. 2011. September Version.
17. Shetty, VH, Shetty, NJ and Nair, DH. Chemical Hair Relaxers Have Adverse Effects a Myth or Reality. *Int J Trichology*. 2013: 1, 26–28.
18. Hoting E, Zimmermann M, and Hocker, H. Photochemical alterations in human hair part II. Analysis of melanin. *J. Soc. Cosmet. Chem.* 1995: 46, 181–190.
19. Goddard, ED, Leung, PS and Padmanabhan, KPA. Novel gelling structures based on polymer/surfactant systems. *J. Soc. Cosmet. Chem.*1991:42, 19–34.
20. Martiny S. Acetylenic polymers for hair styling products. *Int J Cosmet Sci.* 2002:24, 125–34.
21. Rele AS, Mohile RB. Effect of mineral oil, sunflower oil, and coconut oil on prevention of hair damage. *J Cosmet Sci.* 2003: 54,175–192.

GLOSSARY

1. **Gray Hair :** Hair without melanin pigment
2. **Hair Follicle:** An organ and part of the skin below the scalp that produces hair.
3. **Hair Shaft:** The part of the hair that is seen above the skin
4. **Oxidative Stress:** An imbalance between oxidants and antioxidants in favor of the oxidants, potentially leading to damage, is termed 'oxidative stress'
5. **Chronological Aging:** Age of a person measured in years, months, and days from the date the person was born
6. **Androgenic Alopecia: A** common form of hair loss in both men and women
7. **DHT:** Dihydrotestosterone (a derivative of the male hormone testosterone)
8. **18-**MEA: 18-methyl eicosanoic acid (essential hair lipid responsible for hair shine and hair integrity)

PART 3.3.4

MECHANISMS OF CHANGES IN HAIR SHAPE

Dr. Manuel Gamez-Garcia, Ph.D.,

Research Fellow,
Ashland Specialty Ingredients

A note from Meyer R. Rosen, Editor-in-Chief

* This chapter brings to mind a phrase that I hope will stick in your memory for a long, long time. At its heart it is Manuel Gamez-Garcia's unique ability to describe:

The Science of Hair Beauty and the Beauty of Hair Science

ABSTRACT

Changes in hair shape can be categorized as permanent and temporary. They can also be classified as cosmetically desirable and undesirable or by a combination of any of these two categories. For instance, examples of hair shape changes desired permanently are those produced by perm solutions and alkaline relaxers. Examples of desirable temporary changes are those resulting from water-setting, hot irons, and styling polymers. Undesirable permanent shape changes are, on the other hand, those leading to frizzy hair, excessive tangling, and lack of manageability.

This chapter provides an exceptionally detailed look at the development of scientific distinctions based on the integration of polymer physics and chemistry with that of hair behavior and what impacts it in our endless search for beauty.

Whether the changes in hair shape are desirable or undesirable, all of them result from a process consisting of three main steps:

1) the softening of hair, which may involve the breakage of chemical or physical bonds, and/or protein rearrangements in the amorphous and crystalline phases,
2) the mechanical imposition of a new shape, and
3) the fixing or locking of the new shape by the re-formation of broken chemical or physical bonds. In shape changes that are desirable the occurrence of these three steps is induced purposely to create a new shape, whereas in those that are undesirable the three steps occur mostly during hair damage. This chapter will focus primarily on those aspects that are desirable from a cosmetic point of view. Those aspects produced by damage have been reviewed elsewhere (1).

We would point out that technology transfer from the world of polymer physics and chemistry has been of great value in the development and application of "novel" concepts and their use as seminal thinking points for cosmetic hair scientists. We encourage the reader to continue this approach, as much of this type of "new" thinking will open fascinating and productive pathways to novel hair care products.

TABLE OF CONTENTS

3.3.4.1 INTRODUCTION

The key physical properties and mechanistic events related to changes in hair shape can be better understood when we recall that hair is a biopolymer that shares many of the physical and chemical features possessed by synthetic polymers. In fact, we can learn a great deal about hair's mechanical behavior by comparing its properties with those of synthetic polymers having a similar structure. For instance, synthetic semi-crystalline polymers, like hair, possess crystalline melting and amorphous phase glass transition temperatures (2–4).

Furthermore, the composition of hair's architecture is such that it can exhibit two types of physical behavior.

- **One type of behavior is related to the hydrophilic structure of the globular proteins in the amorphous phase.** The protein hydrophilic groups in this structure are capable of forming hydrogen bonds with water. This aspect of the structure makes it highly water swellable and susceptible to plasticization by moisture. It is responsible for the viscoelastic and softening effects produced in hair by water; Max Feughelman refers to this aspect as the "gel structure of the amorphous phase" (6).
- The other type of physical behavior stems from the non-gel structure of the intermediate filaments (IFPs). This structural aspect is comprised of an amorphous network of hydrophobic, and stiffer protein segments. These are covalently cross-linked by disulfide bonds, as well as an ordered arrangement of crystalline proteins regions, which are responsible for both shape stabilization and hair strength.

The entire amorphous phase acts mechanically in parallel with the crystalline phase and gives rise to the unique combination of viscoelasticity and strength typical of hair. This behavior is also found in semi-crystalline polymers and, incidentally, there is a remarkable similarity in the architecture and properties of hair, and a particular type of cross-linked semi-crystalline polymers, namely; those that have been synthesized to behave as shape memory polymers (SMP) (7). These polymers, like hair, also exhibit two and even more types of physical behaviors. These multiple types of behavior result in most cases from the various chemical groups or structures grafted onto main polymer chains introduced with the purpose of storing various temporary shapes (8–11).

As will be discussed later in this chapter, hair, with both its amorphous and crystalline structures, can also act as a shape memory polymer (SMP) and the mechanistic aspects related to changes in its shape can be better understood by using concepts from this field of polymer science. We would point out here that this cross-fertilization of ideas, or technology transfer, is an excellent approach for hair product developers to employ when seeking new ideas.

3.3.4.2 THE SHAPE MEMORY PROPERTIES OF HAIR

a. Definition of shape memory materials

In the scientific literature, C. Liu and C.B. Chun (8) define a shape memory material as follows:

"Shape-memory materials are those materials that have the ability to 'memorize' a macroscopic (permanent) shape, be manipulated and 'fixed' to a temporary and dormant shape under specific conditions of temperature and stress, and then, later, relax to the original, stress-free condition under thermal, electrical, or environmental command. This relaxation is associated with elastic deformation stored during prior manipulation" (2).

Currently, the most rapidly growing area in the field of shape memory materials are shape memory polymers (SMPs), and they can be either purely amorphous or semi-crystalline (12–14). Figure 1 shows a sequence of captions displaying a shape memory polymer changing its shape from a coiled temporary to a straight permanent shape after this event is triggered by elevating its temperature (15). Shape memory polymers can store temporary shapes and can recover their permanent shape by a suitable stimulus, either electrical, chemical, or temperature.

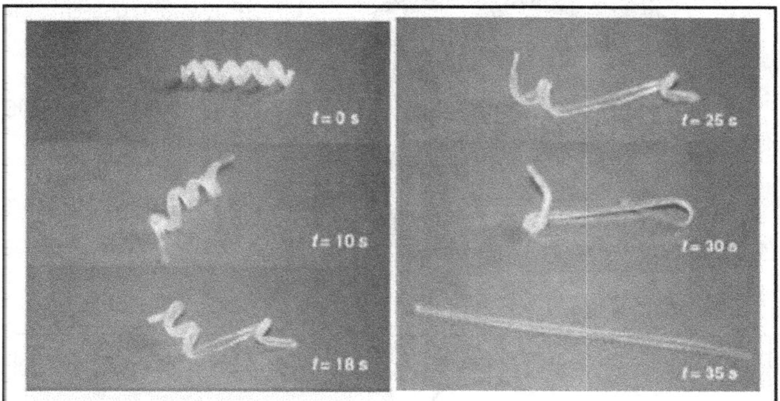

Figure 1) Transition of shape from temporary (spiral) to permanent (rod) of a polymer synthesized from poly-(ε-caprolactone) dimethylacrylate and butyl acrylate (15).

Various scientists working in this field have already listed the main physical requirements for a semi-crystalline polymer to display shape memory properties. According to C. Liu et al., these are as follows (8):

1) a relatively sharp glass transition and/or a high crystalline phase melting temperature that can be used to promptly fix the secondary shape at low temperatures and trigger shape recovery at high temperatures,
2) superelasticity (low loss modulus, high deformability) above the transition temperature that leads the shape recovery and avoids residual strain (permanent deformation) and,
3) complete and rapid fixing of the temporary shape by immobilizing polymeric chains without creep thereafter.

Synthetic polymers with shape memory properties consist primarily of two main features in their chain architecture. These are:

- A primary polymer network with network points, or cross-links that serve as a memory mechanism for the generation of a permanent shape, and
- A structure of secondary groups attached to the main network that serves as memory mechanism for the formation of temporary shapes (8).

These groups can be pendant functional moieties, grafted chains, polymer blocks, interpenetrating networks, or crystalline domains; they act as switches to release the temporary shape when activated by suitable external stimulus (see Figure 1) (7). Moisture, heat, light, and electric fields are examples of external stimulus that can release temporary shapes stored in SMPs with pendant groups or structures sensitive to them (see Figure 2) (8, 9).

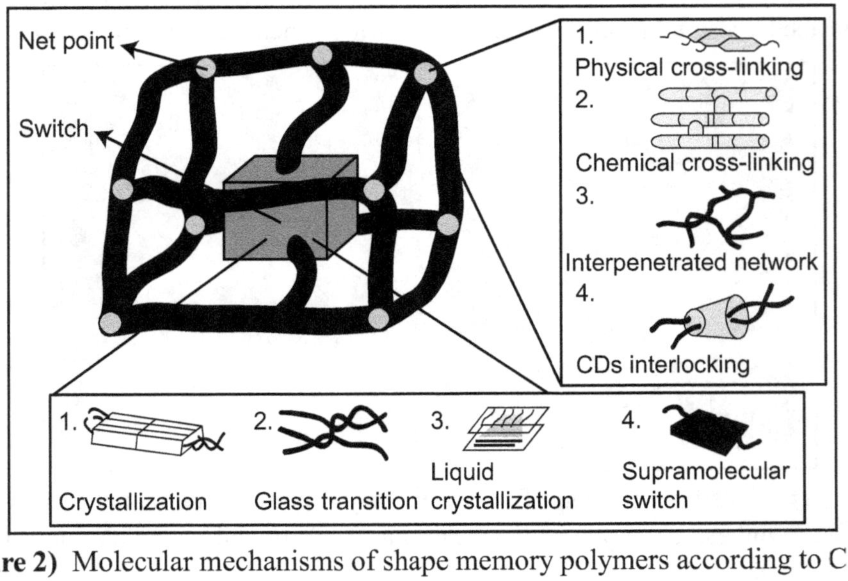

Figure 2) Molecular mechanisms of shape memory polymers according to C. Liu et al. (8)

b. Hair is a biopolymer with shape memory properties.

In the scientific literature, biopolymers such as silk and collagen have also been reported to have shape memory properties, and thus, they have been classified as shape memory materials (16, 17). **Hair is a biopolymer that also behaves as a shape memory polymer**. Clear manifestations of this behavior and properties are the following:

1) hair has a permanent shape,
2) its shape can be changed either temporarily or semi-permanently, and
3) it can "remember" or reverse to its permanent shape when treated appropriately.

Beauticians and cosmetic scientists, aware of these properties, have been creating fashionable hairstyles for years that can be reversed when desired. An example of hair's ability to recover its permanent shape can be seen in Figure 3, where it is shown that a curly temporary water-setting in a woman's hair (Figure 3a) can return to its original straight shape after washing the hair (Figure 3b). Also, Figure 4 displays a sequence of micrographs of a hair fiber recovering its permanent shape from temporary straight to its curly permanent shape.

As in the case of synthetic polymers, the permanent and temporary shape memory sites in hair reside in its crystalline and amorphous phases. In the case of hair, these polymeric entities are of natural origin and located in the macro-fibrils of the cortical cells. These can be listed as follows:

a) a protein crystalline phase forming intermediate filaments which serves as permanent shape memory and is also capable of storing a temporary shape when its crystalline structure unfolds or when it denatures above its melting temperature Tm.
b) a disulfide bond cross-linked protein amorphous phase capable of storing temporary shapes when it becomes soft at the hair's glass transition temperature Tg, or when it undergoes disulfide bond interchange. This structure also contributes to the stability of the crystalline phase, and
c) an extended structure of hydrophilic protein groups located at the surface of globular proteins in the amorphous phase. Its structure forms a gel, is sensitive to moisture, and is also capable of storing a temporary shape.

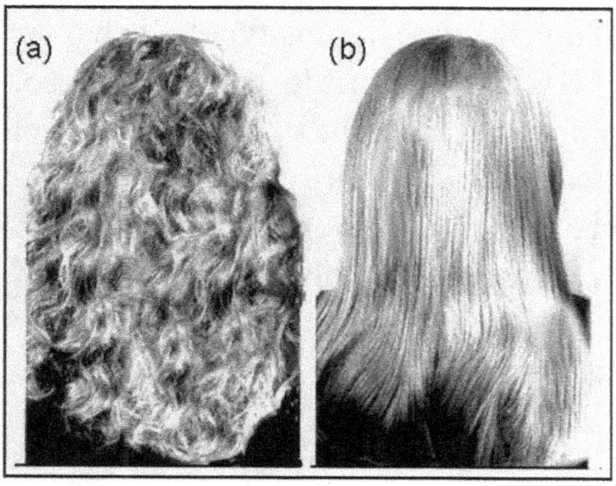

Figure 3) Captions of hair in a woman before (a) and after (b) it recovers its straight shape from a water temporary setting (18).

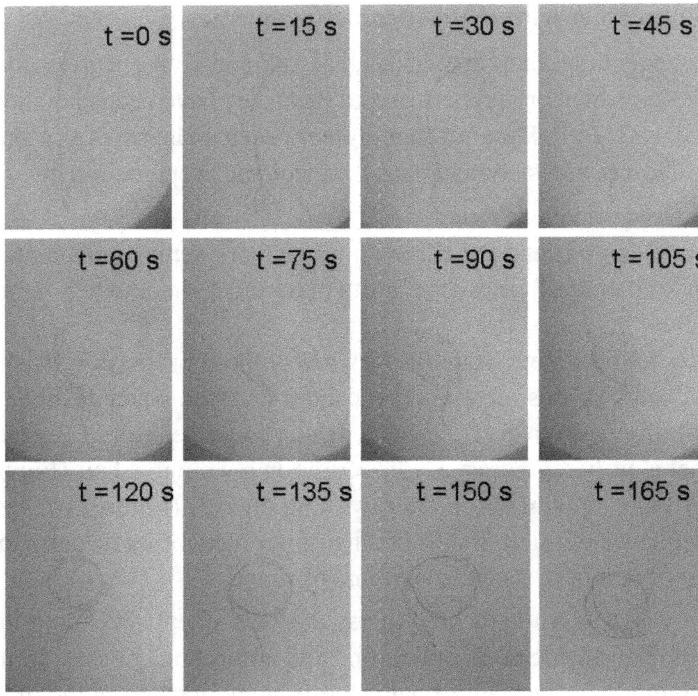

Figure 4) Captions showing sequence of a single hair fiber recovering its permanent shape from a straight temporary shape to a curly shape after water immersion (18).

c. Temporary shape memory in hair

The most common temporary or secondary shapes in hair are stored by physical means. The position of storage is in the protein regions with high levels of hydrogen bonding, i.e., in the soft gel structure of the amorphous phase (6). A typical example of this mechanism is water-setting. The gel structure in hair is ubiquitous in all types of hair and plays a crucial role in most temporary shapes imposed by hair movement and daily grooming practices. It is part of the amorphous phase, and behaves like a material that exhibits variable viscosity depending on the shear rate it is exposed to (i.e., pseudoplastic with a yield stress). This type of behavior can turn hair from very soft and flexible to very hard and brittle and, in doing so, it can virtually lock-in almost any temporary shape in hair. The viscosity of the gel structure depends on the hair's moisture content and, when hard and brittle, it presents a high opposition to the imposition or recovery of any type of shape in the hair. Temporary shapes in hair can also be stored by processes involving vitrification of the disulfide cross-linked amorphous phase and rearrangements of the crystalline phase. A typical example of this is the case of setting hair with hot irons.

The ideal creation of temporary shapes in hair shouldn't involve permanent and irreversible modifications to the protein architecture of hair. This means that after creating a temporary shape, the hair's permanent shape memory should remain intact, i.e., irreversible protein denaturation in crystalline filaments or irreversible breakage of covalent bonds in main protein chains and pendant groups should not be allowed to occur. If these irreversible phenomena occur, the hair may lose part or all of its permanent shape, becoming shapeless, and the imposition of a temporary shape will thus be irrelevant. As will be seen later, when hair is heated above its melting and glass transition temperatures with hot irons, temporary shapes can be created but at the expense of producing some of these unwanted irreversible phenomena.

d. The apparent permanent shape in hair

The hair shape that we normally perceive in our natural hair in everyday life is an apparent shape that results from a number of unavoidable mechanical effects. These unavoidable effects are primarily caused by hair's own weight and by inter-fiber interactions in the hair assembly. Both effects produce a temporary shape that is stored in the gel structure of hair and is always present in our everyday life. It is a form of quasi-permanent water-setting. Therefore, the hair shape that we have in our natural hair is not the "real" hair's native shape, but rather it is a very close representation of it.

We call this close representation an "apparent permanent shape" or temporary shape in equilibrium with the permanent shape. Other factors that contribute to the formation of the "apparent permanent shape" are hair length, relative humidity, and type of hair; i.e., it also depends on whether the hair is naturally straight, wavy, or very curly.

The "real" permanent shape of hair is only manifested when we immerse a single hair fiber in water so that the temporary shape imposed by its own weight and other interactions is released from the gel structure. For instance, experiments have shown that a high percentage of hair fibers from Caucasian origin that appear

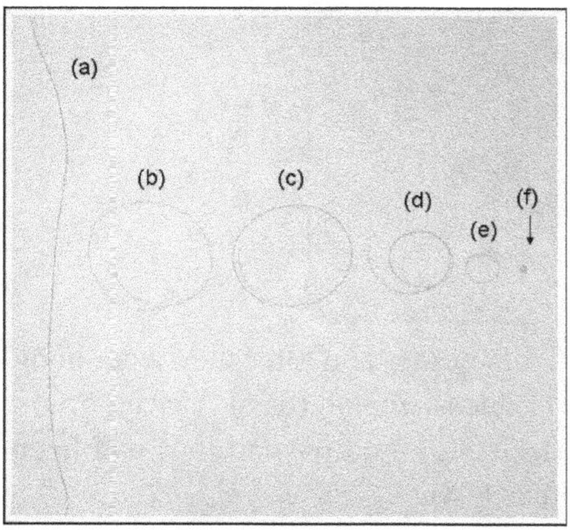

Figure 5) Picture showing six single hair fibers after their shape was equilibrated in water as follows: (a) Oriental, (b), (c), and (d) Caucasian, (e) Mulatto, and (f) of African origin (18).

wavy in shape, regardless of their degree of waviness or curliness, turn into almost perfect circular coils when immersed in water (18)!

We probably have all observed these effects at one time or another upon seeing our own hair fibers floating in a pool of water. These effects are shown in Figure 5 where six single hair fibers from different origins are displayed as follows: (a) Oriental, (b), (c), (d) Caucasian, (e) Mulatto, and (f) of African origin. The shape of the Caucasian and Mulatto fibers was wavy/curly before equilibration in water. Observe in this Figure that the hair fibers of Caucasian, Mulatto, and African origin formed almost perfect circles after ten minutes of water immersion, except for the one of Asian origin. This means that the real permanent shape of most hair fibers that appear wavy in a hair assembly, is actually coiled and circular, and that the wavy pattern results from deformations mostly imposed by their own weight as the fibers hang from the scalp. Another important implication from these observations is that when hair emerges from the follicle, the shape of a high percentage of hair fibers of Caucasian origin is never wavy but rather circular with a predetermined radius of curvature. Thereafter, as the hair fiber grows longer it actually becomes wavy because it is deformed by both its own weight and the interaction with other hair fibers in the scalp.

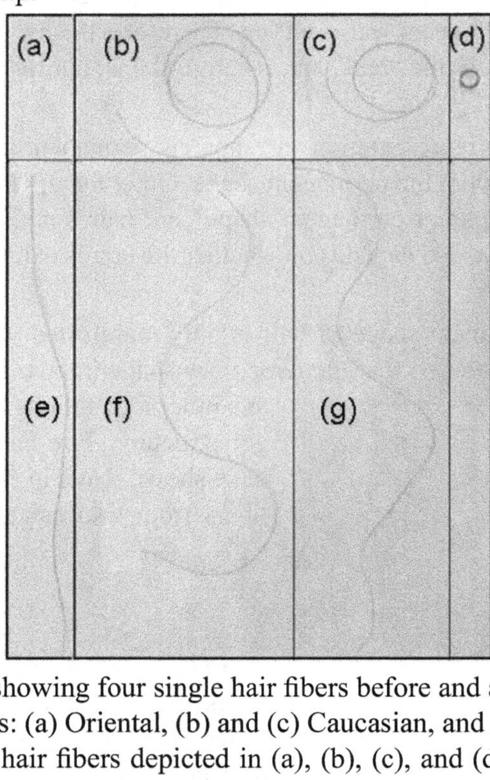

Figure 6) Picture showing four single hair fibers before and after they were hung vertically as follows: (a) Oriental, (b) and (c) Caucasian, and (d) of African origin (12). The shape of hair fibers depicted in (a), (b), (c), and (d) captions had been equilibrated by water immersion for ten minutes (18).

The above-mentioned effects are better visualized in Figure 6 where it can be seen that the circular shapes of two equilibrated Caucasian hair fibers (b) and (c) turn into wavy patterns (f) and (g) as the hair fibers hang. In Figure 4 it can also be observed that the circular coil of an African hair fiber (d) presents a very small tight curly pattern, and does not open its coil upon hanging. The hair fiber of Oriental origin (e) did not change its straight shape very much after being hung.

The observations made on the behavior of African hair are not new and rather confirm what is already known by cosmetologists and beauticians; namely, that hair with a very tight coil is not readily opened by its own weight when hanging from the scalp regardless of its length. The tight curly hair will be opened, however, when we impose a force, either with the fingers or with other devices. As will be seen later in this chapter, hair with very tight curls, such as that depicted in Figure 6d, has a very small radius of curvature, and its modification requires processes that modify a larger number of memory sites in the hair.

The modifications introduced to real permanent shapes in hair by its own weight also explain well-recognized hair shape variations often observed in people's hair when the environmental humidity changes. Higher levels of moisture result in hydrogen bond breakage in the gel structure and, therefore, moisture affects the "apparent permanent shape" of hair.

If the permanent shape is very strong, the hair will recover its real permanent shape, either curly or limp. For instance, people with wavy hair know very well that when the relative humidity is high their hair may become curlier. In contrast, people that have straight or fine straight hair as the real permanent shape may experience a higher level of hair limpness or straightening at high relative humidities. Furthermore, the formation of this "apparent permanent shape" also gives rise to differences in hair shape depending on its position on the head. For the sake of simplicity in the following paragraphs the term "real permanent shape" will be used when referring to hair shapes without any imposed deformation; and the term "permanent shape" will be used to refer to hair shapes in equilibrium.

e. Permanent shape memory in hair

The real permanent shape of hair is cast in the cortical cells during its life cycle through the anagen, catagen, and telogen phases (19–20). It is predetermined genetically and permanently imprinted in the hair follicle by the process of keratinization when the proteins in the amorphous phase are cross-linked by disulfide bonds. Figure 7 shows typical examples of hair with different types of permanent shape. Whether the hair is straight, wavy, or extremely curly, its permanent memory shape essentially resides in the composition ratio of ortho- to para-cortical cells. At the microscopic level, however, the permanent shape of hair is imprinted in the two-phase architectural structure of hair which results from the crystalline keratin micro-fibrils embedded in a highly cross-linked amorphous network of proteins (see Figure 8). More specifically, it is imprinted in the primary, secondary, and tertiary protein structures of crystalline and amorphous phases, chemically and physically stabilized by disulfide and isopeptide covalent bonds and by hydrogen bonds, salt bridges, and dispersion forces. Both protein phases stabilize hair shape and also strengthen the fibers mechanically.

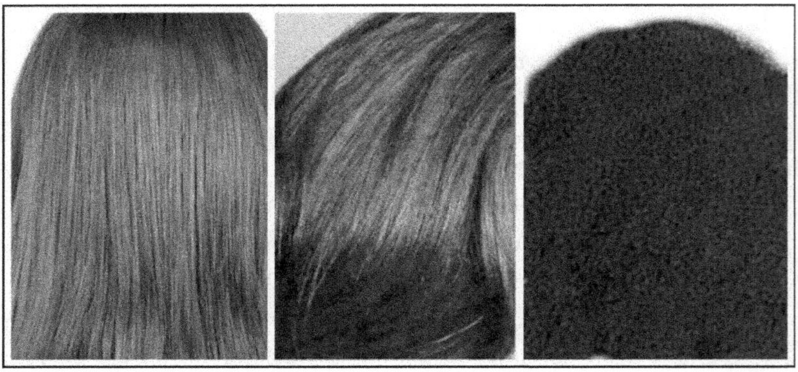

Figure 7) Captions showing three types of natural permanent hair shape as follows: Oriental (left), Caucasian (center), and African (left).

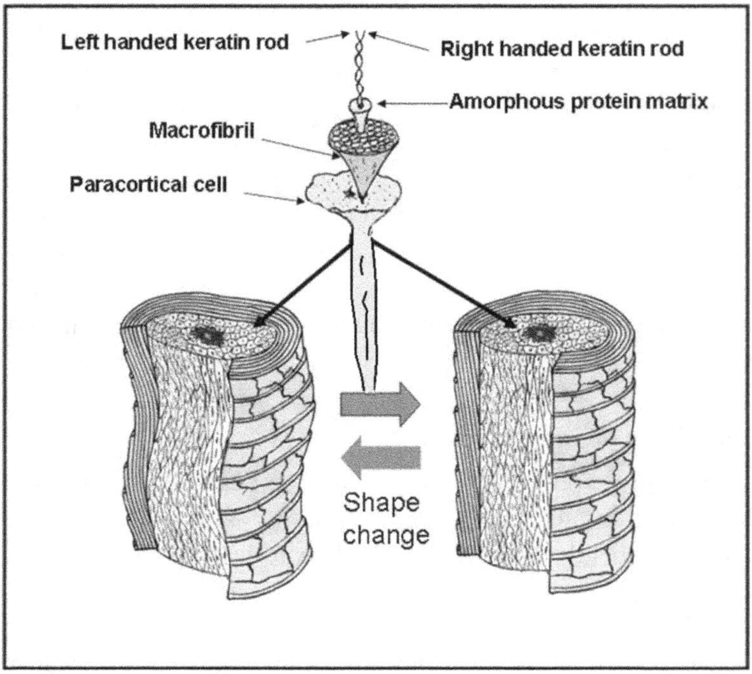

Figure 8) Schematic representation showing two hair fibers with different shape. The permanent shape of hair, either curly or straight, is imprinted in the hundreds of micro-fibrils and amorphous protein networks forming the two-phase protein arrangement in the cortical cells (18).

f. Changes to the permanent shape in hair

Permanent changes in hair shape have very different requirements than those already outlined for temporary shape changes. While temporary changes do not require irreversible modifications to the hair structure, permanent changes do require this process. Irreversible modifications are needed, first, because it is necessary to erase or delete the permanent shape from the memory of hair, and second, because it is necessary to build a new permanent shape in the hair structure when faced with consumer demands and needs. The latter step usually requires irreversible modifications to the crystalline phase, the introduction of new chemical bonds, and the rearrangement of proteins in the amorphous phase. **Thus, permanent changes in hair shape require irreversible modifications to one or two properties of sites where the permanent memory of hair shape resides.**

The irreversible changes may be in the form of chain scission, chemical modification of protein-pendant groups, and breakage of disulfide bonds. They can also involve irreversible protein denaturation, irreversible melting of crystalline regions, or a combination of all these factors (21). Thioglycolate salt solutions and very high pH alkaline creams used in permanent waving and hair relaxers, respectively, involve exactly this type of irreversible protein denaturation. The former is selective to the breakage of disulfide bonds in the protein chains and does not have a strong impact on other chemical bonds. The latter also breaks disulfide bonds but is less specific to them and, it breaks other bonds in the protein chains as well. In addition, the phenomenon also produces irreversible modifications to the crystalline regions and to the whole hair architecture itself (22).

g. Shape reversion

One factor often encountered in treatments geared to produce a permanent change in the shape of hair is that in many instances, they do not produce a real durable permanent change. As a result, there is a partial and gradual reversion to the original fiber shape. Lack of performance of active ingredients, poor formulation design, or poor hair treatment conditions are often the cause of this reversal. Consequently, in the case of permanent waving, various treatments have to be applied periodically to maintain the wavy shape (18). In the case of hair straightening with alkaline relaxers, shape reversion is difficult to correct because after the straightening process, the hair fibers are left weakened due to the high degree of broken covalent and other protein bonds produced by these treatments.

Shape reversion phenomena occurring after permanent waving or alkaline relaxer treatments are usually difficult to explain when using conventional mechanisms of disulfide bond breakage and re-formation. However, the shape reversion processes can be easily explained when it is considered that hair is a shape memory biopolymer with a permanent shape stored in its "memory." As will be discussed later in this chapter, in order to successfully induce permanent changes in hair shape, not only do disulfide bonds have to be broken, but also other chemical and key structural components of the hair memory need to be modified. Otherwise, the induced shape will be semi-permanent and eventually the fibers will undergo shape reversion.

Understanding the shape memory properties of hair can pave the way to optimize processes and produce successful permanent changes in hair shape. Therefore, in the following paragraphs shape memory polymer concepts will be used to review changes in hair shape, and we encourage the reader to use this information as a foundation for innovative thinking in this field.

3.3.4.3 CHANGES IN HAIR SHAPE BY WATER-SETTING

a. The process

Water-setting, or the process of changing hair's shape with water, is by far, among all the temporary setting processes, the easiest to produce in hair. It only entails the use of water and a relatively low-temperature drying process. In order to understand it mechanistically using concepts from the science of SMPs, let us first review the key generic steps necessary to produce shape changes in semi-crystalline polymers (6), and then apply them to hair. Upon thoughtful comparison, polymers also require the same three key steps described above for changes in hair shape:

1) making fluid or softer at least one of the polymer phases,
2) imposing mechanically a new shape followed by stress relaxation in the soft/fluid phase, and
3) immobilizing the soft/fluid phase to lock-in the new shape. In general, temporary shape changes in SMPs also require keeping the polymer structure intact where the permanent shape memory is located (11).

Thus, when we want to impose a temporary shape on a semi-crystalline polymer, or by analogy, in hair, the first requirement is to keep the main polymer architecture intact. To be more specific, in the case of water-setting this implies that the disulfide bond cross-linked protein matrix and the protein crystalline regions should not be modified. Water-setting usually does not produce these modifications except when high temperatures, or large deformations are involved in the production of the temporary shape. High temperatures above 80°C may already start to produce disulfide bond breakage; while deformations higher than 5% already induce alpha to beta transitions in the crystalline phase which may be partially irreversible (23).

b. Physical processes taking place inside hair during water-setting

As outlined in the previous paragraph the imposition of temporary shapes, either in polymers or in hair, requires three main steps (see Figure 9). For the water-setting of hair, step 1 consists of softening the gel structure of the amorphous phase by wetting the hair and allowing water to penetrate into the cortex. This first step will ensure that hydrogen bonds in the gel structure are broken by water. It is important to mention here that when water breaks hydrogen bonds in hair proteins, after step 1 the hair still has all of its covalent bonds intact, and therefore, the permanent shape memory is also unchanged (see Figure 10). As will be seen later, this contrasts with other processes where the hair becomes shapeless and completely loses its real permanent shape. In step 2, once the weak hydrogen bonds are broken, the hair is set into a new configuration with plastic rollers or with the fingers to create the desired new shape, which can be either that of light hair waves or tighter curls.

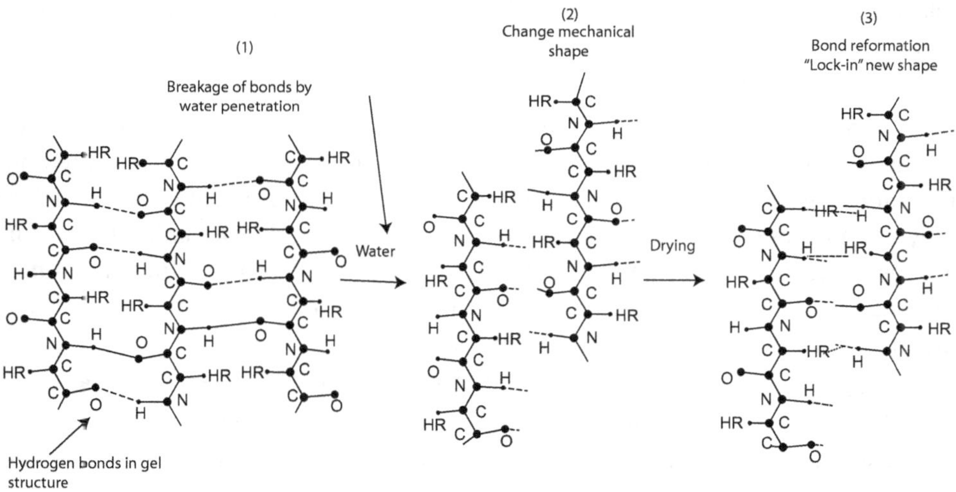

Figure 9) Schematic representation of three steps required to create a temporary shape by water-setting. The three-step process is essentially based on the breakage of hydrogen bonds in the gel structure of hair (step 1), imposition of temporary shape (step 2), and re-formation of hydrogen bonds to lock-in the new shape (step 3) (18).

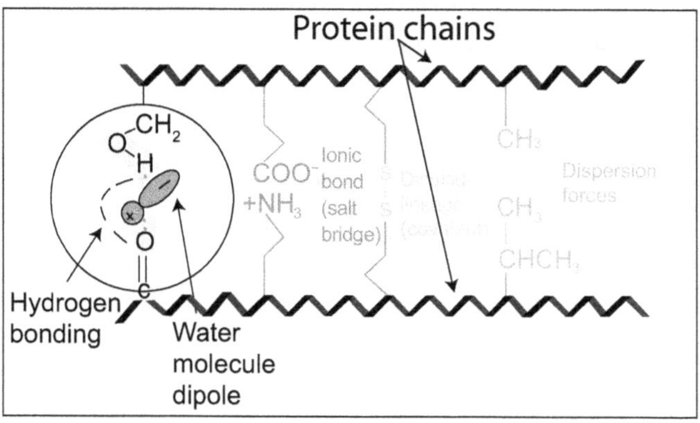

Figure 10) Schematic representation of hydrogen bond breakage by water dipoles during water-setting. Other covalent bonds are not affected.

Finally, in step 3, the hair has to be rapidly dried to extract water molecules in order to re-form the hydrogen bonds in the gel structure. This process will cause hardening of the hair, thereby locking-in the temporary shape and imposing it over the primary hair shape. Drying can be achieved by just exposing hair to atmospheric conditions or it can be accelerated with the aid of blow-dryers. If the drying process is too slow and the hair rollers are removed, the crystalline micro-fibrils and amorphous matrix with its combined elastic force will push for hair to recover its permanent shape and the temporary shape will be lost. Fast drying with blow-dryers will ensure that water is rapidly removed from the gel phase before the hair can elastically recover its permanent shape. In this manner the new shape will be locked-in.

c. Temporary shapes induced by long-term deformations

Another form of water-setting is the one that takes place when hair is subjected to involuntary deformations for extended periods of time at room temperature and high moisture conditions. This situation occurs, for instance, when sleeping, using hats, etc. In these cases the assembly of hair fibers is held in a configuration for various hours, and after freeing the hair from the confined environment a temporary change in hair shape is produced. The phenomenon is caused by stress relaxation in the gel structure of the amorphous phase.

As was previously discussed, the gel phase of the hair is plasticized when the amorphous phase contains moisture. Water from the environment is absorbed in the gel structure and breaks a limited number of hydrogen bonds at protein neighboring sites. When there are no mechanical stresses applied to hair, the broken and unbroken bonds stay in equilibrium. However, when deformations appear as a consequence of imposed deformations, i.e., during sleep, use of hats, etc., broken and unbroken bonds undergo a bond interchange process and the protein chains move to relax internal stresses. This process of internal stress relaxation in the gel structure locks-in the temporary shape that is produced during sleep (bed hair), or with the use of hats, etc. (see Figure 11).

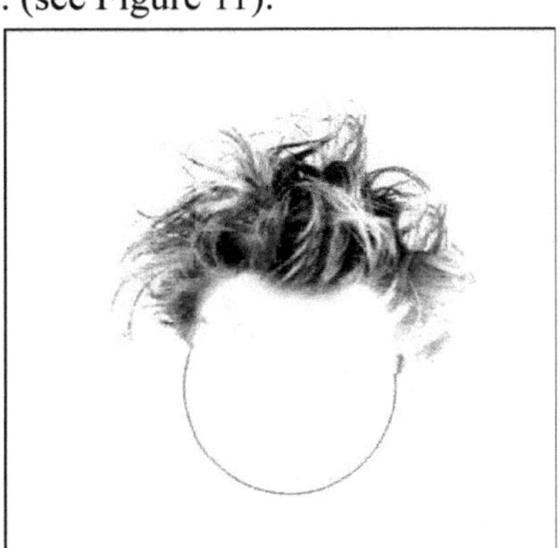

Figure 11) Caption showing typical appearance of bed hair (18)

The imposition of new temporary shapes on hair, either during sleep, use of hats, etc., or during water-setting, will immediately produce internal elastic stresses in the structures where the real permanent shape resides. This occurs primarily in the crystalline regions and in the disulfide protein matrix. These internal stresses will remain there as long as the temporary shape is in place and are needed for the hair to recover its permanent shape. Temporary shapes imposed by water-setting will maintain their secondary character as long as the two following conditions are met. First, the elasticity of the crystalline and amorphous phases does not change, and second, that the gel structure of the amorphous phase remains unchanged. The first condition was previously reviewed and it was referred to as a requirement for superelasticity of the SMPs. This condition is required to ensure that the polymer will always remember its permanent shape. The second condition was also reviewed previously and it relates to the absence of relaxation in the soft phase; it is required to lock-in the temporary shape as long as it is necessary until it is released by an external stimulus.

Shape changes induced by water-setting can, rapidly or almost instantaneously, be reversed by water-wetting. The process of liquid water absorption by hair causes rapid hydrogen bond breakage, softening, and swelling of the gel structure, thereby releasing the temporary shape and allowing the permanent shape to be quickly recovered. If the hair didn't behave like a shape memory biopolymer, it would not remember and recover its permanent shape and would stay deformed like a viscous resin. Thus, water-wetting acts as an external stimulus to quickly release the temporary shape from hair.

d. Limitations of water-setting

Unfortunately, shape changes induced by water-setting in hair are temporary and cannot be maintained as long as we would like nor can they be dormant forever. *It is known, for instance, that shape changes induced by water are slowly recovered even when no water-wetting processes are applied.* Temporary shapes stored in the gel structure are gradually lost because, as has previously been explained by Max Feughelman (6), the gel structure of phase M in hair is viscoelastic, and even at very low moisture contents it will always relax to the Elastic Modulus of the crystalline phase. Thus, all types of temporary shapes induced by water-setting eventually revert back to the permanent shape by a stress-relaxation process and this occurs even under very dry conditions. The process may take months but the shapes will reverse! The memory shape properties of the gel structure in hair are transient, and temporary shapes induced by water-setting cannot be maintained for very long periods.

Another important aspect of water-setting is that, depending on the type of hair, there is a limit on the type of initial shape that can be imposed. This fact becomes more clearly understood when we analyze the following questions:

- How tight can we induce a curl in hair that is very straight, or how straight can we render hair that is very kinky?
- Can this induced curl be achieved just by using a water-setting process? In other words, is it possible to put very tight curls in natural straight hair just by breaking and re-forming hydrogen bonds? Or is it possible to render very kinky hair straight just by breaking and re-forming hydrogen bonds?

Obviously, the answer to the above is no. Everyone who has tried to straighten extremely curly hair just by using water-setting will fail.

This failure can be explained by the fact that the gel structure has only limited mechanical stiffness, and therefore, cannot completely counter the strong elastic recovery forces of permanent shape coming from the crystalline and disulfide cross-linked protein phases. In other words, the gel structure is a weak physical memory and cannot store large changes in hair shape. Thus, the strength and degree of hair curliness is very important in temporary shape changes induced by water-setting. The straightening of extremely curly hair may require additional physical modifications of other, stronger protein structures that store temporary shape. Likewise, this type of reasoning can be applied for the imposition of tight curls in straight hair with water-setting.

According to the ongoing discussion, there appears to be a rule that relates strength of shape change, and number of memory sites required to achieve the changes in shape. This rule *always* prevails when imposing temporary changes in hair shape. In the case of straightening curly hair, the rule is: **the tighter the curl, the more the elements in the architectural sites in hair's memory need to be modified to make it straight.** This means that for any particular type of hair, there is a limit in the degree of shape changes that can be imposed by water-setting. In fact, this is the reason for the use of harsher temporary hair-shaping techniques, other than water-setting, for the straightening of curly hair, such as the use of hot irons and other treatments. As will be seen later in the following paragraphs, the rule of changing shape has important consequences not only for the imposition of temporary shapes but also for engendering those of permanent nature.

3.3.4.4 CHANGES IN HAIR SHAPE BY HOT IRON TREATMENTS

a. Introduction

Changing the hair shape with hot irons is a very old practice. Museums of history already report drafts of hot iron designs made in the 18th century (see Figure 12). Hot irons became popular in the early 1900s for the straightening of extremely curly hair of African origin (24). Later, over the years the application gradually extended to other types of hair to create/enhance stronger curls or to create straight patterns in hair. Currently, there are two main types of hot irons, namely, those of cylindrical shape and those with flat plates (see Figure 13). The use of hot irons with flat plates has become very popular for the straightening of wavy hair. The wanted effects from those who use it nowadays range, in terms of achieving long-lasting behavior—from totally irreversible, or permanent types, to those of long duration and reversible behavior. Most hot iron treatments used today leave only a short temporary change in hair shape. As a result, cosmetic formulators are perennially looking for new hot iron technologies that can extend the persistence and long-lastingness of heat treatments.

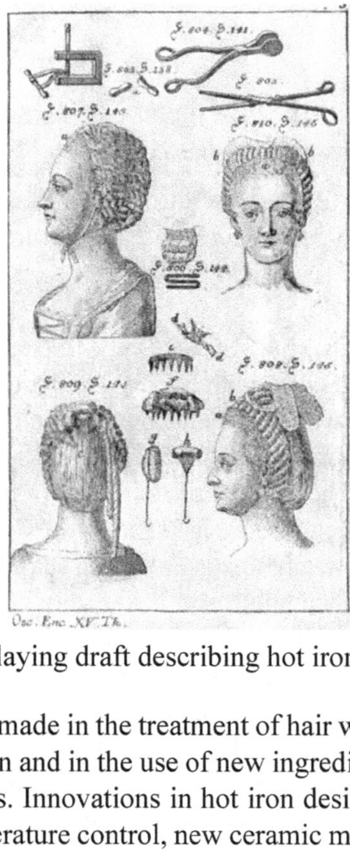

Figure 12) Caption displaying draft describing hot irons used in 1858 (24)

Most of the progress made in the treatment of hair with hot irons has produced innovations in their design and in the use of new ingredients or formulations to aid in the hot ironing process. Innovations in hot iron design comprise, to mention a few: more efficient temperature control, new ceramic materials to improve surface smoothness, better and effective hot iron/hair contact area, use of steam, and the incorporation of infrared heating elements (25). To this end, progress in the area of ingredients and formulations has led to the development of two types of products; namely,

1) those based on the use of polymers geared to enhance shape effects and also to reduce hair damage (26), and
2) those using ingredients that modify or introduce new bonds in hair.

The latter type of products in most cases requires the incorporation of heat to modify the permanent shape memory of hair; either by introducing new cross-links, or by changing the disulfide cross-linking structure of the proteins. Examples of these are the formaldehyde (Brazilean) and sodium bisulfite (Japanese) treatments; both will be reviewed later in another paragraph.

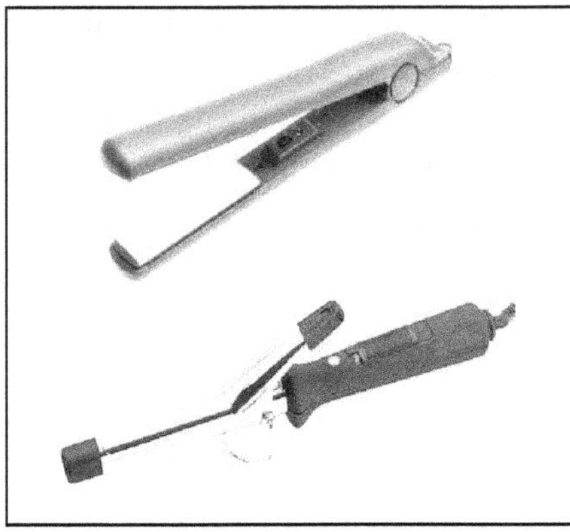

Figure 13) Main modern types of hot irons, flat hot iron (top), and rod hot iron (bottom)

b. The process

A typical hair-straightening process with hot irons consists of the following steps: 1) pre-wash and condition hair with the shampoo and conditioner of choice, 2) dry hair until it keeps about 80% of its moisture content, 2) divide hair into thin swatch sections and then apply the hot iron. The temperature of the hot iron, depending on the type of desired effects, is usually selected between 160 and 230°C. The hot iron is passed two or three times over the hair swatches from root to tip at a speed of approximately one inch/sec. During application the hot iron is held firmly but gently with the hand, so the resulting force of friction will allow smooth sliding over the hair surface, and also, will enhance heat transfer at the interface of hot iron/hair. Excessive force application with the hand should be avoided since this will unnecessarily increase friction at the hot iron/surface interface causing the hot iron to slow down or completely to stop. If this happens the hot iron will damage the hair swatch. If properly used, flat hot irons produce immediate straightening effects in hair (see Figure 14).

Good contact between the hot iron and hair is always necessary for efficient heat transfer. It is important to recognize that heat transfer from the hot iron plates to the hair swatch is always poor because hair, like wool, is a poor heat conductor. Furthermore, because of hair irregularities at the cuticle sheath surface and in view of the formation of air pockets located between hair fibers in the swatch, there is always poor thermal contact between them. This condition causes uneven temperature gradients between hot iron surface and hair swatch. Measurements carried out by placing a thermocouple inside a hair swatch have shown that hair fibers placed in a row 100 micrometers below the hot iron surface always sense at all times an average of 20 to 25°C less than those at the row surface contacting the flat iron plate (27).

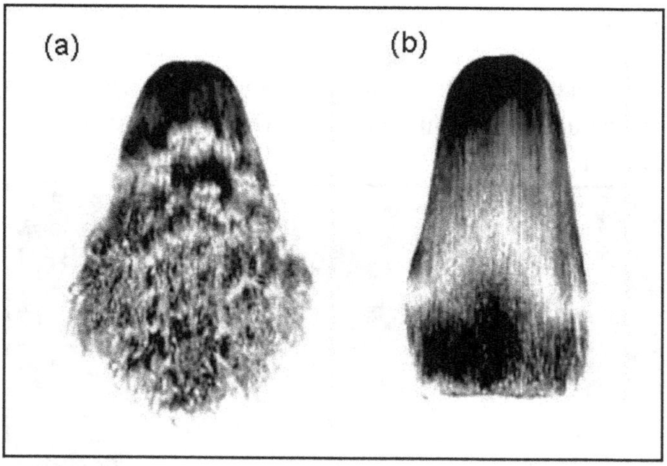

Figure 14) Changes in hair shape before (a) and after (b) treatment with a flat hot iron. The hair shape has been changed from permanent semi-curly to temporary straight.

c. Mechanical action of hot irons

The mechanical action of hot irons on hair is different depending on whether we try to impose a curl on straight hair or whether we try to straighten curly or wavy hair. For instance, if we place a swatch of straight hair in a hot iron of cylindrical shape at 210°C, and press on the hair statically without motion, the hair will acquire a curled shape. In contrast, if we place a swatch of wavy or curled hair between the plates of a flat hot iron at 210°C and let it be there statically without motion, it will not become straight; the action of flattening alone will not lead to changes in hair shape from wavy/curly to straight. For hair to become straight it needs to be in motion so its length can be stretched at least until the curl opens and the hair becomes straight. Thus, there is a big difference in the way the hot iron acts mechanically. This difference depends on whether the change in shape is from straight to curly or from curly to straight. Very curly hair needs a relatively high friction imposed at the interface between the hot iron and the hair surface so the iron plates can stretch and open the curl. In contrast, the process of changing straight hair to curly is not dependent on whether the hair is in motion or not.

Other factors that influence the friction process during the straightening of wavy hair with flat irons are the type of products applied to hair before hot ironing. Hair swatches to be ironed may contain polymers, surfactants, and oils on the surface prior to the ironing process. These ingredients, in particular, include polymers that have been placed there to aid in the styling process. The polymers appear to have an effect in preventing hair damage by eliminating uneven harsh temperature gradients that may create hot spots on the hair swatch (28). Polymers and oils can have, however, a negative effect on the hot ironing process as they can excessively increase or lower the interfacial friction between the iron and the hair surface (34). High levels of friction may cause the hot iron to stop or to produce lifting of cuticle cells and tear them away from the hair (see Figures 15 and 16), while very low friction may reduce the uncoiling of the curl compromising the efficiency of a hair-straightening process (27).

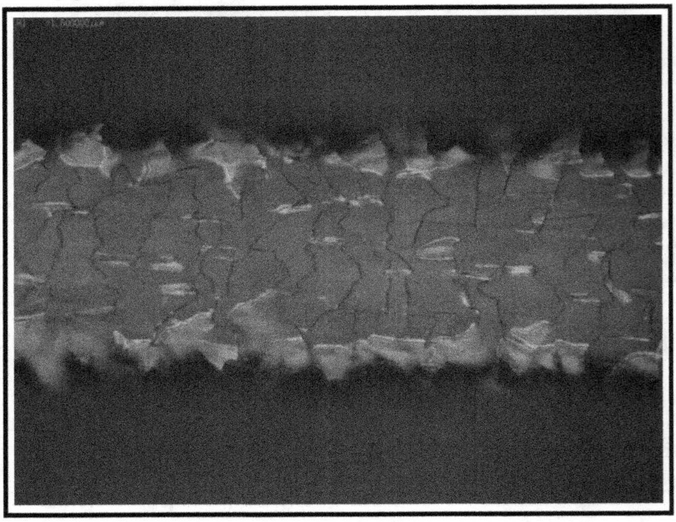

Fig 15) Micrograph of a single hair fiber showing cuticle cell deformation and lifting after treatment with a hot iron at 210°C. The colored sections represent lifted cuticle cells showing patterns of light interference (27).

Figure 16) Micrograph showing fragments on cuticle cells left on plate of hot iron after a hair bundle was treated with a hot iron. Cuticle cell removal was produced by excessive friction at hot iron/hair interface (27).

3.3.4.5 PHYSICAL PROCESSES TAKING PLACE INSIDE HAIR DURING HOT IRONING

a. Water evaporation

Anybody who has witnessed for the first time the application of hot irons to hair is struck by the hissing sound of water vapor or steam coming out of the hair as the hot iron is passed over the hair swatches. At the microscopic level this means that a large quantity of "free" and "bound" water molecules are being rapidly extracted from the protein sites in the amorphous phase. Water-absorbing groups such as amino, carboxyl, and other functional groups capable of forming hydrogen bonds lose their water in this process. As a result, the gel structure of the amorphous protein phase changes from a soft and highly plasticized gel to a hardened amorphous mass.

Experimental observations indicate that rapid water evaporation from hair starts to take place when the hot iron reaches temperatures slightly higher than 100°C. Moreover, if the temperature of the hot iron is maintained at 120°C for 15 seconds while it is in contact with the hair swatch, the hair will be fully dehydrated. This is not surprising since bulk water starts to evaporate rapidly at 100°C. Yet, observations made by scientists in the laboratory and by many stylists confirm that when the temperature of the hot iron is set between 100 and 120°C, it is difficult or almost impossible to efficiently impose a temporary shape on hair, either straight or curly (27).

Furthermore, work carried out in this area indicates that the shape of a wavy hair swatch does not change efficiently from wavy to straight even when the temperature of the hot iron is increased to 150°C. These experiments also indicate that it is not until the hot iron reaches temperatures between 150 and 230°C, that a noticeable and efficient change in shape from wavy to straight starts to appear in hair (27). These observations indicate that the physicochemical processes that are responsible for inducing changes in the shape of hair occur at temperatures ranging between 165 and 230°C, and when the hair is almost fully dehydrated. Incidentally, the only protein processes that take place inside hair within this temperature range are the melting of crystalline proteins and the softening of the amorphous matrix. The relation of these two processes with shape changes in hair will be discussed below.

b. Phase changes and transitions in hair

The thermodynamic transitions taking place in hair when its temperature is increased from 25 to 240°C have been the subject of numerous studies (29–31). Most hair types have been shown to undergo two main thermodynamic transitions, namely a first-order transition associated to the denaturation and melting of its crystalline structure, and a second-order transition associated to the softening or glass transition of its amorphous protein structure. The melting of the crystalline structure in virgin hair occurs at Tm ~ 156°C, and the softening of the amorphous disulfide cross-linked protein phase occurs at its glass transition temperature, Tg ~ 144°C.

The occurrence of these two transitions in most types of hair can be detected and confirmed by Differential Scanning Calorimetry. For instance, in Figure 17 can be seen a typical DSC thermogram showing the endothermic peak related to the melting of the hair crystalline phase. Thus, since the working temperature of a typical hot iron treatment ranges between 150 and 230°C, it is straightforward that both of these transitions take place in the hot iron straightening process. In fact, as will be seen later, the better efficiency in changing hair shape temporarily with hot irons is due precisely to the occurrence of these transitions, as they are the sites with temporary memory properties.

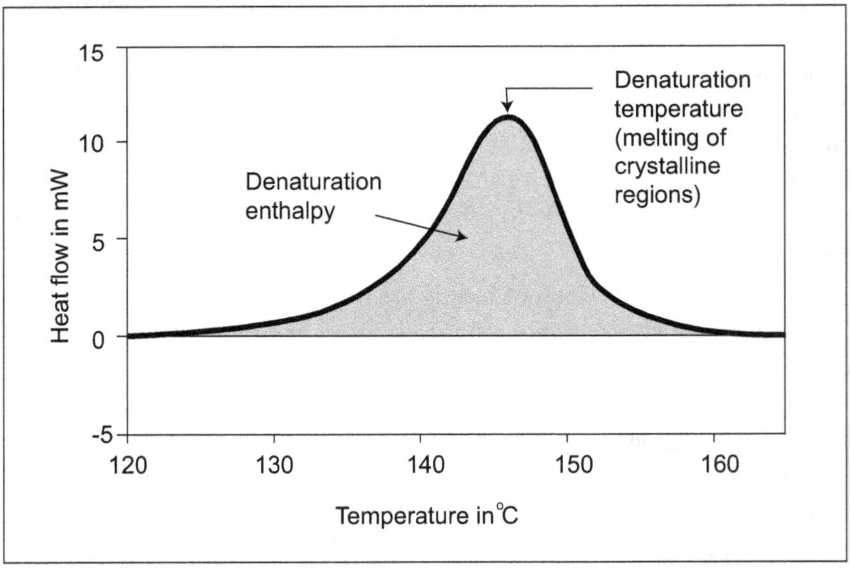

Figure 17) Caption of a typical thermogram obtained by DSC from hair (32).

c. The mechanisms of water and hot iron setting are different.

With the material presented thus far, it is not difficult to anticipate that the mechanism by which hot irons impose a temporary shape in hair is very different from that occurring in water-setting. Setting hair with hot irons does not involve the key and crucial typical step of water-setting, namely that consisting of the breakage of a high quantity of hydrogen bonds to soften the gel structure followed by imposition of the new hair shape.

Setting hair with hot irons involves the formation of hydrogen bonds, but they do not contribute to imposing a new shape. In order to better understand the role of hydrogen bonding during hot iron treatments, let us start by analyzing the role of water on the properties of the gel structure in hair. When water molecules penetrate into the hair structure they adsorb and intercalate on protein-functional sites breaking hydrogen bonds between them. The breakage of these hydrogen bonds renders the gel structure of the amorphous phase softer (6). When the water molecules are removed by evaporation, the internal hydrogen bonds between neighboring protein chains re-form and transform the soft gel structure into a hard viscous gel mass.

Hair swatches to be treated with a hot iron are, however, not required to be wet, for they already contain small amounts of moisture in their gel structure. However, this limited amount of water only breaks a limited number of hydrogen bonds, and therefore, it produces a semi-soft gel structure. When hair tresses with such limited amounts of moisture enter into contact with a flat hot iron at high temperatures, there will be a rapid process of heat transfer into the hair cortical regions. For instance, if after heat absorption, the temperature of the amorphous protein and crystalline phases rises rapidly to levels higher than 160°C, there will be violent evaporation of this limited amount of water, thereby producing the hissing sound typical of hot iron treatments.

At temperatures higher than 160°C the hair will have lost most of its moisture, causing all broken hydrogen bonds to re-form with the consequent hardening of the gel structure. Systematic hair-straightening experiments carried out with Mulatto hair using hot iron temperatures ranging between 110°C and 130°C have shown that hair swatches already become fully dehydrated at these temperatures. Even in the face of full dehydration the process leads to very poor or almost no hair straightening. These observations clearly indicate that rapid hardening of the gel structure attained during hot iron treatments does not allow for an efficient change in hair shape by hydrogen bond re-formation. *In other words, hot iron treatments harden the gel structure of hair before the temporary shape is imposed on it* (27).

d. Hot iron setting: partial denaturation of micro-fibrils and vitrification of the amorphous phase

According to the ongoing discussions, hydrogen bonding does not contribute much to changes in hair shape by hot irons. There are, however, two other important physical phenomena occurring in hair between 130 and 230°C capable of inducing temporary shapes. These are the partial melting or denaturation of the crystalline protein phase at Tm and the softening of the disulfide protein matrix at Tg. Incidentally, both types of phase transitions occur also in cross-linked semi-crystalline polymers with shape memory properties (SMPs) and are commonly used to impose temporary shapes (8). In Figure 18 a schematic diagram explains the mechanism of temporary shape storage by semi-crystalline SMPs. The mechanism involves three key steps:

a) heating the polymer above its crystalline melting and glass transition temperatures to soften the polymer,
b) deforming the polymer to impose the temporary shape, and then,
c) cooling down to lock-in the temporary shape.

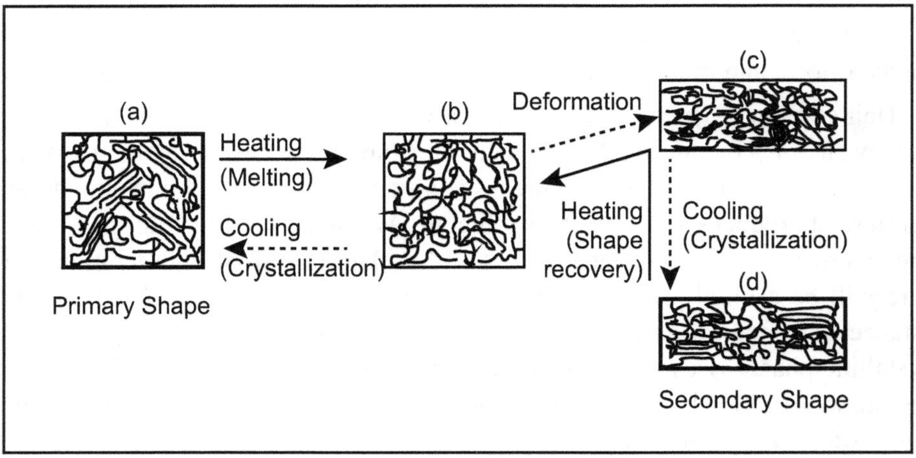

Figure 18) Schematic depiction of three steps needed for temporary shape fixing in cross-linked semi-crystalline shape memory polymers according to C.Liu et al. (8). Step 1 comprises melting of crystalline regions (a), step 2 requires the imposition of deformations to create the temporary shape (b), and step 3 involves cooling of the polymer for the recrystallization to lock-in the new shape (c).

Since hair is also a cross-linked semi-crystalline polymer, it is straightforward that hot irons must store temporary shapes in the hair structure by a similar process. Namely, when the hot iron is set at temperatures above 160°C and passes over the hair, it melts/denatures the crystalline regions and softens the amorphous phase. Then, as the hair is in motion the hot iron plates open the curl by friction and impose the straight shape by mechanical pressure. Once the hair moves out of the hot plates with its straight shape, it cools down. Cooling at room temperature induces a vitrification process of the amorphous phase and also a recrystallization process or a reorientation of crystalline regions (see Figure 19). In this process the molten or denatured crystalline regions and the softened disulfide cross-linked proteins vitrify; while the non-denatured crystalline proteins reorient to comply with the new shape. This process locks-in the new straight shape in hair. Because hot irons use vitrification of amorphous and reorientation of crystalline proteins as processes to store temporary shapes, the stability and durability of the shape is longer than that obtained with water-setting.

It should be mentioned here that the denaturation of crystalline regions at high temperatures in hair is always an irreversible process and, therefore upon cooling, recrystallization of denatured proteins does not occur. Experiments have shown, for instance, that as the temperature of the hot iron rises between 160 and 220°C, the level of irreversible protein melting/denaturation also increases (27, 33, 34). Furthermore, it has been observed that as the level of denaturation increased in this temperature range, and while the hair curl was maintained open under the hot iron, the character of hair straightening shifted from temporary to more permanent (27). These observations clearly indicate that hot irons induce temporary shape changes in hair by a softening and vitrification process of its two protein phases. The amorphous phase locks-in the new shape by a pure vitrification process, while the crystalline phase, by either a reorientation process of the non-denatured crystalline regions or by vitrification of the denatured ones. The straightened shape becomes more permanent in character when the level of denatured crystalline regions that vitrify increases.

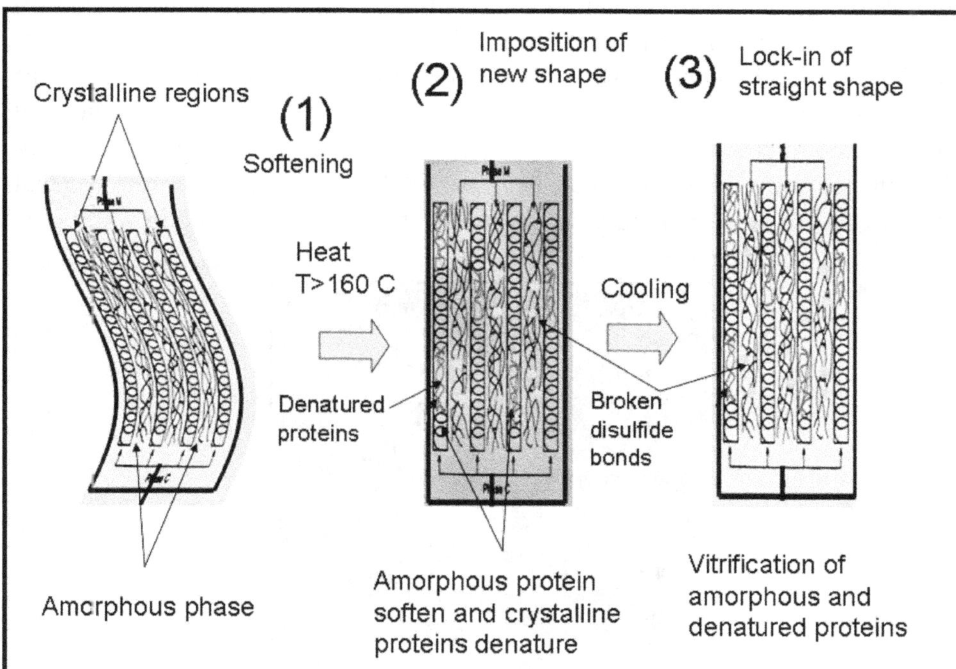

Figure 19) Diagrammatic representation of three steps required for the creation of a temporary shape in hair with hot irons. In step 1 the hair is heated to its Tg so the crystalline regions partially melt irreversibly and the amorphous protein matrix softens, in step 2 a straight shape is imposed on hair, and in step 3 the hair is cooled down to vitrify the amorphous protein regions to lock-in straight shape (27).

The hot iron process could also be detailed as follows: hot irons increase the temperature of hair above its Tm and Tg. This causes the disulfide amorphous protein matrix to soften and become fluid-like while the crystalline regions start to undergo a kinetic melting or denaturation process. The degree of crystalline protein melting will depend, however, on the thermal stability of the amorphous matrix (29). If provisions are taken to reduce disulfide bond scission, then, most of the shape change induced by the hot iron will be temporary and due to vitrification of the amorphous phase and to a reorientation of crystalline regions. However, if disulfide bond breakage occurs readily in the amorphous proteins, the changes in shape will be due to a vitrification of amorphous and denatured proteins and the changes in shape will take a more permanent character (27).

For demonstration purposes Figure 20 shows three hair fibers whose semi-elliptical shape underwent a softening and vitrification process with a hot iron at 220°C. Fiber (a) in Figure 20 shows a pronounced flattening effect on its semi-elliptical shape as a consequence of the softening/vitrification process during hot iron treatment, fiber (b) shows imprints of neighboring fibers, and finally, fiber (c) shows shape flattening due to a similar vitrification process. All these effects indicate that at a certain point during the hot ironing process at 220°C the hair proteins became very soft, viscous, and fluid-like and were able to change their geometrical configuration to comply with the hot iron geometry. Then, upon cooling, the proteins vitrified and reoriented into the new shape. The experiments also showed that these effects are only temporary, i.e., when the fibers are immersed in water they recover their original shape (34).

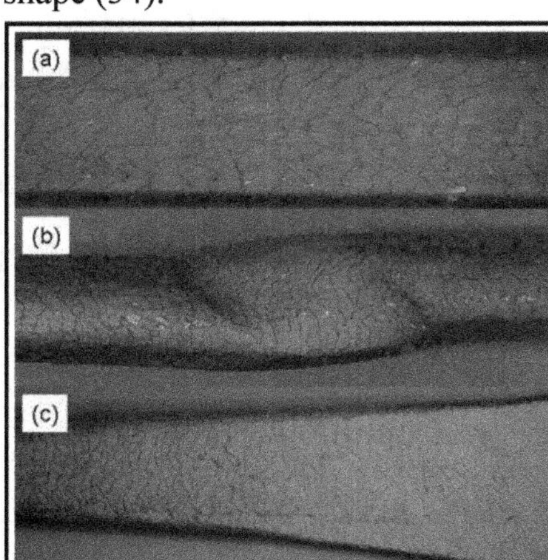

Figure 20) Micrographs of shape distortion produced by 4 cycles of hot irons at 210°C on hair fibers of Caucasian origin as follows: (a) flat shape distortion obtained on a single fiber with a 40 g compression force, (b) imprint left on fiber by neighboring fibers in a hair tress, and (c) deformation left in a fiber selected from a hair tress after treatment with hot iron (34)

Since temporary shape changes induced by hot irons involve only physical mechanisms, the conditions for their recovery also entail physical phenomena. These conditions are met when the protein chains in the vitrified amorphous phase enter into faster motion again. This could be done by increasing again the hair temperature above Tg or when the hair is wet. Thermal motion of main chains in polymers and proteins always occurs at room temperature, and their degree of motion is relative to their Tg. The higher the Tg in a polymer, the slower is the thermal motion of its main chains at room temperature (2). Thus, in theory, temporary shapes induced with hot irons will be very long lasting but unfortunately, the principle of superposition in polymers (2–4) also dictates that the Tg of a polymer can be lowered by a plasticizer, thereby increasing chain mobility.

Let us also remember that water is the main plasticizer of proteins, and it is also the main plasticizer of the gel structure in the hair amorphous phase (5). Even when water cannot penetrate and plasticize the crystalline regions, the effects of water in the amorphous phase have an impact on the orientation and arrangement of the crystalline phase. When the hydrophilic groups of the amorphous phase absorb water the amorphous phase relaxes, and this may result in a reorientation of the crystalline regions storing the temporary shape. The final result is a loss of temporary shape. Thus, even when temporary shapes induced by hot irons are of longer duration than those attained by water-setting, their shape is also lost when the hair absorbs water.

e. Heat transfer from hot iron to hair

It should be mentioned here that because of poor hair thermal conductivity, non-homogeneity of cuticle cell surface, and packing irregularity of hair fibers, not all hair fibers in a hair swatch exposed to a hot iron surface will experience the same temperature. Those hair fibers in contact with the hot iron will certainly be expected to equilibrate rapidly to the hot iron surface temperature. However, those a few millimeters away from the surface will experience a much lower temperature. Systematic experiments using a thermocouple embedded in a hair tress have shown that hair fibers in the middle of a 2 mm hair tress experience ~ 25°C less than those in contact with the hot iron (see Figure 21). Furthermore, additional experiments carried out with hair swatches ~ 1 mm thick and placed on a hot plate at 200°C showed that it takes time for heat to be transferred across a hair swatch into a metallic heat sink to equilibrate temperatures. Once equilibrium conditions are established, the temperature at the hair swatch surface not in contact with the hot plate is always ~ 60°C less than that in contact with the hot plate (see Figure 22).

The simple experiment described above does not represent realistic conditions of hot iron treatments because only one surface of the hair tress is exposed to high temperature. However, the experiment helps us to visualize the time delays needed for temperature to equilibrate across the hair tress. Therefore, we will expect that when a hot iron is passed at 160°C over a hair swatch only those fibers in contact will rapidly equilibrate temperatures with the hot iron; and these fibers will experience melting of crystalline regions and softening of the disulfide cross-linked matrix. Those fibers underneath may not experience this phenomena.

Furthermore, occurrences of the above-described transitions in hair are not only dependent on the position of the hair fibers relative to the hot iron surface but also dependent on the heating rate. For instance, it has been shown that the faster the rate of heating, the higher is the melting temperature of the crystalline regions (29). Since the hot iron is passed swiftly along the hair fibers we would expect, therefore, that if the hot iron temperature is set to 160°C, large numbers of hair fibers will not undergo these transitions. Thus, if we want all hair fibers in a swatch to experience the thermodynamic transitions required, two actions must be taken, namely, 1) to increase substantially the hot iron temperature above 160°C, or 2) to improve heat transfer across fibers. From the practical point of view, only the former action can be easily done and this can be accomplished just by setting the hot iron temperature to higher levels. This analysis helps explain why setting the hot iron temperature in the range of 170–210°C improves substantially the efficiency in hair straightening (27).

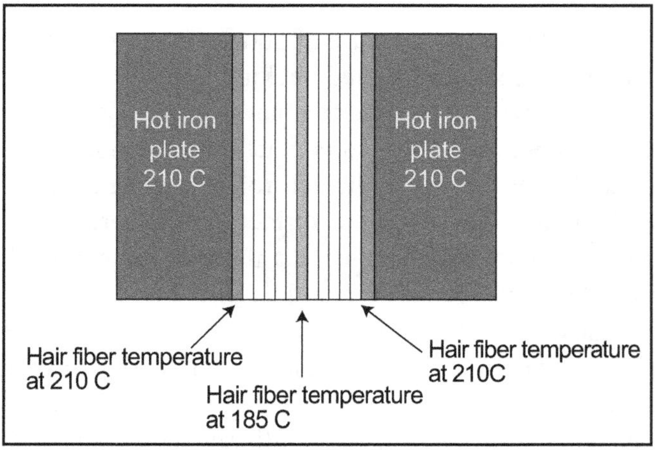

Figure 21) Schematic representation of hair swatch between hot iron plates. The experiments show that hair fibers in the middle section of the hair stress sense temperatures ~20–25°C lower than those at the periphery (27).

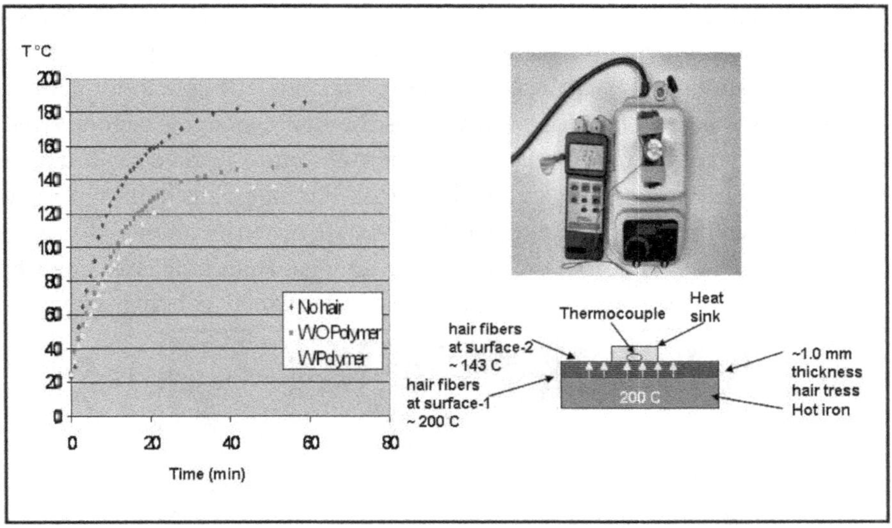

Figure 22) Graph showing variation in temperature as function of time (a) in a thermocouple placed at the top of a hair tress placed on a hot plate (b) an (c). The temperature of the hot plate was preset at 200 C and, then, at t=0 the hair and thermocouple were place on it (27).

f. Unwanted consequences of friction and rising hair temperature above Tm and Tg

Setting temporary shapes in hair with hot irons has advantages over water-setting or any other types of temporary setting. This is true, first, because hot irons introduce stronger changes in shape, and second, because the shapes last longer. In fact, an ideal hot ironing process would occur if the duration of the temporary shape could be controlled at will and the mechanism of shape storage would only involve reversible changes to the amorphous and crystalline phases. Unfortunately, it is very difficult to control water absorption by hair and also to prevent irreversible disulfide bond breakage and other forms of damage that occur in hair at high temperatures. Scientists studying heat damage in hair have reported the occurrence of protein oxidation, cuticle cell lifting/bulging, formation of pores inside the hair (see Figures 23 and 24), degradation of tryptophan, and disulfide bond scission (35–37). *All these effects make the process of flat ironing far from ideal.*

The first cause of damage in hair treated with hot irons comes from the fact that the thermodynamic transitions responsible for storing the temporary shape in hair lead to processes that are not fully reversible. For instance, upon cooling, the softened disulfide cross-linked protein matrix does not return to its original native vitrified state; nor do the denatured crystalline regions recover their original crystalline structure (29). Extensive research carried out in various laboratories has already shown that when hair is heated above its Tm a process of partial irreversible protein denaturation takes place. Lack of full recovery of both amorphous and crystalline phases has been ascribed to various thermal damaging factors. Among these thermal damaging factors the most important one is irreversible disulfide bond breakage. This process causes covalent cross-linking points in the amorphous phase to decrease, thereby producing a different state of vitrification and a process of irreversible destabilization of the crystalline regions. Both processes contribute to a gradual loss of permanent shape and undesirable reduction in hair strength.

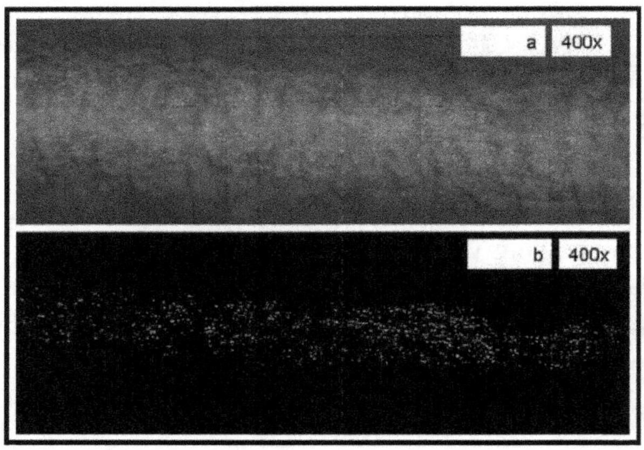

Figure 23) Micrograph of a hair fiber (φ ~ 76 μm) subjected to five treatments of hot ironing showing the presence of pores at a depth of 10 μm inside the cortex (a). By using digital filters in the image, the pores were separated and the remainder of the picture was transformed into a black background (b) (34).

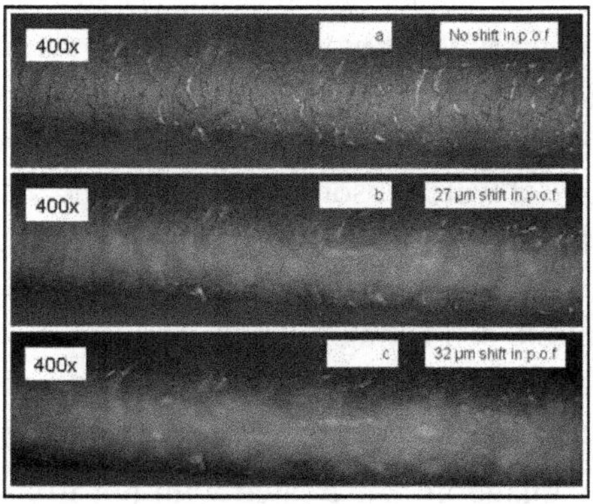

Figure 24) Micrographs of a hair fiber (φ ~ 64 μm) showing image of surface obtained with no shift in plane of focus (11a). Later the plane of focus (p.o.f.) was shifted in 27 and 32 μm, respectively; the white spots in the image are voids with sizes ranging between 3 and 10 μm. The hair fiber was subjected to five hot iron treatments with the hot iron at 190°C and a speed of 0.2 in/s (34).

Cosmetic scientists and formulators are continually working in this area to alleviate these damaging effects and to improve the widely used hot ironing process. Efforts geared into this direction have already resulted in the use of polymers that enhance straightening and decrease damage. Some groups have introduced the use of formaldehyde in hot iron applications. The use of this ingredient in combination with hot irons is very effective in almost permanently changing the shape of hair. However, because of its toxic properties its use has been banned in the U.S. The mode of action of this ingredient will be reviewed later.

3.3.4.6 HAIR SHAPE CHANGES INDUCED BY PERMANENT WAVING SOLUTIONS

a. The Process

The use of thioglycolate salt solutions to chemically reduce or break disulfide bonds in hair forms the basis for one of the most effective methods for permanently changing the shape of hair from straight into a more wavy and curly configuration. Essentially, the process consists of three basic steps that are similar to those already described for other forms of hair setting:

1) breakage of bonds to soften the hair, i.e., in this case the disulfide bonds,
2) imposition of a new shape, and
3) re-formation of bonds to lock-in the new permanent shape.

Breakage of disulfide bonds in hair is carried out by treating hair in a 7–9% solution of ammonium or sodium thioglycolate at a pH of ~ 9.5. Imposition of the new shape is made by winding hair swatches on plastic rollers. Finally, re-formation of the broken disulfide bonds is accomplished by applying a solution or cream containing 3% hydrogen peroxide to reoxidize broken bonds (see Figure 25).

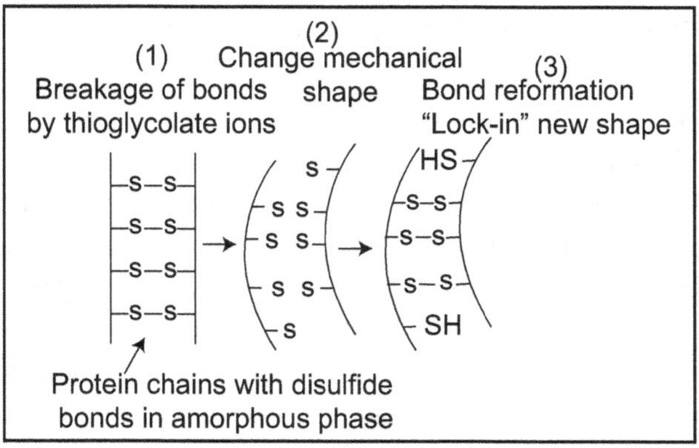

Figure 25) Diagrammatic representation of three steps required for the creation of a permanent shape in hair by permanent waving treatments. In step 1 disulfide bonds are unzipped to erase memory in hair, in step 2 a curly shape is imposed, and in step 3 the broken disulfide bonds are re-formed to lock-in the curly shape (18).

b. Physical and chemical processes taking place inside hair during permanent waving

The role of step one described above in permanently changing the hair shape with ammonium thioglycolate is not just to soften the hair, but mainly to delete the permanent shape in the hair architecture. This process is carried out by the thiolate ion which unzips disulfide bonds in the amorphous structure of hair and produces a certain degree of destabilization in the crystalline regions. Then, once the old shape is partially removed and when the hair is somewhat shapeless, a new shape is introduced in the protein chains by mechanical deformation of plastic rollers. Finally, the new shape is stored in the amorphous protein phase by re-zipping the same bonds in a different configuration by using hydrogen peroxide. Unfortunately, the disulfide breakage and re-formation process modifies only one part of the memory where the permanent shape of hair is stored. Namely, it only modifies part of the tertiary structure of the amorphous proteins. However, it does not modify the crystalline phase nor it does modify the primary and secondary structure of the proteins in the amorphous phase. This means that after the ammonium thioglycolate treatment, there are still shape recovery internal stresses coming from these structures. These stresses will push gradually for the recovery of the original permanent shape in the hair fibers.

Changes in the hair shape memory with ammonium thioglycolate are consequently partial, and will result in a very slow shape reversion process. At the molecular level this process is driven by the recovery of protein conformations to their native state. The forces driving this phenomenon stem from the primary and secondary structures of hair proteins in the crystalline and amorphous phases. It should be mentioned here that the phenomenon of shape reversion is common in a host of denatured proteins and enzymes and, in particular, when it is related to disulfide bonds.

In a famous experiment, C. Afinsen showed that disulfide bond breakage/re-formation in ribonuclease leads to a mixture of denatured and scrambled protein conformations with no enzymatic activity (38). He also observed that the process of protein scrambling by disulfide bond breakage/re-formation was not sufficient for the enzyme to completely lose its shape memory or ability to revert to its native shape. For instance, Afinsen found that traces of mercaptoethanol/urea in combination with the scrambled enzymes in solution were sufficient for the enzyme to reverse and recover its native shape (see Figure 26).

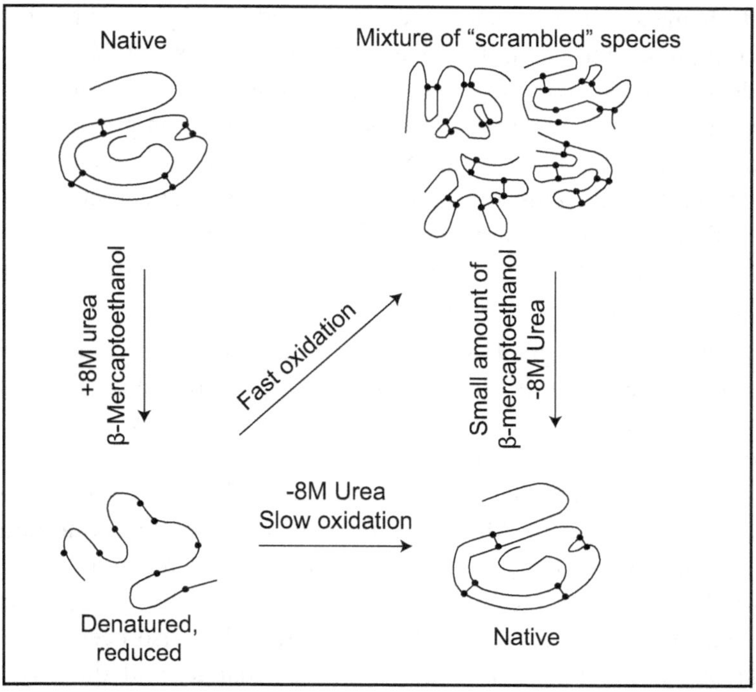

Figure 26) Schematic representation of C. Afinsen's experiment with ribonuclease showing that this enzyme is able to recover its shape even after its disulfide bonds were re-formed with the proteins in a scrambled configuration (38).

It would thus appear that the ability of proteins to recover their native shape is not completely lost when their disulfide bonds are arranged in a different configuration. This particular phenomenon exhibited by proteins helps to explain why the application of treatments that produce only disulfide bond breakage/re-formation in hair are not sufficient to produce irreversible changes in its protein architecture, so that they will support the desired permanent shape changes. Disulfide bond interchange, in combination with recovery stresses coming from the residual memory in the protein architecture of the amorphous and crystalline phases, will be able to drive the reversion process.

From the practical point of view, however, thioglycolate systems are probably the best compromise that can be made between hair damage and persistence in shape changes. Ammonium thioglycolate systems have been shown to produce shape changes that are quasi-permanent and last for months. Certainly, more effective treatments could be designed, but they will probably have to include permanent changes to the primary, secondary, and tertiary protein structures of both the amorphous and crystalline phases. Such a process could be devised but will introduce irreversible damage into other regions of the hair fiber, not to mention the practical loss of recurring business and socialization phenomena that are embedded in the perennial trek to the local cosmetologist. In summary, the process of disulfide bond breakage/re-formation for storing permanent shape changes is not 100% efficient, but it is in a good position as a system because it is very selective to disulfide bonds. It is for these reasons that many scientists working in this field have rather opted for improving the system.

In fact, there is still a great deal of improvement that can be done with these systems. For instance, the disulfide bond breaking/re-formation process is usually assumed to be fully reversible, i.e., it is commonly believed that the amount of disulfide bonds that break can be completely re-formed. Scientists have found that this is not the case and that a small percentage of these bonds always remain permanently broken (39, 40). Much effort has also been dedicated to understanding the effects of temperature, thiolate ions diffusion, and reaction kinetics inside the hair (41, 46). The process of disulfide bond re-formation by means of oxidizing agents such as hydrogen peroxide and other reagents has also been the subject of numerous studies. Effect of fiber diameter on shape changes with these systems has also been the object of concern (43–46). All these studies represent efforts geared to improving the efficiency and effects of the disulfide bond breakage process.

Surprisingly, changes in the crystalline regions after permanent waving have not received much attention and only a few studies have appeared in the literature (47). These studies, however, do not seem to correlate efficiency of shape change with levels of irreversible change in crystalline regions. Certain substances such as urea in combination with ammonium thioglycolate salt solutions appear to enhance destabilization and breakage of hydrogen bonds, apparently improving the efficiency of permanent shape changes, yet their effect on hair's crystallinity has not been reported (48).

3.3.4.7 HAIR SHAPE CHANGES BY ALKALINE RELAXERS

a. The process

The straightening of hair with alkaline cream relaxers belongs to the category of permanent changes in hair shape. It is the most damaging process of all known hair permanent reshaping cosmetic treatments. This is so because during the alkaline straightening process not only are disulfide bonds broken, but also a series of other processes occur that damage the hair architecture. Among these processes are: permanent denaturation of hair proteins, irreversible breakage of disulfide bonds, protein alkaline hydrolysis, protein loses, and excessive swelling of hair (49–51). All alkaline straightening processes are based on the chemical reactivity of the OH ions towards the groups in hair proteins that store the permanent curly shape. The pH of these creams depends on the tightness of the curl, and it ranges between 11.5 and 14.0. As a result, the concentrations of alkaline ingredients in these creams often vary between 1.5 and 3%. Strong chemical bases are used for this purpose and these include sodium hydroxide, lithium hydroxide, combinations of lithium/ sodium hydroxide, and guanidine hydroxide produced *in situ* by the combination of calcium hydroxide and guanidine carbonate.

There are various classifications of cream relaxers in the market. These are known as lye, no-lye, base, no-base, and mix, no-mix, etc. Regardless of their classification, the key active chemical in all of them is always the OH ion. Lye relaxers are those based on sodium hydroxide; no-lye relaxers are those containing any other ingredient than sodium hydroxide. A base relaxer refers to one that needs a layer of petrolatum on the scalp prior the straightening process to protect it from irritation; the no-base relaxer does not need petrolatum separately as it is already formulated in the cream; and finally, a mix relaxer refers to one needing the mixture of two ingredients to produce the OH ions, as is the case of the guanidine carbonate/calcium hydroxide relaxer.

Other types of chemicals used in the straightening of curly hair comprise the use of sodium bisulfite and thioglycolate salts; these systems are referred to as the Japanese and Thio relaxers, respectively. The action of these two ingredients is not based on the action of the OH ions but rather on the reactivity of the sulfite and thio groups. They are more selective to the breakage of disulfide bonds, and as will be seen later, they have advantages and disadvantages over alkaline cream relaxers. A typical salon application of a relaxer consists of three main steps: relaxer cream application, neutralization, and hair conditioning. During the application step the cream is evenly distributed over the selected hair swatches. Almost immediately after application a diffusion of OH ions is triggered from the cream into the hair cortex via the endocuticle and cell membrane complex. As the ions diffuse they start to react with the hair proteins in the amorphous and crystalline phases. Experience shows that 15 or 20 minutes is sufficient for the cream to produce desired hair-relaxing effects.

Relaxer creams in many cases are not designed to reach reaction equilibrium conditions with the proteins in hair. Usually, their OH ion concentrations, which depend on the pKb of the base, are above that required for the hair-straightening process. Consequently, if they are left for longer periods of time on the hair, the effects can be partially depilatory. Thus, as soon as the beautician considers that the hair has been properly relaxed, the cream is rinsed out with water. At this point the OH ions are still reacting with the hair internal proteins; therefore, a neutralization process must be immediately introduced to stop the OH ion/protein reactions. The neutralization process is usually carried out with a shampoo containing citric acid. During this process a strong odor is perceived coming from liberated sulfur. Also, experiments show that the neutralizing solution turns turbid, indicating extraction of protein fragments from the hair structure (52). Because of the high level of damage to the whole hair architecture, a conditioning process is immediately introduced, mainly, to lessen fiber entanglement due to friction effects.

b. Physical and chemical processes taking place inside hair during alkaline straightening

The alkaline reshaping of very curly hair also starts by deleting the hair's permanent shape from the memory located in its architectural structure. In the case of permanent waving this could be done partially by using thio or sulfite compounds to unzip all disulfide cross-linking bonds and allow reorientation of the crystalline regions. The use of these ingredients for the straightening of very tight African-type hair is usually not recommended as it leads to a gradual shape reversion. This happens because disulfide bond breakage alone is not sufficient to delete enough shape memory from the curly hair so the straight shape will resist reversion. The degree of natural curliness in African hair is very tight and strong, and therefore, making it straight requires more changes in its protein chemical structure. This is true, in particular, on sites where the curly shape is imprinted. In other words, African hair was casted from its inception at the hair follicle with a primary, secondary, and tertiary protein architecture complying and supporting very small radius of curvature and also high degrees of fiber elliptical shape (see Figure 27). This means that at the microscopic level the proteins in the amorphous and crystalline phases in these fibers are oriented and chemically bonded to accommodate for these geometries (see also Figure 8).

Thus, in order to attain a complete straightening effect in these curls a sizable amount of shape change or shape deletion is required. If the change in shape were from very tight curly to open curly, the amount of shape deletion in the hair architecture will be less, and this type of mild shape change would not even require the formation of new bonds to lock-in the new shape. However, complete straightening of very tight curly hair requires a higher degree of structure modification; first, because the tight curly shape has to be erased and, second, because the new straight shape needs to be locked-in. It should be recognized that the complete removal of curly shape from a curly hair fiber implies the breakage of chemical bonds that stay irreversibly broken, thus weakening the overall structure of hair. Therefore, the process of introducing a new permanent shape such as in the case of straightening curly hair may require either full reversibility of bond breakage/re-formation, or the introduction of new bonds to stabilize the new shape and also to strengthen the fiber.

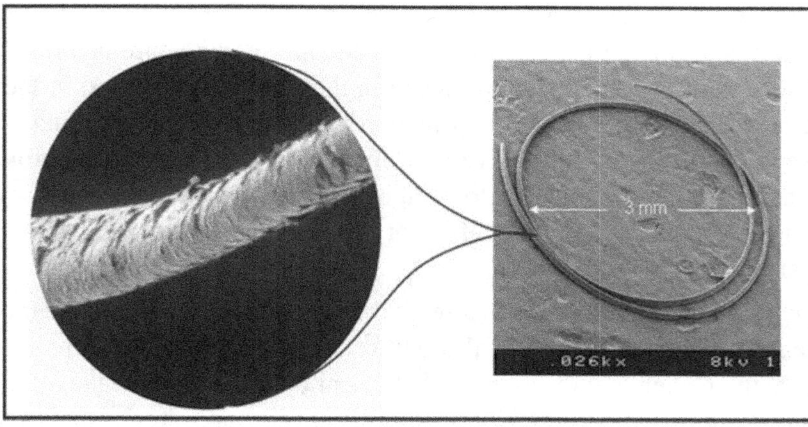

Figure 27) Micrographs of a single fiber of African origin showing tight coil radius of curvature and high degree of ellipticity (18)

As was previously stated, there is a rule relating shape changes and number of sites in memory for curly hair, the rule is: **the tighter the curl, the more the elements in the architectural sites of hair's memory need to be modified to make it straight.** Sizable permanent changes in hair shape always require the annealing of stresses in the internal structure of hair. Otherwise, they will produce strong internal fiber stresses that will drive a shape reversion process. Consequently, large changes in hair shape always need the modification of a higher number of memory sites to eliminate strong reversion forces. The degree of memory deletion process can be outlined in the following manner:

- Weak curls require the breakage of a few disulfide bonds.
- Medium strong curls require a larger amount of disulfide bond breakage.
- Tighter curls require, in addition, denaturation of crystalline regions.
- Very tight curls require all of the above, plus breakage of amide linkages in the proteins as well.

By the same token, the level of chemical and physical stabilization required by the new straight shape increases in the same order.

However, regardless of degree of initial hair curliness, the steps needed to straighten hair with any type of cream relaxer are all the same and almost identical to those required for other changes in hair shape:

1) the softening of hair, which may involve breakage of physical bonds, breakage of covalent bonds, and softening of the crystalline and amorphous regions,
2) imposition of a new shape, and
3) fixing or locking the new shape by re-forming broken chemical or physical bonds, and by rearranging crystalline and amorphous regions.

The role of the first step is not only to chemically soften the hair, but in doing so, also to delete the permanent shape from the hair architecture or memory. In the second step, a new shape is introduced in the shapeless hair, and in the third step, the new shape is stored and imprinted in the memory structure of hair. If we pay close attention to these steps we will immediately realize that the efficiency of changing hair shape, from curly to straight, does not depend only on how much memory is erased but also on how efficient the process of imprinting and storing the new shape is.

In the scientific literature it has already been shown that alkaline creams lead to substantial chemical and physical modifications to the hair structure (53–57). Among the main chemical reactions and physical processes are breakage of weak and strong hydrogen bonds, breakage of salt linkages, and the formation of the following products: lanthionine, cysteic acid, sulfur, and protein fragments. These reactions proceed according to the paths shown in Figures 28 and 29.

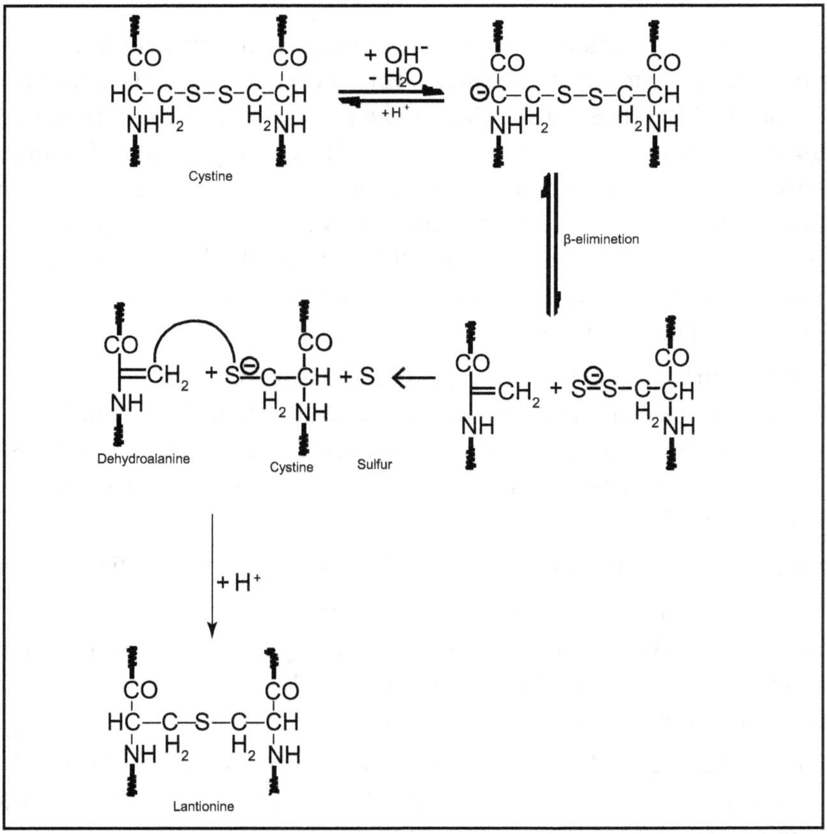

Figure 28) Diagram showing reaction of cystine and OH ions. The reaction takes place during the alkaline straightening of African hair at pHs ranging between 13.5 and 14.0, and it leads to the production of sulfur and lanthionine (32).

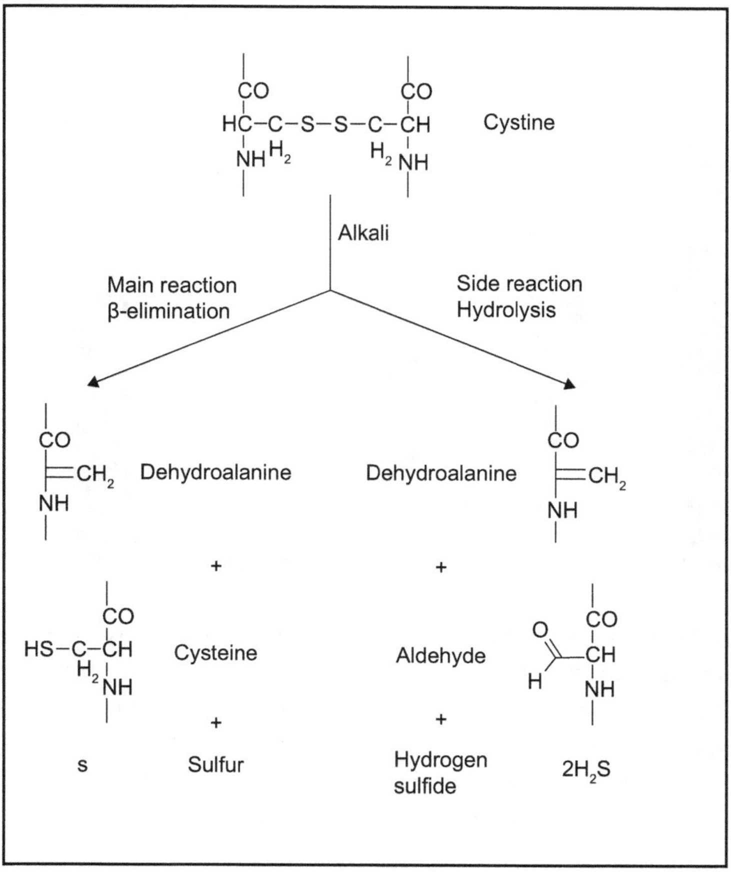

Figure 29) Diagram showing additional reactions of cystine and OH ions occurring in the alkaline straightening of African hair at pHs ranging between 13.5 and 14.0 (32).

Because of the high level of bond breakage, alkaline relaxers also produce high levels of protein denaturation in both the amorphous and crystalline regions. Figure 30 shows typical denaturation enthalpy reductions of various hair fibers subjected to a combination of alkaline and permanent waving treatments. The smaller the bar size in the graph, the higher is the degree of denaturation or disarray in the crystalline regions. All treatments in these experiments showed a decrease in the enthalpy of denaturation and some of them were more pronounced than others (32). Those treated with the alkaline relaxers alone, i.e., with NaOH and No-Lye are more real representations of the irreversible denaturation process taking place in real straightening hair practices, and they show reductions that range between 30 and 50% in their denaturation enthalpies.

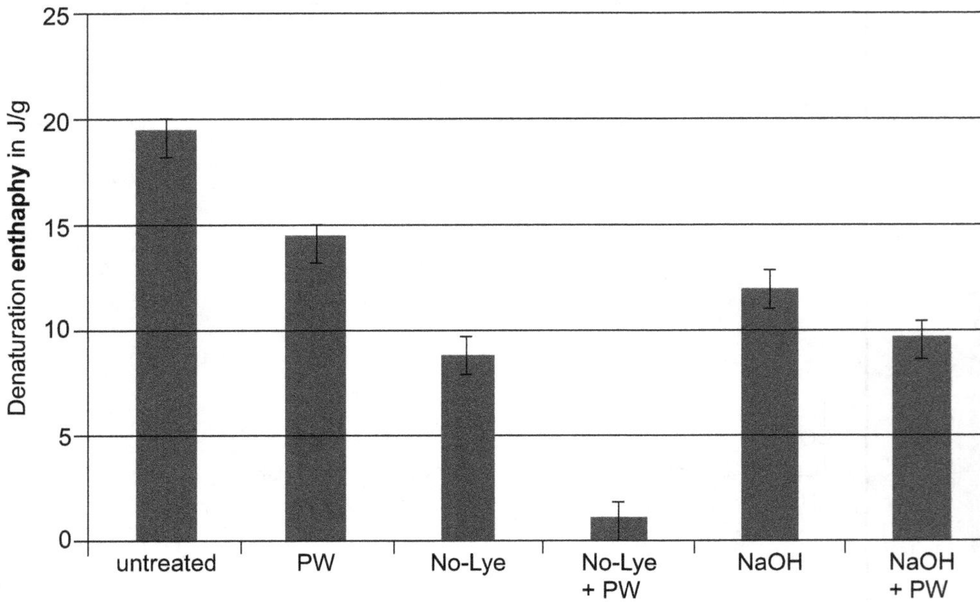

Figure. 30) Denaturation enthalpies of hair fibers after various treatments as follows: Untreated = fiber with no treatment, PW = fiber with permanent waving treatment, No-Lye = fiber treated with No-Lye relaxer, No-Lye+ PW = fiber treated with a combination of No-Lye straightening + permanent waving, NaOH = fiber treated with a relaxer based on NaOH, and finally, NaOH+PW = fiber treated with a combination of a relaxer and permanent waving (32).

This is the reason why alkaline relaxers are very efficient in deleting the permanent shape from the hair architecture—namely, because they modify a large number of hair's physical and chemical features in the protein structures containing the permanent shape memory; i.e. they break disulfide bonds, strong and weak hydrogen bonds, salt linkages, and a certain amount of amide bonds. By breaking all these bonds the OH ions render the amorphous phase extremely soft; in this process the crystalline regions also become scrambled and highly plasticized as well. The hair becomes, therefore, extremely soft and shapeless. The memory deletion process obtained by these effects does not guarantee however the imposition of a new shape, nor the process of locking-in the new shape. For this to happen, new chemical bonds have to be introduced in combination with a process of reconstitution of the hair architecture.

c. Shapeless hair and a new straight shape

As previously discussed, when the alkaline straightening process starts to delete the tight curly shape from the hair memory, the hair fibers gradually become soft and shapeless. The new straight shape is also gradually introduced during the alkaline straightening process by the rubbing of the cream into the hair. The process of new bond formation also appears to occur as the cream is deleting the old curly shape. Experiments have shown, for instance, that if the process of hair straightening is carried out while the hair maintains its coiled shape, the straightening efficiency is less than if the curl is uncoiled and extended (52). Furthermore, if the acid neutralization step is done while the hair is kept in a more straighten configuration the efficiency in straightening also increases (52). These observations indicate, thus, that a certain amount of new bonds, most certainly lanthionine (see Figure 28) (53–59), are gradually introduced while the hair is still reacting with the cream. The straightening efficiency observed during neutralization, on the other hand, is certainly due to a vitrification process of the amorphous phase, and also to a partial reconstitution of the crystalline regions as salt linkages and strong hydrogen bonds re-form upon elimination of the OH ions.

The phenomena of fiber supercontraction and denaturation observed to occur in alkaline treated hair fibers, and reported by many scientists (60–62), cannot explain the straightening process when considered alone. These phenomena are at most manifestations of disulfide and hydrogen bond breakage and also of changes in protein conformation in the crystalline regions. Like the phenomenon of excessive water swelling, they do not impose by themselves the new straight shape or cause the locking-in of the new shape in the hair architecture. Furthermore, in terms of shape changes there are substantial differences between the processes of protein denaturation, supercontraction, and hair swelling. Protein denaturation does contribute to the removal of permanent shape from the hair architecture; while supercontraction and swelling do not, they are physical phenomena associated to destabilization of the protein structure. Protein denaturation per se, however, does not impose a straight shape; nor does it lock-in a new shape.

Currently, there are three main mechanisms that have been proposed to explain the straightening of very curly hair by alkaline creams. The oldest one centers its arguments on the formation of lanthionine as the new chemical bond that is formed during the reaction of OH ions and hair. This bond is proposed to lock-in the straight shape (59–61).

Another mechanism introduced later bases the explanation on the phenomenon of supercontraction. This mechanism essentially proposes that the high level of contraction observed to occur in hair and wool when treated with high pH solutions is responsible for the imposition of the straight shape (60).

Yet, a more recently proposed mechanism suggests that the occurrence of protein denaturation is crucial and that lanthionine and the formation of any other products are just secondary to the straightening process (62). However, when we use concepts from the field of shape memory materials, we realize that the permanent straightening of hair must include the following steps: 1) removal of protein configurations that support the curly shape, 2) imposition of straight shape, and 3) locking-in of the straight shape, either physically or by forming new bonds.

It is quite possible, thus, that the straightening of curly hair by alkaline relaxers occurs by a combination of all three of the proposed mechanisms. Namely, 1) breakage of disulfide and protein denaturation are needed to delete the curly shape from the memory of hair, 2) a certain amount of fiber supercontraction aids during the cream rubbing process to create the straight shape, and 3) lanthionine formation is needed to stabilize the new straight shape.

Finally, it is obvious that the introduction of a straight shape in curly hair needs to be cosmetically acceptable. This means that both the new straight shape and the hair fibers need to have strength so the shape can be maintained to resist external forces without further unwanted deformation or breakage. The hair with the new straight shape has to be able to resist stresses coming from the grooming of hair, i.e., from its own weight and from hair movement produced by combing or styling, either when wet or dried. Experience tells us, however, that relaxer technology still is far from achieving this objective satisfactorily. Currently, many scientists are working to bridge this gap, and it has already been shown that for certain cases, i.e., for medium curly hair, it is possible to impose a straight shape without causing much damage.

These processes involve the introduction of new strong bonds in the protein chains, bonds that are capable of overcoming internal recovery stresses from the old permanent shape. Unfortunately, most of these new technologies are based on formaldehyde. This chemical is known to cause protein cross-linking in proteins and therefore when used in hair it introduces new cross-links in the hair structure (63). Formaldehyde is, however, a potential carcinogen and its use has been banned in cosmetic applications.

Other hair-straightening technologies involving sodium sulfite or thiogycolate salts are more specific to disulfide bonds, but by their nature they are not efficient in fully removing the very tight curly shape from the hair memory. Consequently, later on the hair undergoes total or partial reversion to its curly shape. In summary, it can be said that the alkaline straightening of curly hair by OH ions is characterized by an efficient shape memory deletion process. It introduces a new straight shape, but it falls short of forming new bonds to lock-in the new straight shape so the final hair shape and hair fibers stay strong. We would be remiss if we did not point out that one other area needing research and improvement is the undesirable occurrence of chemical burns on the skin from the highly alkaline processes described above.

3.3.4.8 HAIR SHAPE CHANGES OCCURRING DURING GROOMING PRACTICES

a. Static vs. dynamic changes in hair shape

The imposition of temporary changes in hair shape is always carried out by external means, and depending on the way hair is handled they can be classified into two types: 1) shape changes imposed while hair is under static conditions, and 2) shape changes imposed while hair is under movement. In the first category we find water-setting, permanent waving, and alkaline straightening. All these shape changes are imposed with external devices that force the hair to stay statically or quasi-statically with almost no movement while the new shape is being imposed. By contrast, in the second category, shape changes are also imposed externally, but the temporary shape is imposed while the hair fibers are in a dynamic free or forced intensive movement. Thus, the final shape attained by the fibers is an average shape, and depends on fiber motion in the assembly. These are, for instance, shape changes produced by blow-dryers, combing devices, and by drying towels. In shape changes of the first type, the interaction of fiber to fiber is not important, while in those of the second type this interaction is extremely important as inter-fiber motion in the assembly determines the final average shape. In the following paragraphs we will focus our attention on the latter types of shape change.

b. Friction vs. bending forces in dynamic changes in hair shape

Movement of hair fibers in hair assemblies always occurs by currents of air, head motion, grooming devices, and even when wet hair is allowed to air dry. Because of hair flexibility, length, and motion intensity, the hair fibers bend, flex, and rotate inside the hair assembly. This flexion and rotation imposes instantaneous transient deformations on the fibers and ultimately leads to the formation of transient temporary shapes in the hair assembly. The transient deformations are, however, immediately countered by internal stresses coming from the permanent shape of hair. The hair assembly will stay deformed in a transient state or it will recover its shape depending on whether inter-fiber slippage occurs between fibers.

Ultimately, the degree of fiber inter-slippage will depend on the balance between single fiber bending and its frictional forces. For instance, slippage among fibers can be prevented if the inter-fiber frictional forces are larger than the bending forces. Under these conditions the hair fibers will behave as semi-solid ropes and the contact points between fibers will serve as strong welding joints that restrict inter-fiber movement. This condition occurs for low bending curvatures and high surface frictional forces, or when styling polymers are used. Polymer spot welding and high friction sites restrict fibers form moving and prevent the fibers from slippage when the hair assembly is being deformed.

Conversely, if a high degree of slippage occurs between hair fibers, then, the low surface frictional forces will not restrict inter-fiber movement. Consequently, slippage among fibers will occur and the permanent shape of both single fibers and hair assembly will be rapidly recovered while in motion. This occurs at sufficiently large bending curvatures or when there are relatively low frictional forces at the hair surfaces. These conditions correspond to the case when silicones or efficient conditioners are applied to the hair surface. The final average shape attained by an assembly is dependent on the balance between fiber slippage and friction forces. Figure 31 displays two hair tresses (a) and (b) washed with different shampoos, and showing the effects of these two conditions. Both hair tresses were cut from the same hair batch and were allowed to air dry at room temperature conditions after shampooing. Hair tress (a) was washed with a simple cleansing shampoo, while hair tress (b) was washed with a "2 in 1" conditioning shampoo containing silicone. In Figure 31 it can be seen that hair tress (b) dries with its fibers in a wavy fashion or with a shape that resembles its permanent shape, while hair tress (a) dries into a straight lump. The reason for this is that during fiber movement and drying, fiber inter-slippage in hair tress (b) was dominant and the final hair shape was driven by natural recovery forces.

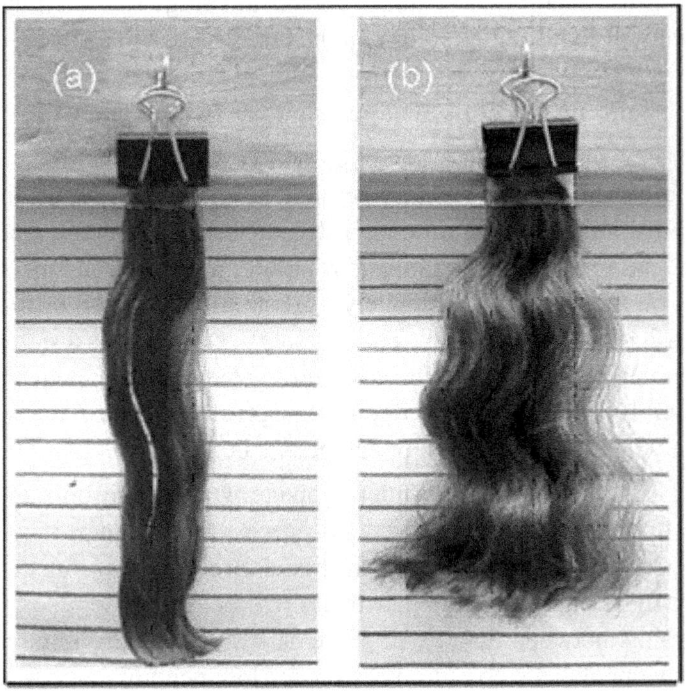

Figure 31) Effect of silicone on the temporary shape of hair after drying. Hair tress (a) was washed with a cleansing shampoo while hair tress (b) was washed with a shampoo containing silicone (64).

Thus, the effect of fiber-to-fiber interaction via surface effects has a strong influence on the acquisition of a temporary shape when the hair is in motion.

Fiber-to-fiber interaction has, therefore, a strong impact on the final shape of the hair assembly. This means that if water-setting is taking place during hair movement, the final shape of the hair assembly will be determined by the interplay between hair inter-fiber friction forces, hair drying rates, hydrogen bond formation in gel-structure, and ability of hair to recover its permanent shape. The role that these processes play in setting dynamic temporary shapes is so important that in the following sections of this chapter their interplay will be analyzed in relation to various grooming practices.

3.3.4.9 HAIR VOLUME AND CHANGES IN HAIR SHAPE

a. Definition of volume

Hair volume can be defined as the effect obtained when a bundle of hair fibers, aligned in synchrony, occupy as a whole or individually a physical space larger than their real nominal volume. Volume in hair is more about the space occupied by the hair bundle than about hair mass or fiber density. The larger the space between fibers or the larger the total volume occupied by the hair bundle, the more volume is perceived (see Figure 32). The definition of volume also includes the ability of the hair fibers to maintain their separate space and shape in synchrony when the assembly of hair fibers is in motion. It should also be perceived when the hair bundle is at rest. These conditions imply that temporary hair shape changes, producing volume should have the strength and elasticity to recover rapidly and in synchrony with shape distortions created during movement. As will be seen later, if this does not happen, the undesirable cosmetic effect will be that of frizzy hair.

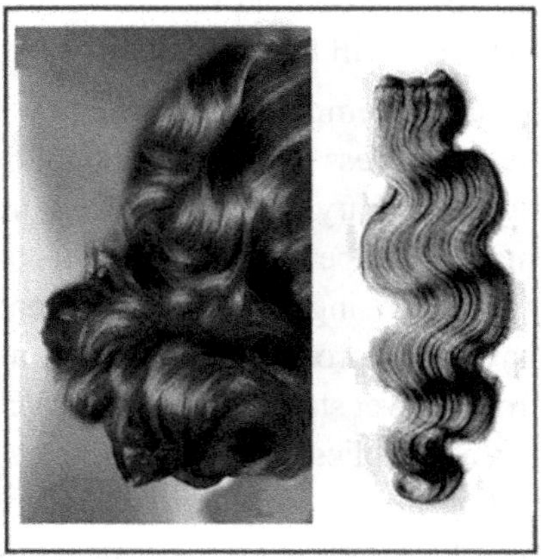

Figure 32) Caption of hair assemblies showing hair volume. The assembly of hair occupies a larger space than it would if each single fiber were shaped straight. Observe also that hair fibers are aligned in synchrony with a particular bundle.

Temporary shape changes in hair that create volume effects can be introduced dynamically while the hair assembly is in movement or also statically. The former is the focus of this paragraph, since the latter belongs to the types of static shape changes already described in previous paragraphs. There are two ways of creating volume by a dynamic process of hair in motion:

1) by imposing a wavy or curved shape in a collective assembly of hair fibers in a synchronized manner while the fibers are in motion. This process usually involves rapid water-setting; and/or
2) by increasing the distance between individual hair fibers, either by creating inter-fiber friction or by using styling polymer films to produce light wavy shapes on smaller hair bundles.

b. Main challenges in creating volume

The creation of hair volume in hair assemblies by any of the procedures described previously always entails hydrogen bond formation, even when polymers or styling resins are used. This means that for all practical purposes, the process of dynamic volume creation has many similarities to the process of water-setting. In water-setting the temporary shape is created statically with plastic rollers, while in the production of dynamic volume the temporary shape is created usually when the hair fibers are in movement. The reason for this is that temporary shapes with volumizing or styling characteristics are commonly created in hair by people after taking a shower, and they are rapidly and conveniently created when the hair is wet and being dried. Therefore, volumizing temporary shapes created by motion are better stored in the hair gel structure of the amorphous phase while the hair is dried. In the following paragraphs of this section, attention will mainly be given to the process of creating hair volume without the use of resins or styling polymers, while the use of styling polymers will be reviewed in a later section.

The main challenge in creating temporary shapes that will result in an increase in hair volume is to coordinate the process of hydrogen bond formation with hair movement in order that an average temporary shape can be captured. Implicit in achieving this is the creation of a temporary shape whose instantaneous strength will be able to resist later shape-recovery forces arising from the permanent shape. While daunting, we note that beauticians have been producing volume in hair just by manipulating hair in motion as it dries from its wet state. As was previously discussed, temporary shapes created by hair fiber assemblies in motion are determined by the interplay between hair inter-fiber friction forces, hair drying rates, hydrogen bond formation in gel-structure, and ability of hair to recover its permanent shape.

In order to better understand the role of hydrogen bond formation and hair movement, let us imagine an ideal and imaginary case of hair volume creation, where the volumizing shapes introduced during hair movement are ideal and will be frozen and stored instantaneously by an extremely rapid process of hydrogen bond formation.

In this ideal process, hydrogen bond formation would be so fast and intense that the instantaneous hair shape acquired during movement would be fixed on hair like a photographic process that freezes a hair shape image while it is in motion. This ideal process would produce a very strong and temporary, rigid pattern of hair volume, somewhat similar to that obtained with the use of styling gels. Such a temporary shape would also resist very well the internal recovery stresses from the permanent shape. Unfortunately, this ideal process does not exist. First, because the rate of hydrogen bond formation by evaporation is slower than the instantaneous shape movement and second, because the instantaneous formation of hair shape during movement depends on the balance between inter-fiber surface friction and shape-recovery forces. Third, and finally, such an ideal process would create a very stiff and static hair pattern that for all practical purposes contradicts one of the main characteristics of hair volume, namely, that of a synchronized hair movement as well. In layman's terms, it is a beautiful thing to watch a woman with long flowing hair shake her head and all of the long tresses move together from side to side. We state this here to bring the reader back, temporarily, to why we have spent such a significant amount of time and scientific research: in the end, all of this technical understanding is intended to bring beauty to hair!

Let's analyze then, a more realistic case; a good example might be that of a head hair assembly with straight shape fibers that are six inches long and belong to a hypothetical subject. After the hair has been shampooed, conditioned, and towel dried, the subject intends to introduce volume by blow-drying. For the sake of simplicity in the analysis, the effect of conditioning ingredients on the hair surface will be omitted. When the straight hair has been wet and towel dried, it still contains about 80% of its internal moisture and, therefore, its gel structure still is very soft because most of its hydrogen bonds are broken.

If at this point the subject introduces motion into the hair fibers, they will be bent and flexed elastically, and the whole hair assembly will be turned into an elastic scrambled irregular pattern. Then, as the subject dries the hair with a blow dryer, he/she forces the hair to move with a brush or a comb to create wavy patterns. As the hair moves and dries, simultaneously hydrogen bonds are formed in the gel structure of each hair fiber, thereby trapping a synchronized wavy temporary shape into their temporary memory. This temporary shape will increase hair volume because the wavy shape of the hair fibers will occupy more space than when the fibers were in a straight shape.

In this simplistic example only two factors affecting the formation of shape were considered. These were the effects of hair drying and hydrogen bond formation. The effects of hair inter-fiber friction, permanent shape strength, and effects of products on rates of drying were not considered. It is easy to foresee, however, that when the fibers enter in motion, the type of shape that will be produced depends on whether the surface is well lubricated or not. It will also depend on the integrity of the hair fibers. It may be that the hair assembly was previously treated with an alkaline relaxer or with other harsh chemical ingredients and thus has a low content of disulfide bonds. In such a case, the instantaneous shape that would form during movement would be very different from that which would have formed had the hair been virgin. Thus, the instantaneous shape that forms during hair movement is also dependent on how strong the real permanent shape is. If the fiber strength and permanent shape are weak, the hair fibers will behave more like viscous fibers and will not be able to recover from instantaneous deformations created by hair movement.

Another factor that was not considered in the prior simplistic analysis is the rate of drying. If the hair contains ingredients on its surface that will retard water evaporation, or if for some other reasons water evaporation is slow, then the process of hydrogen bond re-formation to lock-in the shape in motion will be slow as well. This means that the amount of hydrogen bonds that form at each instant will be so slow that the gel structure will not have the strength to counter the internal shape-recovery forces coming from the real permanent shape. Consequently, the hair wavy pattern produced by hair movement will not be locked-in. For the temporary shape to be locked-in, the numbers of hydrogen bonds that form per second during drying have to be enough to build a hardened mass in the gel structure, so that its strength would be able to counter at any time the internal recovery forces coming from the permanent shape.

By the same token, if the ingredients favor faster drying, then the gel phase in the hair fibers will harden more rapidly, and the wavy shape in motion will be entrapped more efficiently. This analysis explains what cosmetic formulations and beauticians already know, namely, that the types of ingredients applied to hair and the rate of hair drying both have an effect on hair volume. The design of formulations that increase volume thus contain ingredients that in some way or another modify inter-fiber friction, hair drying rates, hydrogen bond formation, or permanent shape.

c. Back-combing and “static fly away”

Back-combing and “static fly away” are two different processes also often used to increase volume. They do not involve the creation of temporary hair shapes by free fiber movement and are based on a different mechanism. Back-combing essentially consists of increasing inter-fiber friction to very high levels by lifting cuticle cells (see Figure 34). The protruding cuticle cells created in this manner interlock the hair fibers at various points. The idea is to totally restrict inter-fiber slippage and movement so the bending deformations introduced during back-combing are maintained. This technique is effective in creating volume; however, it is very damaging to hair. Another way to produce volume in hair is by creating electrostatic repulsion between each hair fiber. Electrostatic repulsion in hair, also referred to as "static fly away" by the cosmetic community, is very common in dried hair, and is due to the buildup of an excessive electric charge in hair. This charge is usually of negative polarity and can also be introduced artificially onto the hair fibers.

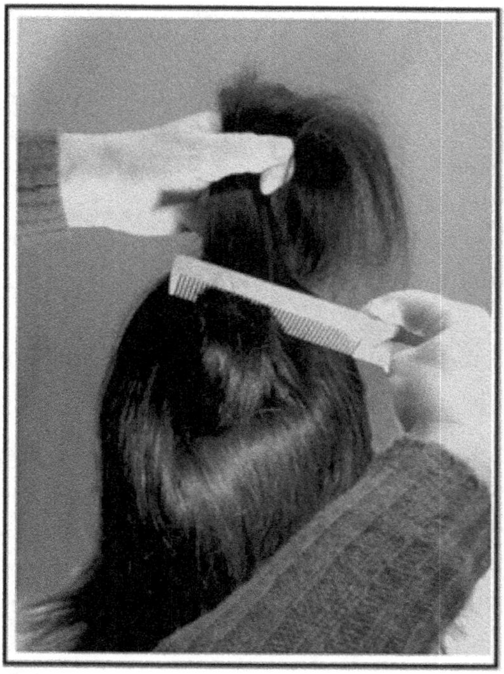

Figure 33) Caption showing process of back-combing ("teasing") to produce hair volume

The process of creating an excess of electrical charge in hair fibers is not a difficult task since hair is an electrical insulator, having very poor electrical conducting characteristics. Therefore, hair, like other electric insulators, is prone to accumulate charges on its surface. Charges are easily transferred from one electrical insulator to another when their surfaces enter into intimate contact. The direction of electric current, or flow of electrons, from one material to another has been studied and categorized for a host of insulating materials and put into a table usually referred to as the triboelectric series (see Table I). Materials at the top of the chart have an excess of negative charges trapped into their structures, and therefore tend to transfer electrons to those at the bottom of the chart. In Table I, it can be seen that hair is below rubber, which is the material often used to make combs. When hair is combed, its surface enters into intimate contact with the rubber in the comb. Electrons are transferred from comb to hair, and thus the hair acquires a negative charge.

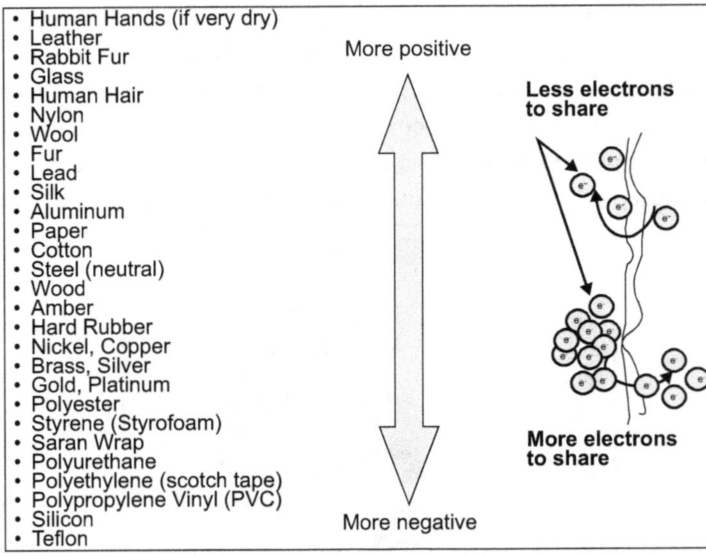

Table I) List of various insulating materials and their position in the triboloelectric series (65).

Since all combed hair fibers acquire the same type of charge, they repel each other, thereby creating a larger distance between them and, ultimately, increasing the hair volume of the assembly. Unfortunately, negative charge in hair does not last long since it escapes via moisture in the hair. Also, the presence of moisturizing ingredients on the hair surface reduces its ability to build up charge. Thus, when hair is highly moisturized, it cannot be charged no matter how many times it is rubbed against the comb. The deposition of certain polymers on the hair surface, however, increases charge buildup and can thus create an apparent effect of volume. The production of "static fly away" to increase volume in hair assemblies is, however, difficult to control as it depends on the rubbing intensity against the comb, i.e., excessive rubbing gives rise to excessive "static fly away." Furthermore, "static fly away" also causes unwanted repulsion or attraction of hair assemblies in proximity, leading to frizzy hair and other unwanted effects (see Figure 34).

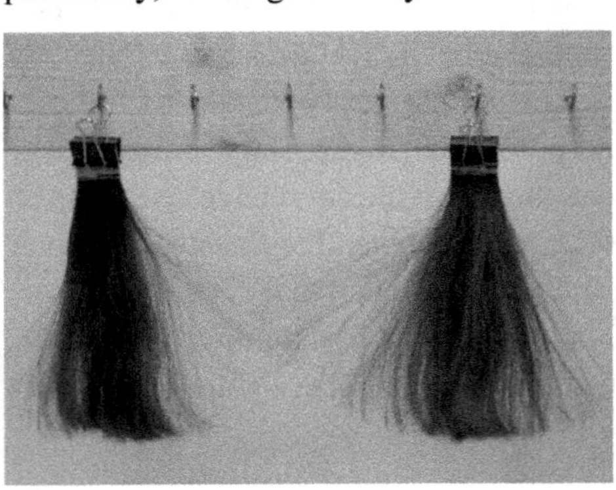

Figure 34) Captions of hair swatches showing effects of "static fly away." There is an attraction between hair fibers of each swatch due to the relative amounts of negative charge in each one, i.e., the hair tress on the right contains a higher level of negative charge buildup (64).

3.3.4.10 FRIZZ IN HAIR AND CHANGES IN SHAPE

Frizzy hair can be defined as the visual aspect of a hair assembly resulting from hair fibers that are positioned geometrically out of synchrony with the remainder of the bundle. The out-of-synchrony effect can be very small or large and can come from a few hair fibers, or almost the whole hair assembly (see Figure 35). The maximum radius of curvature of a frizzy hair fiber separating it from the bundle can be of a few mm or larger (i.e., 1 or 2 cm). Out-of-synchrony effects appear in hair usually immediately after hair drying, and they are more pronounced in hair that has been chemically treated or in hair whose surface has been damaged. In non-frizzy hair, either curly or straight, all hair fibers are aligned in synchrony with their respective neighboring hair fibers. However, in hair with frizz, multiple hair fibers in various sections of the hair assembly separate randomly away from it, forming irregular-shaped curls or waves that are out of synchrony with the rest of the fibers in the bundle (see Figure 35).

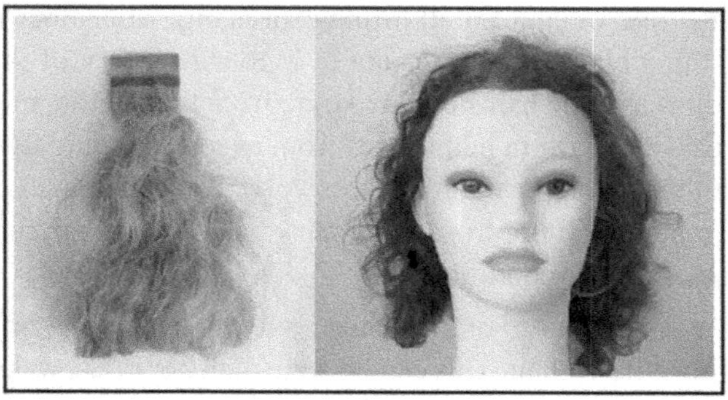

Figure 35) Caption of frizzy hair produced by excess bleaching (left), and by repetitive hot ironing (right). Observe in both cases the large number of single hair fibers that separate out of synchrony from the bundles.

The causes of frizz arise mainly from the inability of hair fibers to recover their permanent shape during or after grooming deformations; i.e., after combing, drying, either by towel, blow-drying, or by hair movement during washing. The inability of hair to recover its permanent shape is caused by damage to the hair structure where the shape memory resides. When this happens, the hair partially or totally loses its permanent shape. Frizz can also be caused by excessive damage to the hair surface. Virgin and healthy hair has its permanent shape memory and also its surface intact. As a result, when the hair fibers are deformed, all of them respond in the same manner. In other words, when they are deformed by motion during grooming practices, they rapidly recover their shape and form an aligned bundle.

In contrast, damaged hair has its memory structures or surface damaged. This damage can be in the form of a partial destruction of disulfide networks in the amorphous phase, or in the form of irreversible denaturation of the crystalline phase. It could be said that hair fibers that present frizz do not remember their permanent shape, and therefore, are partially shapeless. Thus, when damaged hair fibers are deformed, depending on their degree of damage, they respond with shapes that are random and different. For instance, if the various damaged hair fibers undergo excessive stretching or bending during washing, combing, or towel drying, their stretched or bent shape may stay like that or transform into a random shape. The result is that after the hair fibers are dried, their shape is out of synchrony with the remainder of the bundle.

Frizz caused by excessive damage in the cuticle cells of hair fibers is due to very high inter-fiber friction. As was previously discussed, the recovery and final shape in hair fibers during movement is determined by the interplay of the following factors: inter-fiber friction forces, hair drying rates, hydrogen bond formation in gel-structure, and ability of hair to recover its permanent shape. Those hair fibers in a bundle that present high levels of cuticle lifting will not be able to recover their permanent shape after the hair bundle is washed and dried. The reason for this is that high degrees of cuticle cell lifting causes high inter-fiber friction during fiber motion and this phenomenon results in a poor recovery of their permanent shape. Thus, in this case, the hair fibers separate from the bundle, making it appear frizzy. Another cause of frizz in hair comes from excessive static fly away. Typical examples of hair that develop frizz are excessively bleached hair, excessively dried hair, hair often treated with hot irons, and hair damaged during combing/tangling because of a lack of proper conditioning.

Frizz in hair can be reduced or alleviated by temporarily or permanently reconstructing the shape of frizzy hair. This can be done with hot irons, water-setting treatments, or even with treatments that introduce a new shape by re-forming disulfide bonds. When frizz is corrected with temporary treatments such as water-setting or hot irons, the problem is not solved, as the hair fibers will become frizzy again after washing. If it is caused by excessive surface damage, then, frizz can be reduced with treatments that smooth cuticle cells or reduce excessive inter-fiber friction. In many cases, frizz is caused by a combination of damage to the disulfide bond network, damage to the hair surface, and by the appearance of static fly away. In this case, frizz reduction can only be accomplished by a combination of various treatments.

3.3.4.11 BODY IN HAIR AND CHANGES IN HAIR SHAPE

The subjective perception of Body is one of abundant hair that is strong and healthy. It manifests itself during hair movement as a combination of hair mass and hair shape. The closest mechanical descriptor for body is the flexural rigidity of a bundle of fibers. Unlike other mechanical properties that do not take into account shape, flexural rigidity combines Bending Modulus and shape of materials (66). This property recognizes the fact that the same mass of any material is easier or more difficult to bend depending on the way that it is shaped. For instance, it is difficult to make a sheet of paper stand up straight on a surface because it flexes and bends down easily. However, if we fold the same sheet of paper in half it will be able to stand without bending. Thus, just by changing its shape we have changed its flexural rigidity (see Figure 36).

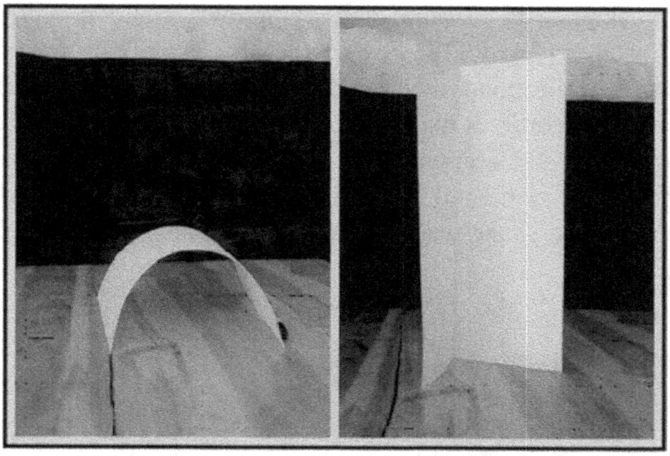

Figure 36) Effect of shape on the flexural rigidity of a sheet of paper. The sheet of paper cannot stand up straight on a surface because it flexes and bends down easily. Observe that after folding it in half the sheet of paper is capable of remaining straight.

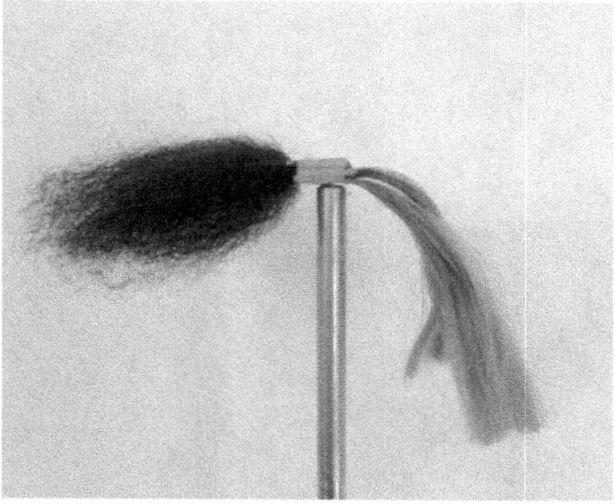

Figure 37) Effect of hair curliness on the flexural rigidity of hair. The bundle in the left with curly hair is able to maintain almost a straight inclination in cantilever without flexing, while the bundle in right with straight hair fibers bends more easily (64).

When we apply these concepts to hair we realize that is easier to flex a hair bundle of very fine hair when its fibers are in a straight fashion, than when a bundle of similar mass has its fibers tightly coiled (see Figure 37). Thus, shaping the fine hair fibers into a coiled configuration allows them to present higher flexural rigidity and higher body. The tighter the coil in hair fibers, the more body the hair assembly has. Furthermore, flexural rigidity in a solid body does not change with movement. However, in a hair bundle, since the hair fibers are not tightly attached to each other, this property may change if the interplay of inter-fiber friction, hydrogen bond breakage with moisture, and drying rates are not properly set for that purpose. For instance, Figure 38 shows two hair tresses with their half-lengths standing up and their tips pointing upwards. The bundle at the left was treated with a solution of cationic particles that increased inter-fiber friction, while the bundle at the right does not contain any product on its surface. The bundle at the left is stiffer than that on the right, and it shows higher flexural rigidity and more body because its pre-formed shape was not allowed to change by the high inter-fiber friction in the bundle.

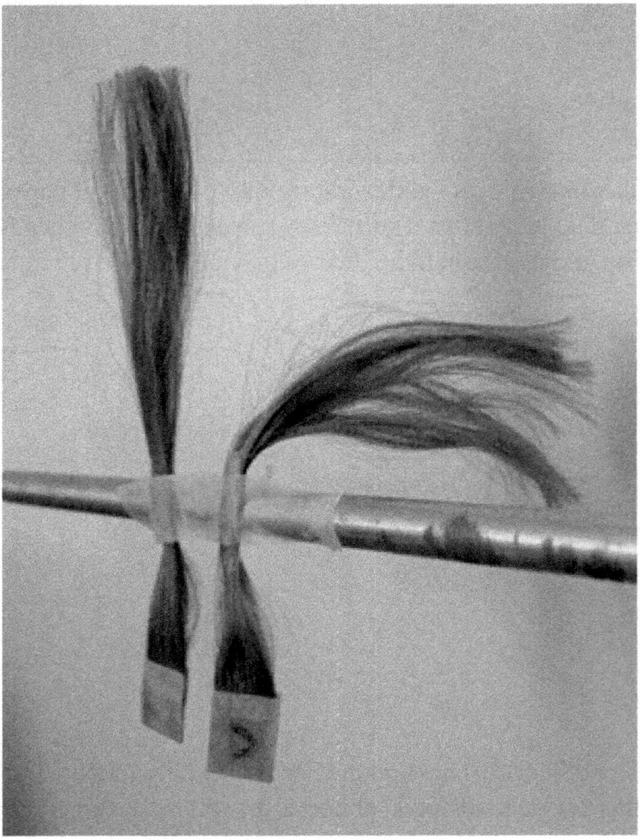

Figure 38) Effect of inter-fiber hair friction on the flexural rigidity of hair. The hair swatch at the left was surface treated with cationic particles and is able to maintain an upward position vertically without any support, while the hair swatch at the right with no treatment bends more easily (64).

Body in hair is, therefore, dependent on the following three properties:

a) hair fiber density, i.e., number of fibers per unit area,
b) intrinsic protein density,
c) inter-fiber friction, and
d) temporary shapes created in hair fibers.

Since cosmetic treatments cannot change properties (a) and (b), in order to increase body, formulators always try to maintain temporary shapes with high flexural rigidity by changing properties (c) and (d). Products that increase body are, therefore, those that can influence and create the formation of temporary shapes with high flexural rigidity, i.e., strong wavy patterns, high inter-fiber friction, inter-fiber spot welding, high drying rates, etc.

3.3.4.12 HAIR SHAPE CHANGES INDUCED BY STYLING POLYMERS

Styling polymers have been used for many years to produce or enhance temporary changes in hair shape and to create fashionable styles that are difficult to achieve by water-setting. The ways to produce these styling shapes vary from beautician to beautician but they can be divided into static and dynamic processes.

Styling static processes involve the following steps:

1) applying a new shape to hair with the help of rollers or other devices while the hair still contains ~ 60–80% of its moisture,
2) applying the formulation containing the polymer,
3) letting the polymer and hair dry, and finally,
4) removing the rollers or devices.

Styling dynamic processes involve, on the other hand, the following general steps:

1) inducing movement in hair fibers with blow-dryers or fingers while the style is being created,
2) applying the polymer as the hair moves to entrap an average shape, and
3) stopping movement and polymer application and letting the hair dry.

From the mechanistic point of view, both polymer styling processes are similar to the static and dynamic water-setting described in previous sections. The only difference is that when a styling polymer is used, these materials are applied to hair via various formulations to produce temporary shapes and/or to enhance their durability. In most cases the mode of action of styling polymers in changing hair shape is external and limited to the production of seam and spot-welding junctions between hair fibers to restrict inter-fiber movement, thereby giving rigidity to the hair assembly (see Figure 39). The polymer by itself does not affect the memory shape or intrinsic structure of hair. In other words, the polymer molecules do not interact with hydrogen bonds, disulfide bonds, or the crystalline structure of hair.

However, formulations used as polymer vehicles may contain water or solvents that penetrate into the cortical cells and enhance or inhibit plasticization of the hair gel structure by breaking or re-forming hydrogen bonds. As will be seen later, these effects are not due to the polymer per se and have an influence on how rapidly the temporary shape is entrapped and locked-in. In the following paragraphs an analysis is made of the influence that polymers have in assisting changes in hair shape. Special attention will be given to how the polymers modify the interplay of hair inter-fiber friction, hair drying rates, hydrogen bond formation in gel-structure, and hair strength to recover its permanent shape.

The effects that formulations have on these processes will also be reviewed but to a lesser extent. Properties and composition of the various polymers used in hair styling applications will not be reviewed here, but for information purposes a list of the most common is given in Table II.

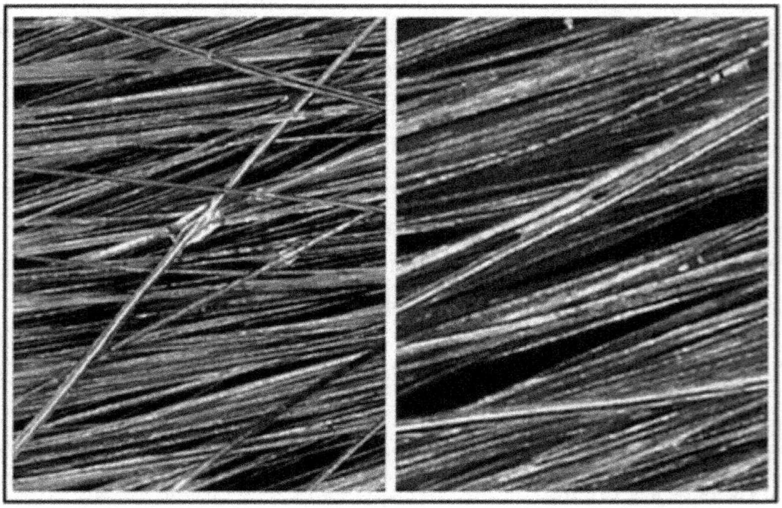

Figure 39) Micrographs of a bundle of hair fibers showing formation of seam and spot welding by polymers (64)

3.3.4.13 ROLE OF STYLING POLYMERS IN CHANGING HAIR SHAPE

As was previously discussed, the water-setting of hair, or the entrapment of a hair shape in movement without polymers, is very simple and controlled mainly by the interplay of hair inter-fiber friction, hair drying rates, hydrogen bond formation in gel-structure, and hair strength to recover its permanent shape. Hair shape entrapment with styling polymers adds, however, various levels of complexity to these factors not only because the polymers play externally a role on hair shape formation but also because the formulations influence the shape.

The added levels of complexity brought about by polymers and formulations are due to the following parameters:

1) rates of solvent evaporation; this will determine how rapid the polymer welding seams and spots dry and harden,
2) hair plasticization by the solvent; mainly when water is used as the solvent,
3) polymer glass transition temperature (Tg); this parameter determines how hard/brittle or soft/ductile is the spot welding, and
4) strength of adhesive joints at the hair/polymer interface. In the following paragraphs a discussion of all these factors will be made in relation to each one of the main formulations used in the styling of hair.

a. Temporary setting of hair with aerosols

In terms of entrapping a hair shape in motion, aerosol formulations are the simplest to analyze because the polymer is usually dissolved in ethanol or in combinations of this solvent with water. The reasons for the simplicity stem from the following facts: 1) the ethanol/water solution produces a very low level of hair plasticization; 2) the solvent mixtures have high rates of evaporation and, therefore, the polymer "welding spots" harden very rapidly, entrapping transient hair shapes efficiently. Thus, provided that the polymer or resin has the appropriate Tg, and that it is properly formulated and delivered from the aerosol bottle, and that the concentration of cationic charge along the polymer chain is sufficient, it will rapidly form welding seams and spots across hair fibers, restricting their motion and thereby entrapping the transient hair shape produced by movement (see Figures 40 and 41).

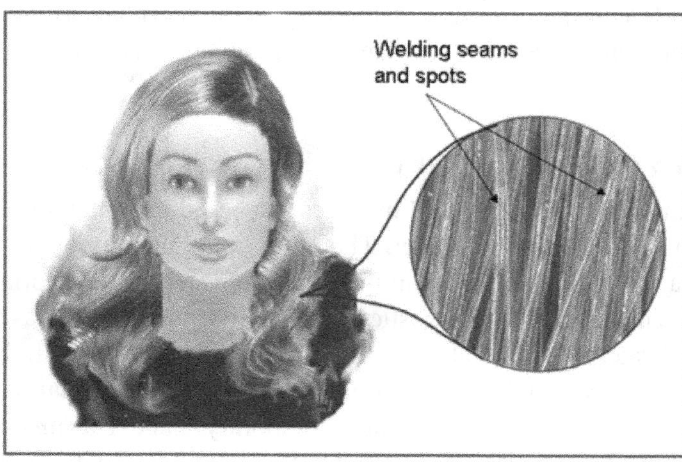

Figure 40) Illustration of hair in mannequin with styling polymer applied (left) and caption showing welding seams and spots (right)

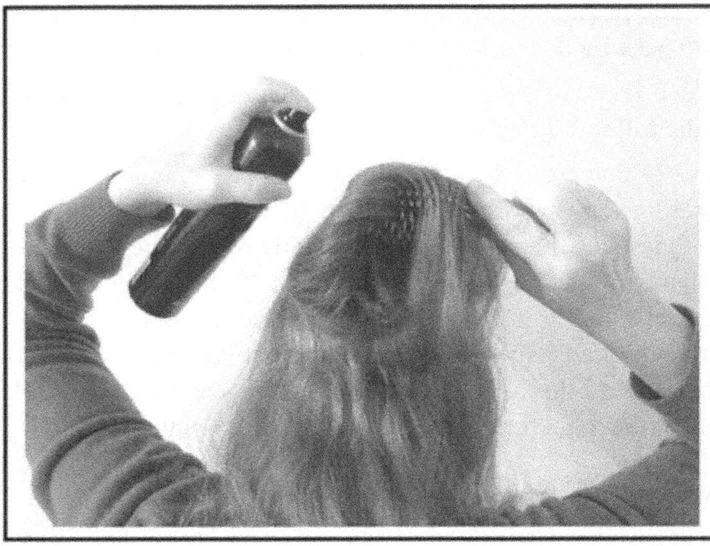

Figure 41) Picture showing action of spraying a styling polymer to entrap shape of hair in motion

Aerosol formulations are also used to enhance temporary shapes produced statically, i.e., when the hair is not in motion. These types of applications do not have the complexities of entrapping an average shape produced by hair motion. The phenomena of fiber-to-fiber slippage, fiber bending, and fiber recovery from instantaneous shape deformations are absent in these cases. Temporary shapes produced under these conditions are preset by any of the methods described before for water-setting or hot irons under static conditions. In these cases the polymers are not used to entrap or capture a temporary shape from hair assemblies that are in motion, but rather are used to enhance long-lastingness of the preset temporary shape.

b. Temporary setting of hair with gels and mousses

Styling formulations like gels and mousses are based on water-soluble polymers and contain high amounts of water. Therefore, they have a double influence on shape formation while the hair is in motion. The water in these formulations diffuses into the hair and partially plasticizes the hair's amorphous phase; meanwhile the polymer/water system is able to provide a certain amount of hold to entrap a temporary shape. With polymer gel or mousse formulations the hair is put into motion with the fingers or a comb to create a temporary shape. During the application step, these formulations are administered to the hair surface with a very high shear rate. Thus, such pseudoplastic behavior results in a low enough viscosity at the high rates of shear to apply easily and effectively, but on stopping the application, the rate of shear goes to zero and the apparent viscosity rapidly increases to a very high value, thereby preventing the hair from recovering its permanent shape. Higher viscosities at zero shear rate (i.e., polymers that form a high-yield stress) are optimal for this approach.

Even when these formulations still contain high amounts of water, they are able to suppress internal hair recovery forces and inter-fiber slippage, providing a transient hold. Once the desired shape is attained the polymer/water system is allowed to dry, and subsequently the polymer hardens, forming "welding spots" and also seams, i.e., points of attachment across multiple hair strands, both of which restrict inter-fiber motion and give flexural rigidity to the temporary shape.

c. Mechanical properties of welding seams and spots

The complexity of hairstyle and hold ultimately depend on the mechanical properties, size, and distribution of welding seams and spots. Properties such as the glass transition temperature (Tg), susceptibility of the polymer to be plasticized by moisture, and adhesive strength at the polymer/hair interface are crucial in the final retention of temporary shape or style hold. Aerosol or sprays produce an irregular distribution of spot welding while gels and mousses yield more uniform welding patterns (see Figure 42). Furthermore, the welding patterns left by gels are, in particular, thicker and more uniform, and this explains why gel formulations, which create high-yield stresses at zero shear rate, are more suitable to create extreme styles. The distribution and amount of polymer that remains after gel application is such that the hair undergoes a transformation from a pure hair assembly to a polymer/hair composite with very different mechanical properties (68–71). The formed polymer/hair composite, depending on the polymer properties, is able to create shapes with very high flexural rigidity that can withstand high levels of relative humidity (see Figure 43).

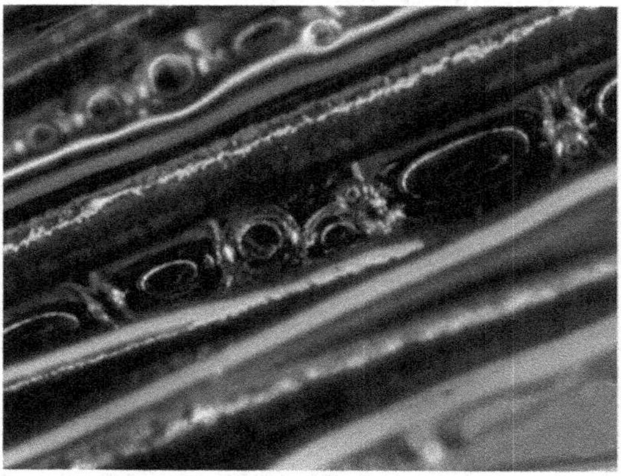

Figure 42) Micrograph of a bundle of hair fibers showing seam welding by a gel formulation.

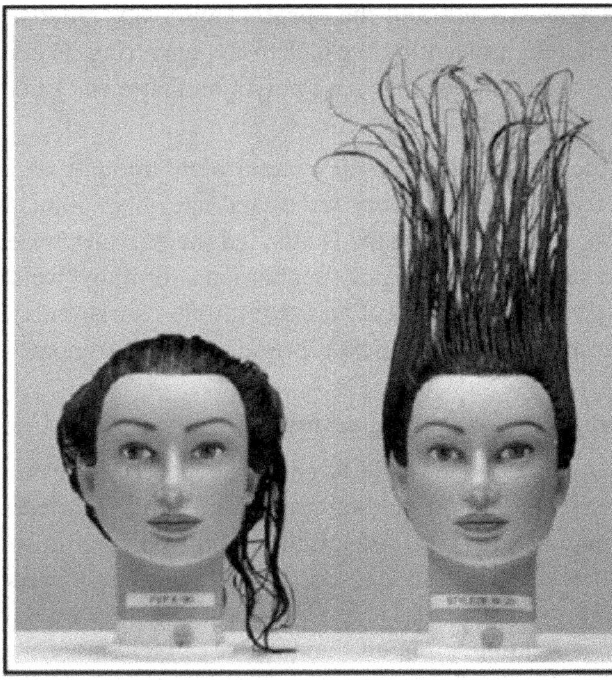

Figure 43) Effect of two gel formulations on the temporary hold of hair after five seconds of water immersion. The hair of the mannequin at the left was treated with a gel containing a polymer with a high Tg and low resistance to moisture, while the hair of the mannequin at the right was treated with a polymer with a high Tg but with high resistance to moisture (67).

d. Effect of polymer glass transition temperature (Tg) on styling

The glass transition temperature of a polymer is a parameter that relates to its viscoelastic behavior. Once the style is set and hair shape has been changed, the polymer welding seams and spots must withstand stress/deformations in the hair assembly arising from head movement and from the hair's own weight. The polymer also has to efficiently counter recovery stresses coming from the memory shape of hair in the amorphous and crystalline phases. These stresses will push the hair fibers for recovery of their permanent shape.

If the Tg of the polymer is too low or if its value decreases because of water plasticization, the spot welding will flow like a viscous "chewing gum" and will not be able to retain the temporary shape (see Figure 44). In contrast, if the Tg is too high the polymer will be very hard and brittle and the seams and spots will break by stress/deformations arising from hair movement. The final effect will be losses in the hairstyle and the production of "flakes" in the hair (see Figure 45).

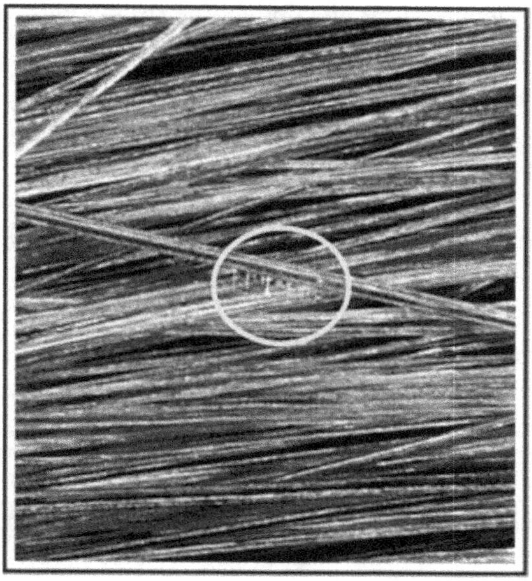

Figure 44) Micrograph showing effects of low Tg in the seam welding of a styling polymer (65).

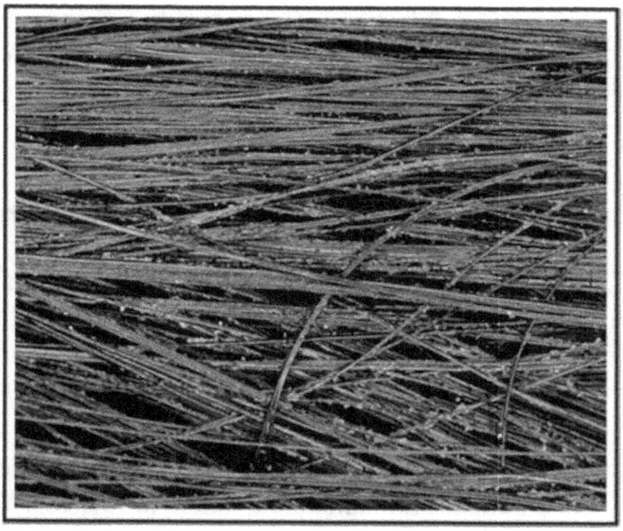

Figure 45) Micrograph showing flaking of a polymer due to a very high glass transition and lack of plasticizer (64).

These two effects are better visualized in Figure 46, where three typical graphs depicting changes in hair Elastic Modulus as a function of temperature are shown. The graphs correspond to three hypothetical polymers (A), (B), and (C) with different glass transition temperatures. In theses graphs, the solid line (a) represents the location of room temperature, the dotted line (b) the glass transition temperature (Tg) of the polymer, and the curved line (c) represents the variation of Elastic Modulus with temperature.

Observe in this graph that when the glass transition temperature (Tg) of the polymer is way above room temperature, i.e., polymer A, the polymer is very stiff, and we will expect that the welding spots and seams will also be very hard and stiff. In the graph at the center with polymer B, the Tg is close to room temperature, and therefore, the seams and spots will be flexible. Finally, in the graph at the right with polymer C, the Tg is below room temperature and the seams and spots will behave extremely soft and will flow viscously. The glass transition of hair therefore has to be properly adjusted so it can provide the necessary hold without having the inconveniences of being very soft or extremely hard.

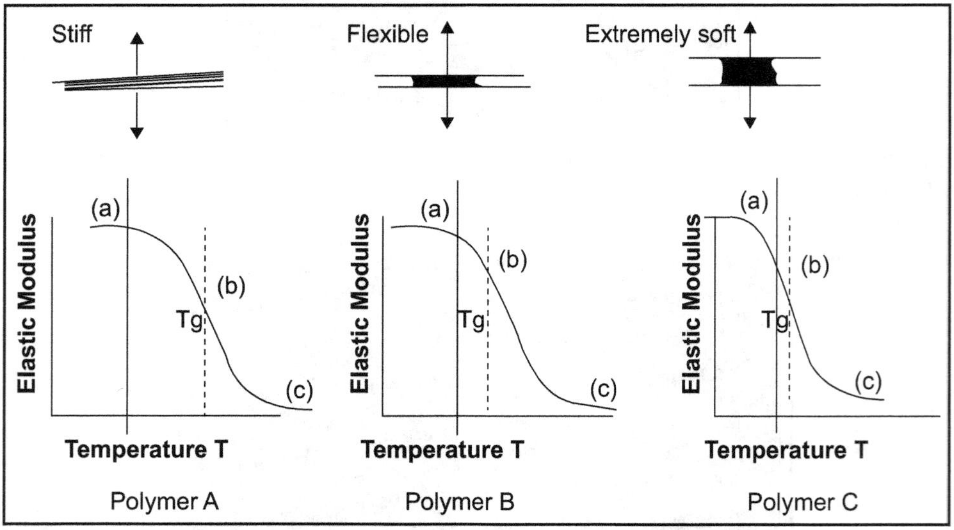

Figure 46) Graphs showing the relationship between Elastic Modulus and Temperature for three polymers with different glass transition temperatures (64).

e. Adhesive strength at the polymer/hair interface

The adhesive strength at the polymer/hair interface of welding seams and spots is another important parameter in maintaining hairstyle (68, 69). The reason for this is that the polymer must be able to counter permanent shape-recovery stresses coming from the disulfide bonds and crystalline regions, and these stresses are transferred from hair into polymer via the adhesive joints. Further, the polymer needs to comply with the strong forces of hair contraction, which are produced during the de-swelling of hair. If the bonding strength of the polymer with the hair surface is weak and breaks, either because of contraction or recovery stresses, then there is no resistance to recovery, and the hairstyle will be lost soon.

In summary, styling polymers help in locking more elaborate hairstyles and temporary shapes, but they also have limitations in terms of the temporary shapes they can induce. For instance, styling polymers, no matter how high their Tg is, or how they are formulated, may not be able to straighten extremely curly hair, or vice versa, they may not be able to produce tight curls in very straight hair. The reason for this is, again, that the polymer cannot counter the strong recovery forces coming from the permanent shape stored in the hair's memory. *Styling polymers can however contribute substantially to attaining these changes when combined with other treatments, i.e., with hot irons or other chemical treatments.*

The styling polymers used currently also have limitations in terms of complying with increasing demands of performance and with restrictions in the use of volatile organic compounds in aerosol formulations. These issues have put a lot of pressure on polymer designers and formulators to create novel ingredients that can meet performance and regulatory issues. New polymers are required to be completely soluble in water and/or at least to be partially soluble in it. This task represents a major challenge because in terms of performance, styling polymers are required to resist plasticization by moisture. Polymer synthesis scientists have responded to these challenges by creating polymers with particular pendant groups and domains that appear to provide water solubility and yet are able to transform into hydrophobic materials once they cast into dried films. The field of polymer innovations is vast and most certainly in the years to come there will be a solution to all these issues. Examples of some of these styling polymers are shown in Table II below.

Gels	**Styling Polymers – Sprays**
PVP Polyvinylphrrolidone	Octylacrylamide/Acrylates/Butylaminoethyl Methacrylate
VP/Dimethylaminoethylmethacrylate Copolymer	Copolyme
PVP/ DMAPA Acrylates Copolymer	VA/Crotonates/Vinyl Neodecanoate Copolymer
Hydrolyzed Wheat Protein/PVP Crosspolymer	Acrylates Copolymer
VP/VA Copolymer	Acrylates/Dimethicone Copolymer (Elasteesse)
Vinyl Caprolactam/VP/	Digylcol/CHDM/Isophthalates/SIP Copolymer
Dimethylaminoethylmethacrylate Copolymer	Octylacrylamide/Acrylates Copolymer
Acrylates Copolymer	Ethyl Ester of PCM/MA Copolymer

PVM/MA Copolymer
Polyquaternium-4
Polyquaternium-11
Chitosan
Chitosan PCA
Polyacrylate- 3
Mousses
Polyquaternium-4
Polyquaternium-11
Hydrophilic Polyester Polyurethane
PVP
VP/VA Copolymer
VP/Dimethylaminoethylmethacrylate Copolymer
PVP/ Acrylates/Lauryl Methacrylate Copolyme
Hydrolyzed Wheat Protein/PVP Crosspolymer
Acrylates/ Allyl Methacylate Copolymer?
Acrylates Copolymer
Polyquaternium-37

(Table II) List of main hair styling polymers

Acknowledgments

The author would like to thank Linda Foltis for her helpful discussions and support during the writing of this chapter. Thanks also to Ashland, Inc. for providing the opportunity and resources to carry out this task.

REFERENCES

1) M. L. Tate, Y. K. Kamath, S. B. Reutsch, and H.D. Weigmann, Quantification and prevention of hair damage, J. Soc. Cosmet. Chem., 44, 347–371, (November/December 1993)

2) L.H. Sperling, "Mechanical Behavior of Polymers" in Introduction to Physical Polymer Science, eds. John Wiley and Sons Inc, New York, pp. 503–547, (1992)

3) I. M. Ward, J. Sweeney, Mechanical Properties of Solid Polymers, Publisher: John Wiley & Sons Inc, December, 2012

4) R.P. Kambour and R.E. Robertson, CH. 11, in "Polymer Science", by A.D. Jenkins, ed. North Holland Publishing Co., Amsterdam, (1972)

5) D.V. Istrate, "Heat Induced Denaturation of Fibrous Hard α-Keratins and their Reactions with Chemical Reagents", PhD Thesis, Aachen University, 2011

6) M. Feughelman, "Mechanical Properties and Structure of alpha-Keratin Fibres; Wool, Human Hair, and Related Fibers", Published by University of New South Wales Press, 1997.

7) T. Cheng. A. Romo-Uribe, and P.T. Mather, "Two Way Reversible Memory in a Semi-Crystalline Network", Macromolecules 2008, 41, 184–192

8) C. Liu, H. Qinb, and P. T. Mather, "Review of progress in shape-memory polymers", J. Mater. Chem., 2007, 17, 1543–1558 | 1543

9) Jinlian Hu, Chapter I, "Advances in Shape Memory Polymers", The Textile Insitute, WP: Woodhead Publishing

10) J. Diani, P. Gilormini, C. Fredy, and A.R. Ingrid, "Role of Viscoelasticity in Predicting the Shape Memory Effect of Polymers",Chapter 12, in Experimental and Applied Mechanics", Volume 4, Conference Proceedings of the Society for Experimental Mechanics Series 2013, pp 97–104

11) K. Gall, CM Yakacki, Y. Liu, R. Shandas, N. Willett, KS Anseth, "Thermomechanics of the shape memory effect in polymers for biomedical applications" J. Biomed. Mater Res. A. 2005 Jun 1; 73 (3): 339–48.

12) M. Behl and A. Lendlein, "Overview of Shape Memory Polymers", in Shape Memory Polymers and Multi-functional Composites", Eds. J. Lend and S. Du, CRC Press Taylor and Francis Group LLC, Boca Raton, Florida, 2010.

13) J. Ivens, M. Urbanus, C. De Smet, "Shape recovery in a thermoset shape memory polymer and its fabric-reinforced composites", Polymer Letters Vol.5, No.3 (2011) 254–261

14) H. Huang, J. Hu, Y. Zhu, "Shape-memory biopolymers based on β-sheet structures of polyalanine segments inspired by spider silks", Macromol. Biosci. 2013 Feb; 13 (2) : 161–6.

15) Lendlein, S. Kelch, „Shape-memory polymers“. Angew. Chem. Int. Ed. 41: 2034–2057, (2002).

16) O. Emile, A. Le Floch, and F. Vollrath, “Biopolymers: Shape memory in spider draglines”, Nature 440, 621 (30 March 2006)

17) P. J. Skrzeszewska , L. N. Jong , F. A. de Wolf , M. Stuart, and J. van der Gucht, “Shape-Memory Effects in Biopolymer Networks with Collagen-Like Transient Nodes”, Biomacromolecules, 2011, 12 (6), pp 2285–2292

18) M. Gamez-Garcia unpublished results

19) S. Thibaut, P. Barbarat, F. Leroy, B.A. Bernard, Human hair keratin network and curvature, Int. J. Dermatol. 2007 Oct; 46 Suppl 1:7–10

20) B.A. Bernard, Hair shape of curly hair, J. Am. Acad. Dermatol. 2003 Jun; 48 (6 Suppl) S 120–6

21) C. Robbins, “Chemical and Physical Behavior of Human Hair” 5th. Ed. Springer-Verlag, New York, 2013, pp. 211–206

22) C. Robbins, H.D. Weigmann, S. Ruetsch, Y. Kamath, Failure of intercellular adhesion in hair fibers with regard to hair condition and strain conditions, J Cosmet Sci. 2004 Jul-Aug; 55 (4): pp. 351–71.

23) L. Rebenfeld, H. D. Weigmann, and C. Danzizer, Temperature Dependence of the Mechanical Properties of Human Hair in Relation to Structure. J. Soc. Cosm. Chem. 17, 525–538 (1966)

24) 19) In Krünitz Encyclopeida of Economics, 1858, 11:41, 27 October 2007

25) 25) WO 2010123966 A2, Infrared emitting hair roller and methods of use

26) Y. Zhou, etal, “Investigation of thermal Damage of Hair from Hot Flat Ironing and the Thermal Protective Effects of Cosmetic Pretreatments”, presented at 26 th Congress of the IFSCC in Argentina, September 20–23, 2010.

27) M. Gamez-Garcia, “ Hair Setting With Hot Irons and Heat Activation”, SCC Scientific Seminar, June 2–3, Las Vegas 2011

28) R. McMullen and J. Jachowicz, “Thermal Degradation of Hair I. Effect of Curling Irons”, J. Cosmet. Sci. 49, pp. 223–244 (July/August 1998).

29) D. Istrate, C. Popescu, M. Möller, Non-Isothermal Kinetics of Hard α-Keratin Thermal Denaturation, Macromolecular Bioscience, Volume 9, Issue 8, pages 805–812, August 11, 2009

30) P. Milczarek, M. Zielinski, M. L. Garcia, The mechanism and stability of thermal transitions in hair keratin, Colloid and Polymer Science, November 1992, Volume 270, Issue 11, pp 1106–1115

31) F.J. Wortmann, M. Stapels, R. Elliott, L. Chandra, The effect of water on the glass transition of human hair. Biopolymers. 2006 Apr 5;81(5):371–5.

32) J. M. Quadflieg, Fundamental properties of Afro-American hair as related to their straightening/relaxing behavior, PhD Thesis, Aachen: Rheinisch-Westfälischen Technischen Hoch- schule, 2003.

33) A. Dussaud, B. Rana, and H. T. Lam, Progressive Hair Straightening Using a Hot Iron: Function of Silicones, J. Cosm. Sci., 64, 1–13, March/April 2013

34) M. Gamez-Garcia, "Heat Damage to the Cortex and Cuticle Sheath of Human Hair Produced by Hot Appliances, Cosmetic Science Technology, 2011, pp. 119

35) M. Gamez-Garcia, Void and pore formation inside the hair cortex by a denaturation and super-contraction process occurring during hair setting with hot irons, J Cosmet Sci. 2011 Mar-Apr;62(2):109–20.

36) M. Gamez-Garcia, "The Cracking of Human Hair Cuticles by Cyclical Thermal Stresses", J. Soc. Cosmet. Chem., 49, 141–153 (1998).

37) S.B. Ruetsch and Y.K. Kamath, "Effect of Thermal Treatment with a Curling Iron on Hair Fiber", J. Cosmet. Sci., Vol. 55. pp. 13–27, (July/August 1998).

38) A. Szilagyi, J. Kardos, Sz. Osvath, L.Barna, and P. Zavodszky, Protein folding. In Handbook of Neurochemistry and Molecular Neurobiology, Eds. A. Lajtha and N. Banik, Volume 7, Chapter 10. pp. 303–344. Springer, 2007

39) T. A. Evans, T.N. Ventura, AB Wayne, The kinetics of hair reduction, J Soc Cosmet Chem. 45, 279–99 (1994).

40) R. Hellingotter, Permanent Waving of hair; in The Chemistry and Manufacture of Cosmetics, 2nd, ed., M De Navarre, ed. Orlando: Continental Press, 1167–227 (1975)

41) R. E. Reed, M. DenBeste, F. L. Humoller, Parrnanent waving of human hair; The cold process, J.Sco. of Csmet. Chem. 1–109–22– (1948)

40) J. G. Gumprecht, K. Patel, R. P. Bono, Effectiveness of reduction and oxidation in acid and alakline permanent weaving, J. Sco. Cosmet. Chem. 18, 717–32, (1977)

42) K. H. Herman, Hair Keratin, Reaction penetration and swelling of mercaptan solutions, Trans. Faraday Soc. 59 1633 (1963)

44) M.A. Manuszak, E.T. Borish, R.R. Wickett, The kinetics of disulfide bond reduction in hair by ammonium thoglycolate and dithio-glycolic acid, J. Soc. Cosmet. Chem. 47 49–58 (1988)

44) N. E. Yin, R. H. Kissinger, W. S. Tolgyesi, E. M. Cottington, The effect of fiber diameter on the cosmetic aspects of hair, J. Soc. Cosmet. Chem 28 139–50 (1977)

45) S. Ogawa, K. Fujii, K. Kaneyame, K. Arai, and K. Joko, "A curing Method for Permanent Hair Straightening Using Thioglycolic and Di-thioglycolic Acids', J. Cosmet. Sci., Vol. 51, pp. 379–399, (November/December 2000).

46) L. J. Wolfram, "The Reactivity of Human Hair. A review", in Hair Research, Ed. By Orfanos, Montagna, Stuttgen and Springer-Verlag, Berlin Heidelgerg 1981

47) F. J. Wortmann, C. Popescu, G. Sendelbach, Effects of reduction on the denaturation kinetics of human hair, Biopolymers 600–605 (2008)

48) M. Feughelman, A comment on "Bending relaxation properties of human hair and permanent waving performance", J. Sco Cosmet Chem 42 129–31 (1991)

49) E. Tolgyesi, F. Fang, Action of Nucleophilic Agents on Keratin; in Hair Research, Springer Berlin, eds. CE Orfanos, E Montagna, G. Stuttgen, 1981, pp. 116–122

50) R. S. Asquith, P. Carthew, The Competitive Addition, Reaction of Dehydroalanine Residues Formed during the Degradation of Wool Cystine Residues, J. Text. Inst., 64:10 19

51) A. Syed, H. Ayoub and A. Kuhajda, Recent advances in treating excessively curly hair, Cosmet Toil 113(9) 47–55 (1998)

52) M. Gamez-Garcia unpublished results

53) John Halal, Hair Structure and Chemistry Simplified, 4th ed. Milady Thomson Learning

54) A Syed, A Kuhajda, H Ayoub and K Ahmad, African-American Hair: Its physical properties and differences relative to Caucasian hair, Cosmet Toil 110(10) 39–47 (1995)

55) J Menkart, LJ Wolfram and I Mao, Caucasian hair, Negro hair, and wool: Similarities and differences, J Soc Cosmet Chem 17 769–787 (1966)

56) A. N. Syed and H. Ayoub, Correlating Porosity and Tensile Strength of Chemically Modified Hair, Cosmetics & Toiletries magazine/57

57) S. S. Thakur, and P. Balaram, Characterization of Alkali Induced Formation of Lanthionine, Trisulfides, and Tetrasulfides from Peptide Disulfides using Negative Ion Mass Spectrometry, American Society for Mass Spectrometry, 2009,
58) S. H. Feairheller, M. M. Taylor, D. G. Bailey, 35S-Sulfide incorporation during alkaline treatment of keratin and its relation to lanthionine formation, Adv Exp Med Biol. 1977;86B:177–86.
59) M. J. Horn, D. B. Jones, S. J. Ringel, "The isolation of lanhionine from human hair, chicken feathers and lactablbumin, J. Biol Chem. 138 141–49, (1941)
60) M. Wong, G. Wis-Surel, and J. Epps, "Mechanism of Hair Straightening", J. Soc. Cosmet. Chem., 45, 345–352 (November/December 1994)
61) A. Syed, Hair Straightening, in Chemistry and Manufacture of Cosmetics, Volume II, Formulating, 4th, ed. M Schlossman, ed, Carol Stream: Allured Pub. 337–385 (2008)
62) F. J. Wortmann, J. Quadflieg, L. J. Wolfram, "Mechanistic aspects of African hair relaxation", presentation at Hair'S 11, Irsee, Germany, Sep. 6–8, 2011.
63) E. Hinton, A Survey and Critique of the Literature on Cross-linking Agents and Mechanisms as Related to Wool Keratin. Textile Research Journal, p. 256, (1974).
64) M. Gamez-Garcia unpublished results
65) K. L. Kaiser, Electrostatic Discharge, CRC Press, Taylor & Francis Group, Boca Raton, Florida, 2006, pp. 2–5
66) S. Timoshenko, G.H. MacCullough, Elements of Strength of Materials, D. Van Nostrand Company, Incorporated, 1940
67) Ray Rigoletto, internal Ashland Mannequin Water Dunking Test
68) J. Jachowicz, Dynamic Hairspray Analysis III, Theoretical Considerations, J. Cosmet. Scie., 53, 249–261 (September/October 2002)
69) D. W. Rafferty, J. Zellia, D. Hasman, J. Mullay, Polymer Composite Principles Applied to Hair Styling Gels, J. Cosmet. Sci., 59, 497–508, (November/December 2008)
70) D. W. Rafferty, J. Zellia, D. Hasman, J. Mullay, The mechanics of Fixatives as Explained by Polymer Composite Principles", J. Cosmet. Sci., 60, 251–259, (March/April 2009)
71) R. Rigoletto, J. Albanese, S. Wossene, S. Subramanian, N. Clements, "Polyquaternium-69: A New Fixative Polymer with Enahnced Styling Benefits", Cosmetic Science Technology 2007.

HAIR CARE

PART 6.9

FORMULATING WISDOM CATEGORY BY CATEGORY

Hair's original purpose was to provide body coverage and warmth—the first line of the body's defense against the environment. Hair has evolved to provide minimal protective function but becomes highly important in the areas of appearance and hygiene.

Composed of nonbiologically active protein, the hair has many unique and important properties—flexibility, extendability, insolubility (to normally experienced solvents), and adaptability (to changes in length, style, color, etc.). Hair grows at approximately 0.25–0.33 inches per month. Unlike living skin, hair cannot repair itself—whatever damage occurs remains until the hair is lost naturally by shedding, is cut, or breaks off.

The products developed for hair care serve multiple purposes—cleaning, conditioning, treating, coloring, etc. The following is a description of the categories involved in hair care.

PART 6.10

SHAMPOOS
INGREDIENTS, FORMULATION AND EFFICACY EVALUATION

Author
Carrie Shipley
Applications Scientist
Grain Processing Corporation

ABSTRACT

When formulating a successful shampoo, there are many components and interactions to take into consideration. This chapter will begin with Section I by introducing some of the basic ingredients used in the formulation of shampoos as well as what differentiates some of the types of shampoos on the market. The subsequent section will discuss the actual cleansing mechanism of shampoos and the effects that shampoos and surfactants have on the hair. Section III introduces a few of the factors used to evaluate a shampoo formulation as well as some of the key attributes that need to be taken into consideration when evaluating a shampoo's performance. The final section wraps up with a brief look into the future trends of the shampoo industry.

TABLE OF CONTENTS

INTRODUCTION

It would seem that modern day shampoos have come a long way from the first commercial shampoos that were introduced in the early 20th century, and in many respects, they have. Modern formulations have become more personalized, less harsh, and tend to follow certain consumer-driven trends. On the other hand, shampoos cannot stray far from their origination because design designates them to do one primary function: clean the hair and scalp.

When formulating a successful shampoo, there are many components and interactions to take into consideration. The surfactant system may seem to be the most important part of the formulation due to the primary functionality of a shampoo. It is very important to use a carefully chosen blend of surfactants that will deliver the appropriate detergency, lather, and wetability to a formula, but this should not delineate from the importance of the other ingredients in a shampoo formulation. Consumers have certain expectations from their shampoos. They expect a certain viscosity and rheology as well as other benefits such as good combability, shine, and manageability.

In the following sections, this chapter will outline some of the basic ingredients used to formulate different types of shampoos as well as examples of starting formulas. A detailed explanation of how these ingredients clean the hair and scalp as well as the effect that they can have on hair will be discussed. The final sections focus on evaluation components for shampoo formulas as well as for performance attributes and end with a brief look into the future of the shampoo industry.

SECTION I: TYPICAL SHAMPOO INGREDIENTS

6.10.1 SURFACTANTS

The surfactant component of a formula provides many basic functions to a shampoo. Not only do these ingredients provide the cleansing mechanism for the shampoo, but surfactants also provide the foaming, contribute to the formulation rheology, and also play a large part in the safety of the shampoo. Foaming properties have to be adequate, both in quantity and quality, for the consumer to consider a shampoo to be adequate. Foam does not equal quality to a formulator, but to a consumer, copious amounts of rich foam are a basic expectation for a good shampoo.

Shampoo formulations usually consist of primary as well as secondary surfactants. The primary surfactants are responsible for the main cleansing mechanism in the formula as well as the foaming and some of the viscosity control. Secondary surfactants are usually gentler than the primary surfactants but by themselves do not have the best foaming or cleansing properties. These surfactants are usually added to help boost the foaming and detergency as well as reduce irritation caused by many primary surfactants. Most primary surfactants in shampoos (not including baby shampoos or special formulations) are anionic or negatively charged molecules, while most secondary surfactants are nonionic (have no charge), amphoteric (can be positive or negative depending on pH), or cationic (positively charged).

Anionic Surfactants

Alkyl and alkyl either sulfates are the most commonly used primary surfactants in the majority of shampoos on the market. These surfactants are excellent cleansers and foamers. They are cost effective and can easily be thickened with sodium chloride, which makes them a popular choice for many shampoo formulations. Most mainstream formulations contain some combination of alkyl and/or alkyl ether sulfate with sodium lauryl sulfate (SLS), sodium laureth sulfate (SLES), ammonium lauryl sulfate (ALS), and ammonium laureth sulfate (ALES) being the most prevalent.

The lauryl and laureth sulfates are produced by a sulfation reaction using mostly C_{12} fatty alcohols. This chain length is chosen to maximize the foaming and wetting traits of the final surfactant. Various mixes of C_{12}–C_{14} chain lengths are commonly used but will vary depending on the manufacturer [1].

As stated above, SLS and ALS are excellent foamers and cleansers, but many of the 12 carbon chain-length fatty alcohols can cause irritation to the scalp and eyes and have some solubility issues. This is reduced by the reaction of the fatty alcohols with ethylene oxide (EO) prior to the sulfation process, producing SLES as well as ALES. The higher the degree of ethoxylation, the more soluble the compound as well as the higher the reduction of irritation is seen. SLES is usually reacted with an average of two moles of EO while ALES is commonly ethoxylated to an average three moles of EO.

The lauryl and laureth sulfates are sometimes used by themselves but are most commonly used in combination with each other. Lauryl sulfates by themselves produce a creamier foam with smaller bubbles while laureth sulfates produce better flash foam. When used in combination, they complement each other. When deciding between the sodium and ammonium salts, ALS/ALES produce a slightly higher amount of foam and can be easier to thicken, but care has to be taken when using these surfactants because they can release free ammonia at higher pH values.

Although most mainstream shampoos will have some sort of alkyl or alkyl ether sulfate combination as their primary surfactant base, alpha olefin sulfonates (AOS) rank second in use [2]. The alpha olefin sulfonates are usually 14 to16 carbons in length and are comparable to SLS and SLES in foaming capacity (in the presence of sebum). AOS is easily solubilized and contains very little color or odor. It is stable over a wide pH range including lower pH systems, which is a benefit over the alkyl and alkyl ether sulfates. In lower pH formulations, alkyl and alkyl ether sulfates can be hydrolyzed. AOS is usually not used in premium shampoos because it has been reported to leave a harsher feel than the lauryl or lauryl sulfates and is also harder to thicken. Due to AOS surfactants containing a sulfonate group instead of a sulfate group, these surfactants can be formulated into sulfate-free formulas.

Other Anionic Surfactants

Sulfosuccinates. Sulfosuccinates contain both a carboxylate and a sulfonate group and are often used in combination with alkyl and alkyl ether sulfates in mild shampoo formulations or as part of a surfactant combination in baby shampoo formulas. The addition of a sulfosuccinate surfactant helps reduce eye and skin irritation, improves the lather, and contributes some conditioning benefits.

N-Acyl Methyltaurates. N-acyl methyltaurates (AMT) are the fatty amides of methyltaurines. They are noted for their low irritancy and are claimed to protect hair against cuticle damage. This class of surfactants finds limited usage in shampoos because of poor solubility and foaming performance, especially in hard water [3].

Sarcosinates. N-acyl sarcosinates are produced by reacting a fatty acyl chloride with N-methylglycine. These secondary surfactants do not lather well and tend to form precipitates in hard water, but are extremely mild. They can be used in combination with other anionic surfactants to reduce eye and skin irritation as well as provide some conditioning properties. The two most common forms of this surfactant that are used in shampoos is cocoyl sarcosinate and sodium lauryl sarcosinate [4].

Isethionates. Acyl Isethionates are condensation products of fatty acid chlorides and the sodium salt of 2-hydroxyethanesulfonic acid. They are very mild to the scalp and hair and produce a creamy, soap-like lather in both soft and hard water. They hydrolyze easily at low and high pHs. They have limited solubility at room temperature and so are not used in clear formulations [3].

N-acyl polypeptide condensates (protein derivatives). This class of surfactants is produced by the condensation of fatty acid chlorides and low-molecular-weight protein hydrolysates. Most often the cation is either potassium or triethanolamine, and the acyl group is a cocoyl moiety [3]. These surfactants have poor flash-foaming properties but produce a creamy, tight lather. They are stable in hard water, very mild to the eyes and skin, and have some conditioning attributes, but can be susceptible to bacteria [5].

Nonionic Surfactants

Although the detergency of nonionic surfactants is equal to, and in many instances superior to, that of anionic surfactants, nonionics are generally not used as primary surfactants in shampoos. This is due to inferior foaming characteristics, which result from their large surface area per molecule and the lack of charge on the surface films in nonionic foams [1]. However, nonionics are used extensively in a secondary capacity as foam modifiers, viscosity builders, emulsifiers, solubilizing aids, and in some case, conditioning agents.

Alkanolamides

One of the most common classes of nonionic surfactants is the fatty alkanolamides. They are produced by the condensation of a mixture of a primary or secondary alkanolamine with a fatty acid or derivative. The ratio of the amine to fatty acid yields differing products. The 1:1 condensates, referred to as “superamides,” are much more prevalent in shampoo formulations. Products derived from different fatty derivatives and different condensation ratios carry the same name, and wide variations in the chemical composition and performance of Alkanolamides from different manufacturers is not unexpected [3].

Alkanolamides are used for foam stabilization as well as viscosity enhancement, but care has to be used when choosing the alkanolamide to formulate with. Many formulators shy away from formulating with cocamide DEA or diethanolamine due to the potential for free amine production, which can form carcinogenic N-nitosamines. Many formulators will use Cocamide MEA (monoethanolamine), which is the monomer form. The foam stability is comparable to that of the DEA form, but the MEA form will build slightly higher viscosity.

Amine Oxides

Another widely used class of nonionic surfactant, the amine oxides are prepared by the oxidation of tertiary amines with hydrogen peroxide. The N-O bond is highly polarized, and at below-neutral pHs, amine oxides become protonated, which allows them to take on cationic characteristics such as conditioning and anti-static benefits. At pH 7 and above, the molecule is nonionic. The performance of an amine oxide can be compared to that of an alkanolamide. Amine oxides are best known for their ability to enhance foam characteristics and stabilize lather as secondary surfactants [3].

Alkyl Polyglucosides

One of the newer nonionic classes of nonionic surfactants are the alkyl polyglucosides. These can be considered hybrids combining properties from nonionic and anionic surfactants. They are prepared by reacting corn starch glucose with a fatty alcohol. The result is group of surfactants that are good foamers, have good detergency and wetting properties, and are toxicologically safe and biodegradable [1]. They are mostly used as secondary surfactants to help reduce irritation from the primary surfactant.

Polyethoxylated Surfactants

These surfactants represent the largest group of nonionics and include fatty alcohols, the ethoxylated derivatives of alkylphenols, fatty esters, and diglycerides. They have poor foaming power but are excellent cleansers, which makes them unusable in many shampoos as a primary surfactant. When used as secondary surfactants, both polysorbate-20 and PEG-80 sorbitan laurate can greatly reduce eye irritation caused by anionic surfactants and will not affect the foaming attributes

[1]. It is because of these reasons that these nonionic surfactants are usually formulated into baby shampoos.

Amphoterics

Amphoterics can be divided into two groups based on their pH response. The first group contains the carboxylated imidzoles and N-alkyl betaines. This group is zwitterionic at pHs at and above their isoelectric points and cationic at lower pHs. The second group contains the sulfobetaines and phosphobetaines, which are zwitterionic as the anionic portion is dissociated at all pHs [1]. The amphoterics have a very low irritation potential and are almost completely nonstinging to the eyes. These surfactants are compatible with a wide range of other surfactants and can be formulated into many different types of shampoos including baby shampoos. For instance, they are often found in conditioning shampoos due to their compatibility with quaternary compounds.

It should be noted that true amphoterics actually contain dual functional groups in the same molecule that allows them to exist in nonionic, cationic, as well as anionic states depending on pH. Betaines exist only in their nonionic and cationic states, depending on pH [1]. Betaines function as excellent foam boosters and viscosity enhancers when utilized as secondary surfactants, having good water solubility over a wide pH range [3]. Cocamidopropyl betaine is the most widely used example of this type of amphoteric surfactant and is often used in amide-free formulas as well as baby shampoos.

Cationic Surfactants

For several reasons, the use of cationic (positively charged) surfactants in shampoo formulations is more limited than that of other surfactant classes. They are generally not as effective detergents due to their ability to strongly bind to the hair's negatively charged surface. Their foaming properties are inferior to those of anionics. Furthermore, because they are not efficiently removed during rinsing, the hair is left more hydrophobic with the cationic's hydrophobic tail extending from the surface. This results in increased attraction of oily soils to the hair. Therefore, their use (at low levels) has been limited to their hair conditioning, lubricating, and antistatic benefits [3].

6.10.2 RHEOLOGY AND VISCOSITY MODIFIERS

Surfactants are fundamental to the formulation of a shampoo, but the rest of the ingredients should not be overlooked. Many of these ingredients play an important role in how a shampoo is viewed by the consumer. A surfactant blend diluted in water cleans just fine, but the average person won't be convinced of this. The consumer is conditioned to look for certain attributes in a shampoo, and much of the initial perception of a shampoo's cleaning ability is dependent upon the rheology and viscosity of the formula.

Shampoo rheology and viscosity are difficult to discuss independently. Rheology and viscosity are not interchangeable terms, but rheology, or the flow properties of a product, cannot be determined without taking into consideration viscosity or thickness, of non-Newtonian fluids such as shampoos. Viscosity modifiers have their own rheology, which must be taken into consideration when used to thicken because they are going to lend some of these rheological characteristics to the final formula. Some of the common viscosity modifiers are going to be discussed as well as the rheology they contribute to the final shampoo formula.

Salts

The most common way to add viscosity to a surfactant system is by adding a salt. While salt is not necessarily a viscosifier in the same means as the other reagents that will be discussed, salts are one of the most common substances often used in conjunction with other agents (salt-responsive thickeners), to control viscosity and modify rheology in anionic and nonionic surfactant systems. Sodium chloride is a commonly used monovalent salt in this process, but multivalent salts can be used also and are more effective since they contribute more ionic strength to the solution. Divalent salts such as calcium and magnesium chloride are not used as often because they tend to precipitate out and raise the cloud point of a shampoo formula. Ammonium chloride is another commonly used multivalent salt and is very effective, but pH and concentration have to be taken into consideration, especially if using an ammonium-based surfactant. Free ammonia can be given off if formulated above a neutral pH.

Salts themselves do not provide the thickening mechanism but in conjunction with surfactants, they promote a thickening of the surfactant system. Surfactants contain molecules with hydrophilic as well as hydrophobic portions. When specific surfactant concentrations are introduced to water, micellular structures are formed. These structures have hydrophilic or polar heads that orient themselves together in the water, while the hydrophobic tail regions sequester themselves in the center of the structure away from the water. These micelles are constantly moving and rearranging themselves. When salt is added to an anionic, nonionic, or some anionic-amphoteric surfactant systems, the charge density of the solution is lowered; this allows the micelles to pack more closely together, forming micellular agglomerates. These large agglomerates are what increase the viscosity of the shampoo. This mechanism does not work exactly the same in every formula. The salt-thickening response depends on the type and concentration of surfactants as well as the type of electrolyte used. Solution temperature and initial charge density of the formula also has to be considered [9]. Most surfactants already contain a small amount of free organic salts, so there is already some electrolyte present in the system, which can affect the amount of salt needed.

Salt addition is not always a simple way to thicken a surfactant system. Too much salt can create a phenomenon called "salting out." A small amount of electrolyte (usually between 0.1 and 3%) is needed to thicken most systems. Salting out happens when the maximum electrolyte balance has been reached and the amount of free electrolyte starts to interfere with the micelle structure. The charge density is then lowered and the micelles begin to repel each other, which dramatically decreases viscosity. The proper amount of electrolyte can be determined by plotting a salt curve using increments of 0.1% electrolyte and then taking a viscosity measurement [10]. It is important to stay on the upside of the curve in order to achieve maximum results. The ideal amount of salt will provide a Newtonian rheology to a shampoo formula. Too much salt can also create an undesirable rheology, which can be stringy and pituitous.

Alkanolamides

Foam-stabilizing agents such as alkanolamides (i.e., cocamide DEA, MEA) are discussed earlier in this chapter under the surfactant section. These agents are often added to shampoo formulas not only to create longer-lasting foam and a tighter structure, but also to build viscosity and modify the rheology of a shampoo formulation. These are salt-responsive thickeners. They will add a pseudoplastic rheology and provide thickening by interacting with the surfactant micelle [11]. This interaction shifts the salt curve, allowing less salt to be used to achieve maximum viscosity.

Acrylic Acid Polymers

Another group of commonly used viscosity builders and rheology modifiers used in shampoos are the acrylic acid polymers. This group includes, but is not limited to, carbomers, and acrylate crosspolymers and copolymers. Acrylic acid polymers are high-molecular-weight synthetic polymers that have the ability to swell in aqueous solutions. This swelling of the high-molecular-weight polymer is what provides the thickening mechanism. They cannot swell, however, without being neutralized by a base that converts them to their salt form. This can be done by the addition of NaOH, NH_4OH, or KOH. Acrylic acid polymers are very efficient thickeners that impart a highly pseudoplastic rheology. These polymers are normally compatible with most surfactants including cationics, but most have some amount of electrolyte and pH sensitivity [11].

Gums

Gums are frequently used to modify viscosity and rheology in shampoos. There are many gums available, but only a few that are commonly used in shampoo formulations. One of the most common, nonmodified gums used is Xanthan. Xanthan is enzymatically produced from the bacteria Xanthomonas campestis and is considered a natural thickener/rheology modifier. It is compatible with anionic and nonionic surfactants and also with most mono- and divalent salts. When used in very small amounts (0.1–0.5%), it provides sufficient thickening and a pseudoplastic flow [11]. When used in excess, Xanthan can have a very negative impact on rheology. The solution can turn to a soft gel upon standing and the flow becomes very elastic.

Gums can be modified to create certain characteristics, enhance solubility, or create a specific rheology. Cationic and hydroxypropyl guar (HP guar) are examples of modified guar gum. Cationic guar is substituted with a quaternary ammonia compound. The cationic portion of the molecule is substantive, so it creates a conditioning feel while the guar portion provides the thickening and rheological attributes. The HP guar is hydroxypropylated, which provides better pH and electrolyte stability.

Corn Starches

Using corn starch is another way to thicken a shampoo while controlling the rheology. Unfortunately, unmodified corn starch is rarely used as a viscosity control agent in personal care products due to its unmodified characteristics. Unmodified dent corn will retrograde and form opaque gels, and it also imparts a high viscosity during processing, which makes it hard to work with. Waxy corn, which is also a base commonly used to make corn starch, won't retrograde to the same extent as a dent corn–based starch due to its high amylopectin content, but it has a very stringy, uneven flow that is not favored for a shampoo. Most corn starch that is used for rheology modification is chemically and or physically modified. These modifications (primarily hydroxypropylation) help create starches with increased clarity, less retrogradation, lower gelatinization temperatures, greater pH toleration, and the ability to help with foam stability due to increased film-forming capabilities. The addition of modified starch to a shampoo formula can add a short, thixotropic rheology to a shampoo and will enhance spreadability.

Corn starches are made up of small granules that swell when hydrated. This mechanism is what causes an increase in viscosity. When added into a solution containing a high amount of surfactant such as a shampoo, the surfactant can interfere with the swelling of the granules by grabbing up the available water, causing a decrease in normal viscosity development as well as an upward shift in the gelatinization temperature. The situation is dependent on the starch base as well as the type of surfactant used. This may be linked to the amount of amylose contained in the starch granule [12]. Waxy maize starches with very little if any amylose tend to see less of this phenomenon, whereas dent-based starches which contain roughly 24% amylose will see this decrease in viscosity. For the shampoo formulator using corn starch as a viscosity/rheology modifier, it is important to know this when formulating. As a rule of thumb, waxy-based corn starches will contribute higher viscosity with less usage but can have a slightly longer texture, dent-based corn starches require a higher usage but will contribute a shorter, smoother texture. Corn starches can also be used to thicken most cationic-based surfactants where some of the other viscosity modifiers fail.

Cellulose Derivatives

Cellulose derivatives are often used for viscosity control and rheology modification, but much like corn starch, are used in their modified form. Cellulose derivatives can be modified to be more or less hydrophilic as well as pH and electrolyte tolerant. Some of the most frequently used modified cellulosics are methylcellulose, hydroxypropyl methylcellulose, and hydroxyethylcellulose. They provide a pseudoplastic rheology and are typically used at 0.5–1.5% [11].

Modified Polyethylene Glycols

Modified polyethylene glycols (PEG) are nonionic thickeners that provide different rheologies depending on the R-group that is attached to the basic chemical structure. The R-groups can consist of either a fatty alcohol, a glyceryl ester, or a propylene glycol. Of these polymers, the most commonly used PEGs for shampoos are the stearic acid esters of polyethylene glycol, typically PEG-150 distearate. The number associated with the PEG denotes the number of PEG moles in the polymer. PEG-150 distearate is a high-molecular-weight polymer that is compatible with most surfactants as well as pH, and is temperature stable, which imparts a shear-thinning rheology to a shampoo formulation [11].

Others

Some of the other viscosity modifiers used in shampoos are clays such as bentonite, hectorite, and magnesium aluminum silicate. They impart a thixotropic rheology to a formula by swelling to produce viscosity. This group of thickeners can also be used to stabilize colloidal or pearl systems in shampoos as well as for stability in anti-dandruff shampoos.

6.10.3 OTHER SHAMPOO INGREDIENTS

Opacifiers and Pearlizing Agents

Opacity or pearlescence can be imparted to a shampoo by several different types of raw materials. Ethylene glycol stearate, glyceryl stearate, and cetyl or stearyl alcohols are frequently used with alkyl sulfates. These materials are incorporated into the surfactant solution at temperatures above their melting points and then crystallize upon cooling, producing a pearlescent appearance. The opacifying effect is dependent on the crystal size, distribution, and reflectance [3].

Antioxidants/Sequestrants/UV absorbers

Traditionally, antioxidants are included in shampoo formulations to avoid oxidation of unsaturated components such as vegetable oils and oleic acid derivatives. Typical antioxidants used are BHT, BHA, and tocopherol [3]. In some newer formulations, antioxidants have taken on a more modern role and have been marketed as helping to provide healthier hair by fighting free radicals. The antioxidants used in these shampoos are more often of the "superfruit" type.

Sequestering agents are included in shampoos to prevent the formation of insoluble metal ions, which can be formed in the presence of hard water. These ions can create a film on the hair, making it appear dull. The sequestering agent binds with the metals ions to form soluble complexes. Typically, EDTA and its salts, citric acid, or polyphosphates are used.

UV absorbers are not used in shampoo to the same degree and traditional sense as they once were. UV absorbers such as benzophenone are still used to protect formulations in clear packages against color fading or discoloration upon prolonged light exposure, but most shampoos manufactured today are contained in opaque packaging. When discussing UV absorbers in the present sense, most shampoo manufacturers market them as a protectant for the fading of hair color from light exposure. In order for a UV absorber to work in this way, it has to be water soluble as well as substantive to the hair. There are newer compounds available that combine quaternary ammonium compounds with UV filters to create this type of protection (multifunctional ingredients). One such ingredient is cinnamidopropyltrimonium chloride, which can be found on the ingredient statement of some shampoos and conditioners claiming color protection [6].

6.10.4 FRAGRANCE

Fragrance has become an increasingly important aspect of a shampoo formulation. The ability of a fragrance to influence consumers' perception of a shampoo should not be underestimated. The fragrance also serves the purpose of covering any base odor in the formula, particularly as the product ages. The level of fragrance incorporated into a shampoo formula above that necessary to cover base odor depends primarily on the intended shampoo market. The fragrance must be compatible with the shampoo formula, it should not adversely affect viscosity or stability, nor should it induce irritation. Factors affecting fragrance selection include evaluations of the residual fragrance left on the hair following shampooing in addition to assessments of the fragrance in the package and during use [3].

6.10.5 PRESERVATIVES

Preservatives are essential components of a shampoo formulation to protect against microbial growth. Among the potential sources of microbial contamination are water supplies, improperly cleaned manufacturing equipment, and raw materials [3].

There are generally three types of commonly used preservatives: parabens, formaldehyde donors, and MIT (methylisothiazolinone) systems. All have been under public fire for one reason or another, but all usage is highly regulated by each country's government.

Parabens include the esters such as methyl, ethyl, and propylparaben. These are very active against fungi and are weaker against gram-negative bacteria. They are also only active in the water phase of a formulation and can be inactivated, either partially or fully, by strong hydrogen bonders such as polysorbates, cellulose derivatives, and proteins [7].

Formaldehyde was once a common preservative in cosmetic and personal care formulations, but is rarely used in its raw form due to its carcinogenic link. It is banned in the EU as well as in Japan. The formaldehyde donors (DMDM hydantoin, quaternium 15, imidazolidinyl urea, diazolidinyl urea) tend to give off a small amount of free formaldehyde, but it is in a much lower quantity and since they are effective in such small percentages, these preservatives are used in place of formaldehyde. The formaldehyde donors all have their different strengths and weaknesses, but most perform the strongest against bacteria and the weakest against fungi. Formaldehyde-releasing preservatives should not be used with protein derivatives as they are inactivated during condensation with the free amino groups.

MIT can be used alone or in combination with other isothiazolinones such as chloromethyl isothiazolinone. These are broad-spectrum biocides that perform well against both bacteria and fungi [7].

Other Additives

Many modern shampoos have additives that take them beyond the basic cleansing shampoo and suggest additional cosmetic benefits. Some of these additives include proteins such as hydrolyzed wheat protein, hydrolyzed silk or collagen, vitamins such as panthenol and biotin, moisturizers and humectants, oils and botanicals. All have been marketed as an added benefit to the hair and scalp. These are normally added at such small percentages that there is some question of their actual benefits.

6.10.6 TYPES OF SHAMPOOS

Basic Cleansing

The basic cleansing or clarifying shampoo formula is formulated to remove substantive residues from styling products as well as provide a deeper cleaning than some of the other formulas. They are usually formulated with higher levels of anionic surfactants to boost the cleaning potential. The following is a typical basic formula for a cleansing shampoo:

Cleansing Shampoo

Ingredient	% wt/wt
Sodium laureth sulfate	25.0
Cocamidopropyl betaine	7.0
Cocamide MEA	2.0
Fragrance	0.7
Preservative	0.5
Citric acid	q.s. pH 5.5–6.5
Sodium chloride	q.s. viscosity
Water	q.s. to 100

Mild/Baby

Baby shampoos and other mild formulas (children's shampoos) are formulated for gentleness, especially to the eyes. To achieve this, these products are formulated with higher levels of nonionic and amphoteric surfactants, which are less irritating than the alkyl and alkyl ether sulfates. As mentioned before, the presence of ethylene oxide reduces the irritation of the anionic surfactants, so Polysorbate 20 and PEG-80 (20 and 80 moles of ethylene oxide respectively) are often used as anti-irritants in baby shampoos.

Baby Shampoo

Ingredient	% wt/wt
PEG-80 sorbitan laurate	12.0
Sodium trideceth sulfate	5.0
Sodium lauroamphoacetate	5.0
PEG-120 methyl glucose dioleate	2.0
Cocamidopropyl hydroxysultaine	1.0
Fragrance	0.7
Preservative	0.5
Water	q.s. to 100

Source: Reference [3]

Conditioning/Two-in-One

Most shampoos on the market today have some type of conditioning agent in them even if they are not labeled as an actual two-in-one shampoo. This helps to improve the wet combability, and adds softness and shine to the hair. These formulas are more complex than a typical basic or cleansing shampoo since most of the conditioning agents are not soluble in water, and an emulsion has to be made (usually oil in water), which will require the addition of some type of emulsifying agent.

Silicones such as dimethicone, dimethiconol, amodimethicone, and dimethicone copolyol are frequently used in these types of formulas. Silicones provide light conditioning by forming a thin film on the surface of the hair. This type of conditioning is less than that seen by a separate conditioner, but is sufficient to improve aesthetics over that of a shampoo without a conditioner.

A number of non-silicone conditioning agents have been used in shampoos, either alone or as secondary conditioners in two-in-one formulations. Because of their compatibility with anionic surfactants, cationic polymers such as polyquaternium-10 and polyquaternium-7 are sometimes used in these types of formulas. Normally, these two cationic polymers can be very substantive to the hair and can form deposits, but due to complexes that are formed with the cationic polymer and anionic surfactant, this deposition is greatly reduced [1].

Below is an example of a two-in-one formula from U.S. Patent 6,007,802 [13] containing polyquaternium-10 and an anionic surfactant as well as a dimethicone.

Conditioning (Two-in-One) Shampoo

Ingredient	% wt/wt
Ammonium laureth sulfate (3 EO)	14.00
Cocamidopropyl betaine	2.70

Ingredient	% wt/wt
Polyquaternium-10	0.15
B8/C10 diester of adipic acid	0.30
Cocamide MEA	0.80
Cetyl alcohol	0.42
Stearyl alcohol	0.18
Carbapol 981	0.50
Dimethicone	1.00
Fragrance	0.37
DMDM hydantoin	0.37
Color solution (ppm)	64
Water	q.s. to 100

Source: Reference [2]

Anti-Dandruff

In the United States shampoos and non-shampoos containing an anti-dandruff agent are considered drugs. Similar controls over these preparations exist in other legislative areas. Active anti-dandruff ingredients that can be used in the United States, as well as claims that can be made, are governed by the FDA under 21CFR358 subpart H. There are only a few active ingredients approved for use in the U.S. See Table 29.1 for the list of ingredients as well as the approved percentages.

Table 29.1. Anti-Dandruff Ingredients

Active Ingredient	Allowable Usage (%)
Coal tar	0.5–5.0
Salicylic acid	1.8–3.0
Sulfur	2.0–5.0
Selenium sulfide	1.0
Zinc pyrithione	0.3–2.0
Ketoconozole	1.0
Climbazole	1.0–2.0

Source: 21CFR358.D.2013

Most anti-dandruff agents are water-insoluble so that when the hair is rinsed after shampooing, the insoluble particulates remain on the hair and scalp for further treatment. This insolubility makes the actives harder to formulate with. Anti-dandruff agents can be difficult to suspend due to high specific densities, but much work has been done to improve formulations so that many now contain milder surfactants and conditioning agents.

The Sulfate/Amide-Free Shampoo

Trends come and go in the personal care world, but shampoo manufacturers must succumb to the consumer. Sulfate- and sometimes amide-free shampoos have become more mainstream in the last few years. Once only seen in specialty salons, they are now seen on the common store shelves. As consumers begin to pay more attention to ingredients in the products they use, certain ingredients come under scrutiny; surfactants containing sulfates are one of them. Sulfate-free shampoos are not always easy to formulate because the surfactants can be harder to thicken and may not foam as well as other conventional surfactants. ALS/ALES and SLS/SLES are used because of their excellent foaming and cleansing properties as well as their low cost. They are easy to thicken with electrolytes or other conventional thickeners and are readily available. Surfactant companies are constantly coming out with new surfactants to meet the needs of the formulator. The following is an example of a sulfate- and amide-free shampoo formula.

Amide- and Sulfate-Free Shampoo

Ingredient	% wt/wt
A. Water	31.72
Disodium laureth sufocuccinate (40%)	27.68
Cocamidopropyl betaine	17.89
Ammonium cocoyl isethionate (30%)	13.92
Lauramine oxide	4.83
PEG-30 glyceryl cocoate	1.00
Polyquaternium-7	0.60
B. PEG-120 methyl glucose dioleate	1.91
C. Preservative	0.05
D. Citric acid (adjust final pH 6.0–6.5)	0.40

Source: Reference [13]

Shampoos with Cosmetic Benefits

Most mainstream shampoos sold on the market today have some sort of cosmetic benefit tied to them. Cosmetic benefits can range from the simple addition of a humectant for moisturization to the claim of added volume, increased shine, strengthening, or revitalizing. These shampoos have become very popular as the consumer has grown to expect more from a shampoo than just basic cleansing. Below is an example of a volumizing shampoo.

Volumizing Shampoo

Ingredient	% wt/wt
A. Water	24.50
B. Polyquaternium-4	0.25
C. Sodium chloride	2.50
D. Water	26.27
E. Sodium laureth sulfate (28% active)	42.90
F. Cocamidopropyl betaine (30% active)	3.34
G. DMDM hydantoin	0.24
H. Citric acid	q.s. to pH 6.0–6.5

Source: Reference [13]

SECTION II: HAIR-CLEANSING MECHANISM

This chapter has discussed the basic ingredients that are involved in the formulation of a shampoo as well as the different types of shampoos that are commonly formulated. This next section is an excerpt from chapter 29 of *Harry's Cosmeticology 8th Edition* that does an excellent job explaining how shampoos carry out the cleansing mechanism as well as their effects on hair.

The surfactants play the leading role in cleansing mechanism, so an understanding of how surfactants carry out their hair-cleansing function is necessary in order to assess the relative cleaning efficiencies of different surfactants and surfactant combinations. It is also important for determining how best to balance, in a formulation, the often-conflicting aims of optimum cleaning, foam, viscosity, actives deposition, mildness, and so forth.

The epicutical of hair is substituted and coated with material responsible in large part for the observed hydrophobicity of untreated hair surfaces. Because of their protein composition, however, these surfaces can also contain charged hydrophilic sites. For virgin hair, the observed isoelectric point is near 3.67, which ensures that the hydrophilic sites on this hair will carry a negative charge at the ordinary pH level of shampoos. The combination of negative charge and the hydrophobicity affects not only the type of soils and actives that bind to the hair but also the ease with which different soils are removed from the fiber surface.

Most consumer-bought shampoos are not going to be used on virgin hair. Most modern hair succumbs to numerous cycles of chemical treatment as well as exposure to sunlight. This will affect the cleaning mechanism of a shampoo due to the fact that the distribution of negatively charged sites on untreated hair is uneven, increasing from root to tip. This is a result of exposure to sunlight, which oxidizes cystine in the hair to cystine S-sulfonate and cysteic acid. In addition to oxidation by sunlight, hair can also be chemically oxidized as a result of perming, bleaching, or permanent dyeing. These treatments, all of which include oxidative steps, convert cystine to cysteic acid. The degree of resultant negative charge is generally greater than that from sunlight oxidation. In many cases after sufficient treatment, the entire hair surface can be converted from a hydrophobic to a hydrophilic character. This, of course, also affects deposition and removal of materials on the hair surface.

6.10.7 CLEANING OF SOLID PARTICULATES

For studies of hair-surface cleaning, it is convenient to divide possible soils into two types: solid particulates and oily or liquid deposits. Particulate soils can come from the environment or from hair care products. Examples of the latter include many anti-dandruff agents, while the former include carbon particles in the form of soot, clays, or rubber abraded from automobile tires.

In general, solids soils adhere to the hair surface through ionic or van der Waals forces. The ease of removing these soils from a surface in water depends on the relative affinities for each other of the water, soil, and substrate. A hydrophobic particle, for example, would be much easier to remove from a hydrophilic substrate than from a hydrophobic surface. This can be seen in the equation for the work of adhesion, Wa, which is defined as the free-energy change per unit area involved in removing a solid particle from a surface to which it is adhered:

$$Wa = \gamma PW + \gamma HW - \gamma PH$$

In the above equation, γ is the interfacial tension between any two surfaces, P represents the particle, H represents the hair surface, while W represents water. For hydrophobic particles, γHW would be larger and γPH would be smaller for hydrophobic surfaces than for hydrophilic substrates. The resultant larger work of adhesion indicates again that hydrophobic particles are more difficult to remove from hydrophobic than from hydrophilic surfaces.

Anionic and nonionic detergents can effect removal of particles from hair surfaces by adsorbing to these substrates with their hydrophobic portions in contact with surface and their hydrophilic heads oriented toward the water. This reduces γHW and, therefore, Wa. Similarly, binding of surfactant to a hydrophobic soil reduces γPW, effecting an additional decrease in the work of adhesion.

A more effective cleaning mechanism than the preceding results when anionic surfactants adsorb to solid particles and the surfaces to which they are adhered. Such adsorption effectively deposits negative charge on both soil and substrate, facilitating soil removal as a result of mutual charge repulsion. Since nonionics cannot impart a charge potential on surfaces, they are not in general as effective as anionic surfactants in cleaning soils.

6.10.8 CLEANING OF OILY SOIL

The second major class of soils found on hair is hydrophobic, or oily, soil that is liquid, at least at cleaning temperatures. Examples include sebum from the scalp, which is mostly liquid at body temperature; silicones, oils and waxes from hair care products; and lipids from skin cells. There are a number of possible detergency mechanisms for these types of soils, including rollback, emulsification, solubilization, and mesophase formation. These are discussed in the following sections.

Rollback Mechanism

The expression for work of adhesion in the previous section applies to oily soils as well as particulates. As with particulates, the more hydrophobic the liquid soil, the more difficult it is to remove from a hydrophobic substrate. Also as with particulates, detergents can effect soil removal of oils by adsorbing to the hair surface. In this case, the increased affinity of the surface for water permits the water to displace the oil droplet and simply roll it up. This process is termed the rollback mechanism. This mechanism is described quantitatively by Young's equation, which for aqueous systems is written as:

$$\gamma HW = \gamma HO + \gamma OW \cos \theta$$

where γ is the interfacial tension between two phases, H represents hair, *O* represents the oil phase, and W represents water. θ in the above equation is the contact angle between the soil and the hair surface; the lower this angle, the greater is the contact between the two phases.

It is implicit in Young's equation that adsorption of a surfactant to the hair surface, which lowers γHW, will increase the contact angle of the oil droplet. For sufficiently large increases in γHW, θ will increase to 180°, and the oil droplet will spontaneously separate from the hair surface. In practice, application of mechanical work during shampooing—for example, flexing and rubbing of hair—will help to completely remove those soils. Increased temperature also aids in soil removal, facilitating droplet roll-up by reducing soil viscosity and also by increasing rates of surfactant adsorption. These temperature effects are particularly important in view of the short cleaning times involved in the shampooing process.

Solubilization of Soils

The rollback process is the most important soil-removal mechanism for products that are highly diluted during cleaning, so that surfactants are present primarily in the form of monomers.

If surfactant concentration is sufficiently high during use, then soil removal can also proceed via solubilization. This is accomplished by surfactant aggregates called micelles, which form above a certain concentration termed the critical micelle concentration, or CMC. The surfactants in micelles are arranged so that the surfactant heads form a hydrophilic surface in contact with the water, while the tails are lined up in the micelle interior, forming a hydrophobic core.

Micelles solubilize soils by incorporation into the micellular structure. More polar soils are incorporated near the hydrophilic heads, while hydrophobic soils end up deep in the micelle interior. Kinetic investigations on fatty acid solubilization indicate that solubilization begins by diffusion of micelles to the soil surface, followed by surfactant adsorption onto the soil and incorporation of soil into the surfactant aggregate. The process ends by desorption of the soil containing micelle and diffusion away from the surface. The latter two steps were found to control the rate of the solubilization process. The critical micelle concentration for most anionic shampoo is about 5×10^{-3} M surfactants. It can be seen that in a shampoo containing 10–20% sodium lauryl sulfate, most of the detergent (98–99%) is present in the form of micelles. Even if the shampoo is diluted tenfold upon application to wet hair, as much as 88% of the surfactant is still in the form of micellular aggregates. The possibility exists, therefore, that solubilization is a major factor in shampoo cleaning.

As with rollback, soil removal by solubilization is greatly increased through rubbing and flexing of hair (mechanical work) and increasing temperature. More work needs to be done to precisely determine the contribution of solubilization in the hair-cleaning process.

Emulsification, Penetration, and Mesophase Formation

Emulsification and mesophase, or liquid crystal, formation are two important mechanisms that can be involved in removal of soil from hair. Emulsification involves the breaking down of an oily soil into smaller particles that can form a stable suspension. It requires a low interfacial tension between the oily soil and the bath medium, which may be accomplished by adsorption of shampoo surfactant onto the soil surface. Mechanical work also helps in breaking up of the soil.

Amphiphilic compounds in soils, such as fatty alcohols or fatty acids, can greatly aid the emulsification process by interacting with the shampoo detergent to spontaneously emulsify the soil. Since the shampooing process is short, emulsified soils need be suspended for only a few moments.

Phase diagrams of detergents, water, and certain polar salts such as fatty acids and alcohols can contain large regions that flow easily and are composed of a liquid crystalline phase. Such mesophase formation with amphiphiles, or oily soils containing amphiphiles, constitutes another important mechanism for soil removal from hair.

6.10.9 EFFICACY OF SOIL REMOVAL BY SHAMPOOS

The soils most commonly found on hair originate from three sources: secretions from the body, residues from hair care products, and deposits from the environment. The first type of soil is composed mostly of sebum from the sebaceous glands. Residues from hair care products include hairspray resins and various conditioning materials, while environmental soils include particulate matter from soot, clays, rubber from automobile tires, and so forth.

The efficiency of shampoos in removing these soils and the types of mechanisms by which such removal is carried out depend on a number of factors, including the nature of the soil, the state and condition of the hair surface, and the particular surfactant or combination of surfactants employed in the shampoo. In the following sections the principles of cleaning of different soils by shampoos will be discussed.

6.10.10 CLEANING OF SEBUM

Sebum is probably the single most important soil found on human hair. It is composed of a mixture of lipid materials that are secreted into the follicular duct by the sebaceous glands. The emerging terminal scalp hair is coated with sebum, and mechanical actions such as combing and rubbing against pillows ensure that the sebum becomes distributed more or less evenly over the entire hair surface.

Sebum, which is almost completely molten at body temperature, lubricates the hair, giving it (when not present in excess) a smooth, moisturized feel. Hair with too much sebum on the surface, however, becomes limp and clumped together and is perceived by consumers as dull, dirty, and greasy. Moreover, because it is sticky, the presence of sebum leads to further soiling as a result of adhesion of airborne particulates and other material with which it comes in contact. In addition, sebum can act as a binder, cementing many soil particles together.

Detergents do not penetrate hair appreciably during the relatively short times involved in shampooing. As a result, cleaning of soils such as sebum by shampoos is confined primarily to the hair surface. Internal lipids, however, do not appear to contribute to consumer-perceivable soiling effects. Thus Robbins found that the same quantity of internal lipid (as much as 9% of the total hair weight) could be extracted from both oily and dry hair, indicating that the oily feel of the hair was entirely due to surface sebum. Because of its composition and physical state, sebum can potentially be cleaned from hair by any of the cleaning mechanisms presented in the previous sections. Sebum can be removed from hair by a rollback mechanism. Sebum is also subject to removal by emulsification and mesophase formation. Finally, since the concentrations of surfactants during cleaning are generally well above the surfactant CMCs, sebum can also be cleaned from hair by solubilization.

The relative importance of these mechanisms in cleaning sebum from hair is not identical and more than one cleaning mechanism can certainly operate simultaneously. In any case, the multiplicity of possible cleaning mechanisms for sebum might lead one to expect that shampoos would be very effective in removing sebum from hair. This expectation is supported by much of the literature: a number of studies have demonstrated that anionic surfactants at normal shampoo concentrations can clean surface lipids effectively. Effective cleaning of lipids by anionic surfactants was also reported, and gas-chromatographic techniques were used to measure percent removal from hair of the various components of an artificial sebum. Table 29.2 lists some of the results from this work. It can be seen that the more polar fractions of the sebum, such as free fatty acids, were removed from hair to a greater extent than the less polar fractions, such as paraffin. In other words, hydrophobic soils, like paraffin, have a greater affinity for the hydrophobic hair surface than do more polar deposits and are therefore more difficult to remove.

Sodium laureth-2 sulfate (SLES-2) is seen in Table 29.2 to remove sebum fractions from hair more effectively than ammonium lauryl sulfate (ALS). One reason for this may be related to higher adsorption of SLES-2 than of SLS, which would favor increased removal of sebum by the rollback mechanism.

Table 29.2. Sebum Cleaning by Surfactants

Sebum Component	**% Removal by SLES-2**	**% Removal by ALS**
Triglycerides	94.7	94.6
Free fatty acids	96.2	97.1
Spermaceti wax	96.2	84.6
Squalene	98.4	87.6
Paraffin	95.2	80.8
Average % removal	**95.9**	**85.9**

Source: Reference [3]

6.10.11 CLEANING OF QUATERNARY AMMONIUM COMPOUNDS

Conditioners are used to increase ease of hair combing, reduce flyaway, and improve the feel of the hair. The most widely used conditioning agents in commercial products are quaternary ammonium compounds. These compounds are generally used in combination with lipid conditioners such as long-chain alcohols.

Two of the most widely used quaternary conditioners are stearalkonium chloride (SAC) and cetrimonium chloride (CTAC). Other important quats include steartrimonium chloride, dicetydimonium chloride, and tricetylmonium chloride. The most important lipid conditioners include cetyl and stearyl alcohols. Concentrations of cationic surfactants in commercial conditioners are generally on the order of 1–2%, while lipid concentrations are equal to or greater than those of the quats.

Conditioners are generally used at pH levels above the isoelectric point of hair, that is, on negatively charged fiber surfaces. Quaternary ammonium compounds, by virtue of their positive charge, are therefore substantive to the hair surface. Treating hair with these compounds results in a hydrophobic coating that is soft and easy to comb. The binding to hair of quaternary compounds has been found to increase with increases in the hydrophobic chain length and number of chains. This hydrophobic dependence indicates that van der Waals forces play an important role in the deposition of quats on hair.

Deposition of quaternary conditioners on hair is also a function of the degree of negative charge on the hair surface. Compared to virgin hair, bleached hair, which has a more negatively charged surface, retains more than twice the amount of stearalkonium chloride.

Table 29.3. Detergent Cleaning of Stearalkonium Chloride

Treatment	SAC (mg)/g Wool	Detergent (mg)/g Wool
1% SAC	6.68	--
5% ALS	--	1.94
1% SAC/5% ALS	4.58	4.09
5% SDES-2	--	1.94
1% SAC/5% SDES-2	2.52	2.12

Source: Reference [3]

Many quats deposited from conditioning products have been reported to build up over time, indicating that removal of these materials from hair may be more difficult than is the case for sebum. One reason for this is simply the strong electrostatic attraction between the positively charged quats and the negatively charged hair surface. Another reason is that, since quaternary ammonium conditioners are solids, they are not subject to removal by the rollback mechanism. In addition, the positive charge on quats interferes with the mechanism for particulate soil removal, that is, the introduction of negative potentials on soil and substrate as a result of adsorption of anionic surfactant.

Solubilization is a possible mechanism for cleaning of quaternary conditioners. Reich and coworkers have shown, however, that, at least for SAC and CTAC, solubilization by lauryl and laureth sulfates is ineffective. Instead, cleaning with these surfactants results in the formation of insoluble surfactant:quat complexes that are dulling and difficult to remove from hair.

Reducing the hydrophobic chain length of the cleaning surfactant to ten carbon atoms results in formation of more soluble surfactant:quat complexes, which can be more readily cleaned from the hair. Thus washing deposited SAC with 5% sodium deceth-2 sulfate (SDES-2) resulted in higher removal of the deposited conditioner.

The above findings apply to cleaning of the pure quaternary conditioners; cleaning of deposits from fully formulated conditioners lead to improved removal by ALS.

Despite increased quat removal from a fully formulated conditioner, insoluble complex formation between SAC and ALS still occurs. This is evidenced by the increase in deposited ALS measured after cleaning the residue with this surfactant.

6.10.12 CLEANING OF POLYMERIC RESIDUE

Several types of polymers can be found on hair as a result of use of hair care products, including hairspray resins, silicone conditioners, and cationic conditioning polymers. The ease of removal of these polymers from hair depends on several factors, including charge, molecular weight, structure, nature of side chains, and so forth. In the following sections, the ease of cleaning of several important examples of hair care polymers will be discussed.

Cationic Conditioning Polymers

Several cationic polymers are available commercially that provide conditioning benefits, especially increased ease of wet combing. Important examples include polyquaternium 10, a quaternized hydroxyethylcellulose polymer; polyquaternium-11, a copolymer of vinylpyrrolidone and dimethylaminoethyl methacrylate quaternized with dimethyl sulfate; polyquaternium-16, a copolymer of vinylpyrrolidone and quaternized vinylimidazole; polyquaternium-7, a copolymer of diallyldimethylammonium chloride and acrylamide; and polyquaternium-6, a homopolymer of diallyldimethylammonium chloride. As a result of their cationic nature, these conditioning polymers are substantive to hair.

Deposition on hair fibers has been claimed to be an inverse function of charge density, an effect that has been explained by noting that the greater the charge density, the lower the weight of polymer needed to neutralize the total negative charge on the hair.

Polyquaternium-10 is quite substantive to hair, resisting complete removal by SLS even after exposure to detergent for as long as 30 minutes. Similar results were obtained in cleaning experiments with radio-tagged polyquaternium-10. First, as with monofunctional quats, deposition of polyquaternium-10 was found to increase with increasing negative charge on the hair. Thus bleached hair was found to bind more than 2.3 times the amount of polyquat as did untreated hair. In addition, bound polyquaternium-10 was found to be difficult to remove: only 43% of the polyquat could be removed from wool swatches in a single washing with SLS.

Reducing the charge density on the polyquaternium-10 led to more complete cleaning. Thus in a single SLS wash, 75% of this polyquaternium could be removed from wool swatches. Results similar to the above were obtained with polyquaternium-7, which was found to be about as resistant as polyquaternium-10 to removal from wool substrates. The difficulty in cleaning these polymers does not appear to be related to formation of insoluble conditioner:detergent complexes, as was the case with SAC and CTAC. This is evidenced by the fact that cleaning polymer-treated wool with SLS was not observed to result in detergent buildup, even after several cycles of polymer/detergent treatment. It is concluded, therefore, that the difficulty in cleaning polyquats is most likely related to the multiple points of attachment between the polymer and the keratin surface. In order to clean these polymers, it is necessary to break all the points of attachment at the same time, a more difficult proposition than the elimination of the single point of attachment between a small molecule and the hair surface.

Fixative Residue

The holding properties of styling products such as hairsprays, mousses, gels, and setting lotions are provided by various polymeric resins. These materials are generally neutral or negatively charged in order to facilitate removal from hair. Typical examples include the copolymer of vinyl acetate and crotonic acid, the ethyl ester of the copolymer of polyvinyl methyl ether and maleic anhydride (PVM/MA), the copolymer of polyvinyl pyrrolidone and vinyl acetate (PVP/VA), and the copolymer of octylacrylamide/acrylates/butylaminoethyl methacrylate.

The ease of cleaning of hairspray resins was measured using the radio-tagged ethyl ester of PVM/MA. A single washing with 10% SLS resulted in removal of 89%

of the deposited resin. This is also consistent with the expectation that noncationic fixatives would be easier to remove from hair than positively charged polymers.

Dimethicone Residue

As was stated in the introduction, the active ingredient in most two-in-one shampoos is dimethicone, a hydrophobic polymer (polydimethylsiloxane), which is commonly found in many conditioners.

As was the case with fixative resins, little has been published in the literature on the ease of removal of dimethicone. One quantitative study, however, was performed by Rushton and coworkers, who used electronic spectrum for chemical analysis (ESCA) and atomic absorption measurements to study buildup and cleaning of dimethicone. ESCA measurements by Rushton indicated a dimethicone buildup of roughly 35% after five washings of virgin hair with a commercial two-in-one shampoo. After five washings, however, no further buildup was observed. In addition, Rushton found that more than 90% of deposited dimethicone could be removed by a single wash with a commercial shampoo.

6.10.13 EFFECT OF SHAMPOOS ON HAIR

The immediately preceding sections dealt with cleaning of soils by shampoos. Shampoos are also involved in damage of hair, either directly, through removal of structural components of the hair fiber, or indirectly, through removal of protective deposits on the hair. These processes are discussed in the following sections.

Direct Damage by Shampoos

Studies in the literature have indicated that the nonkeratinous regions of the hair, which include the endocuticle, or inner portion of the cuticle, and the cell membrane complex are susceptible to damage by surfactant molecules.

These and additional experiments indicate that exposure to shampoos can have a deleterious effect on hair structure over time. The extent and consequences of these effects are unclear, especially since preexisting damage may render the hair more susceptible to surfactant damage.

Indirect Damage by Shampoos

The use of shampoos can damage hair indirectly as a result of fiber abrasion occurring when hairs are rubbed against each other during cleaning. More important to the damage process, however, is the removal of sebum from the fiber surface during shampooing. This is because sebum acts as a natural lubricant for hair; removal of this material increases damage from grooming, due to chipping, fragmenting, and tearing away of cuticle cells, and it should be attributed to combing and brushing.

Figure 29.1 shows an example of the damage than can occur from grooming. This rather extreme example was induced by washing a tress of virgin hair with a cleaning shampoo and then combing it 700 times while wet. It can be seen that cuticle damage is widespread, with noticeable loss of some cuticle cells and extensive lifting of others from the hair surface. Repeated grooming of the hair gradually erodes the cuticle cells, with the greatest loss occurring at the tips of the hair. Eventually all of the cuticle cells can be lost, exposing the cortex and resulting in a split end. An example of such splitting is shown in Figure 29.2.

Damage to Chemically Treated Hair

Permanent waving, bleaching, and oxidative dyeing can result in significant damage to the hair. In addition to causing tensile damage, all of these treatments oxidize the surface of the hair, resulting in a considerable increase in surface friction. This subjects the hair to increased grooming damage because sebum is easier to clean from an oxidized hair surface, while combing forces are increased as a result of increased friction.

Chemically treated hair is also subject to increased water swelling and penetration by different materials as a result of reduced disulfide cross-linking and damage to nonkeratinous regions of the hair, including the cell membrane complex. Increased uptake of surfactants can, of course, lead to direct damage as a result of increased extraction of structural components of the hair fiber.

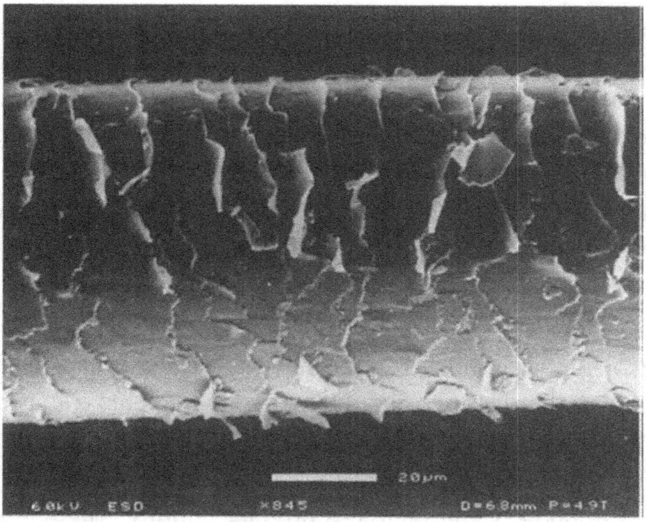

Figure 29.1. Combing damage resulting from washing a hair tress with a cleaning shampoo and then combing 700 times while wet. The scanning electron micrograph (SEM) is typical of hair taken from the combed tress. Note raised and chipped cuticle cells, and areas where cells have been completely torn away.

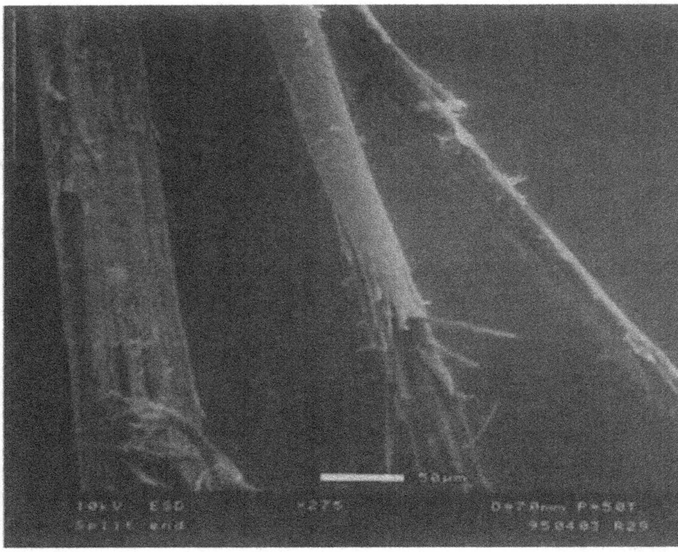

Figure 29.2. SEM photograph of a split end. Note the structure in the exposed cortex.

SECTION III: SHAMPOO EVALUATION

Formula Evaluation

Along with testing on actual hair, the shampoo formula itself needs to be tested for certain attributes. One of the most important tests a formula must make it through is shelf stability. Accelerated testing in different temperature/humidity extremes is usually used to evaluate the stability of a formula. Foam height and density is another very important attribute, but before it is tested on tresses, the actual foam height needs to be measured. The last formula attribute that needs to be taken into consideration is the ease of manufacturing. If the formula is not scalable, it is not marketable.

Stability

Products going on the store shelves should have at least two years of shelf life. During this time period, the shampoo should not see appreciable changes in viscosity, color, or fragrance. Multiphase products should not separate and there should be no precipitation seen.

Accelerated aging tests are run to test product stability. These tests are usually run at temperature extremes to simulate warehouse storage or shipping conditions. There are no standard accelerated aging tests for hair care products, so most manufacturers develop their own. A typical shampoo accelerated aging test suggests oven storage at 40°C and 50°C for three to six months as well as 25°C for a year.

Samples should be packaged in glass as well as the packaging that the shampoo would be sold in. The products should also go through one or more freeze/thaw cycles to evaluate the effects of lower temperatures [2].

Foam Height/Density

Foam is a very important attribute of a shampoo. Consumers will evaluate a shampoo based on the quality and quantity of the foam produced even though most shampoos have much more surfactant in them than actually needed to clean the hair. Strong abundant foam is directly related to the cleaning mechanism of a shampoo according to the average consumer.

There are various tests to measure the foaming potential of shampoos in the absence and presence of lipids. One very simple test is by shaking a known concentration of the shampoo formula in a graduated cylinder for a set amount of time. The foam height is then measured after shaking.

Manufacturing Ease

When formulating a shampoo, the ease in which it is manufactured or scaled up must be taken into consideration. A complex formula opens up more opportunity for production error. Order of addition, viscosity adjustments, mixing equipment, as well as heating capacity all need to be thought out carefully when transferring a formula from lab or pilot scale to manufacturing scale.

Evaluation of Shampoo Performance

A stable formulation is just the beginning for a shampoo formulator; performance of the shampoo ties together the entire gamete of consumer-driven traits that a formula must exhibit. These can be tested in a laboratory on tresses and if all goes well, the formulas can be tested by trained cosmetologists using half-head test methodology. This type of testing does not involve consumer evaluation, but is useful because it eliminates the differences seen in various hair types. Finally, once the shampoo passes all laboratory and half-head testing, it can move on to consumer testing. This is usually carried out in salons or at cosmetology schools with salons. Only after consumer approval for efficacy and safety, should the formulas go to market.

The following sections introduce some of the important attributes that are looked at when evaluating a shampoo's performance.

Ease of Application

This attribute is related to shampoo viscosity. A shampoo should be viscous enough to remain in the palm of the hand during pouring, but should easily disperse over the hair during application.

Lather

It is important for the foam height of the shampoo to be checked before it is added to hair, but the lather needs to be evaluated on tresses also. This should take into consideration the speed and amount of lather generated, the quality as well as the stability on hair. An extension of lather generation is lather rinsability. Water hardness, temperature, and rinsing rate all need to be taken into account when rinsing is evaluated, as well as any residuals left on the hair once rinsing is complete.

Wet/Dry Comb

Combing ease can be defined as the ease of aligning hair fibers in a parallel arrangement with a comb. Evaluations of combing ease, especially on wet hair, are often used as the primary assessment for the broader consumer attribute of hair conditioning, which also includes hair softness and lubricity. Hair fiber properties that improve combing ease are increasing stiffness, diameter, and cohesion; and decreasing curvature, friction, length, and static charge. Studies have indicated how different types of hair treatments can affect combing ease. Shampoos can affect several of these properties depending on the particular formulation. For instance, high-cleaning shampoos can make the hair more difficult to comb by removing sebum and oily soils that can lubricate the hair, while conditioning shampoos can deposit materials on the hair that decrease friction and thereby make the hair easier to comb [3].

The ease of combing attribute includes ease of snag removal and ease of comb slip on both wet and dry hair. Methods to evaluate combing ease include both qualitative combing of tresses combined with statistical evaluation of the results and quantitative instrumental methods. Instrumental methods involve the measurement of combing forces on tresses following treatment using an Instron or Diastron tensile tester [3].

Luster/Shine

Luster or shine is a very important aesthetic property to the consumer. Aging hair, chemical treatments, buildup of styling products, use of heated styling tools, as well as certain shampoo ingredients can all add to the dulling process. Shampoos that claim to add shine have a great market advantage as consumers associate this added shine or luster to creating healthy strong hair.

There are many instrumental methods as well as subjective evaluations that can be used to evaluate shine or luster on hair. No matter which method is employed, there are several factors that need to be taken into consideration when substantiating a claim for luster or shine enhancement: fiber straightness, degree of alignment of the hair, as well as hair color.

Volume/Body

The consumer attribute of body is both a visual and a tactile hair property indicative of fullness and volume combined with springiness and bounce. The effects shampoos have on hair body are formula dependent. For instance, deep-cleaning shampoos containing higher amounts of anionic surfactants can provide an increase in body by removing surface oils that weigh down hair. These types of shampoos can be marketed as volumizing or shampoos for fine/thin hair. Alternatively, shampoos containing materials than can build up on the hair can reduce hair body [3].

Several instrumental methods have been developed to evaluate parameters associated with hair body. These approaches measure changes in fiber friction, stiffness, curvature, diameter, weight, cohesion, and length. Treatments that increase the hair's curvature or diameter increase the frictional forces between fibers, or make the hair stiffer will increase body; those that increase the cohesion between fibers or weigh them down will decrease hair body [3].

Manageability

Manageability is a measure of styling ease and style retention. It is a complex consumer attribute that is difficult to assess by any one hair parameter or method. It has been suggested that evaluators consider three types of manageability: style arrangement manageability, style retention manageability, and flyaway manageability (static control). These properties can be assessed best by using a control treatment. As with other attributes, the effects that a particular shampoo has on manageability can vary. Any assessment of manageability is further complicated by factors involving the type of hair, humidity, and style [3].

Fragrance

Fragrance may not be a performance attribute for a shampoo formulation, but its importance cannot be overlooked. The effects that fragrance can have on a shampoo go far beyond that of formulation compatibility. The lasting power and acceptability of a fragrance needs to be taken into consideration before a formulation goes to market.

SECTION IV: FUTURE TRENDS IN SHAMPOOS

Consumer demand directs the mainstream shampoo market, which is why it is important for the formulator to stay abreast of any upcoming or lasting trends.

Natural and Biodegradable Ingredients

As stated before, consumers are becoming more aware of what they are putting on their bodies, as well as what is being done to the environment. Consumers perceive natural or naturally derived ingredients to be milder and safer than their synthetic counterparts as well as more eco-friendly. Ingredients that have chemical-sounding names are usually not deemed natural by the average consumer, so cosmetics and personal care items are trending more toward naturally derived ingredients and simplicity on the label. The biggest problem plaguing the formulator is that natural ingredients are sometimes hard to work with and don't necessarily function the same as the synthetic or chemically modified ingredients. Yet the consumer expects the natural shampoo to have the same attributes as a regular shampoo.

Many shampoo manufacturers have come out with "natural" product lines. These formulations may not be all-natural, but many contain biodegradable surfactants as well as botanicals and oils to replace some of the synthetic ingredients used in their regular formulas.

Anti-Aging Benefits

It is no secret that the anti-aging trend has taken over the cosmetic world. Staying young, or at least the perception of staying young, has spilled over into the hair care industry. As hair gets older, it gets coarser, the color fades; it becomes thinner and loses some of its natural luster. Shampoos are being manufactured that have anti-aging benefits that claim to help combat some of the issues hair goes through as it ages.

The "Free" Shampoo

Whether it be sulfate-free, amide-free, paraben-free, or silicone-free, there will always be the consumer demand for some type of "free" shampoo. These trends cycle and depend highly upon which ingredient is the hot topic of the moment. Even though the type of "free" shampoo can have a short life span and are of the specialty type, these shampoos have made it from being seen only in salons, to the mainstream store shelves.

Dry Shampoos

Although not necessarily a shampoo in conventional terms, the dry shampoo, once popular in the 1970s, is making a strong comeback, especially in European countries. This type of shampoo is not only brought back for its convenience factor, but also to satisfy the growing number of people who worry about the consequences of shampooing every day.

Dry shampoos are simple formulas consisting primarily of a corn or rice starch, which is used to absorb oils from the scalp and hair. Most modern dry shampoos also contain some sort of conditioning agent so that they don't leave the hair stiff like the very first formulas did. The problem facing this type of "shampoo" is that the starch used for these shampoos is white, so it is not very adequate for use in very dark hair.

REFERENCES

1. Mirajkar, Yelloji-Rao K., Application of Surfactants in Shampoos, Chapter 8 in *Handbook of Detergents*, Zoller, Uri ed., CRC Press, 2008, 151–180
2. Tarng, Jiashi J. and Reich, Charles, Shampoos and Conditioners, Chapter 10 in *Liquid Detergents*, Lai, Kuo Yann, ed., CRC Press, Boca Raton, FL, 2005. 377–449.
3. Reich C and J Chupa, Hair Shampoos, Chapter 29 in *Harry's Cosmeticology, 8th Edition*, Reiger, M. ed., Chemical Publishing Company, New York, 2000.
4. Wong, Michael, Cleansing of Hair, Chapter 3 in *Hair and Hair Care*, Johnson, Dale H., ed., Marcel Dekker, Inc., New York, 1997.
5. Panda, H., Cosmetics for The Hair, Chapter 6 in *Herbal Cosmetics Handbook*, Asia Pacific Business Press, Delhi, India, 2004.
6. Dalrymple, Damon M., Tommey, Ann B., Kortemeier, Uta, Multifunctional Ingredients in Hair Care Products, Chapter 3 in *Multifunctional Cosmetics*, Schueller, Randy and Romanowski, Perry, ed., Marcel Dekker, Inc, New York, 2001.
7. Steinberg, David C., Common Preservatives, Chapter 2 in *Preservatives for Cosmetics: Second Edition,* Allured Publishing Corporation, Carol Stream, IL, 2006.
8. A course on Hair Care Technology Symposium, Instructed by Colleen Rocafort, Joseph Dallal and John Bozza. Presented on August 24–26, 2010. Glenpointe Marriott, Teaneck, NJ.
9. Romanowski, Perry, Why does salt thicken Shampoo?, www.chemistcorner.com/why-does-salt-thicken-shampoo/.
10. Schueller, Randy and Romanowski, Perry, *Beginning Cosmetic Chemistry,* second edition, Allured Publishing Corporation, Carol Stream, IL, 2003, 217–226.
11. Clarke, Mary T., Rheological Additives, Chapter 4 in *Rheological Properties of Cosmetics and Toiletries*, Laba, Dennis, ed., Marcel Dekker, Inc, New York, 1993.
12. Hossain, Md. Mohsin, Interactions Between Starch and Surfactants by Ternary Phase Diagram, *Canadian Journal on Scientific and Industrial Research*, May 2012, Vol. 3, No. 4, 246–253.
13. Kozlowski, Angela C., Formulary in *Cosmetic and Toiletries Hair Care: From Physiology to Formulation*, Allured Publishing Corporation, Carol Stream, IL 2003, pg 556, 559.

GLOSSARY

viscosity – thickness of a liquid or resistance to flow.

rheology – the study of the flow of liquids.

anionic – negatively charged ion.

nonionic – does not have a positive or negative charge.

cationic – positively charged ion.

amphoteric – can act as a positive or negative ion depending upon pH.

zwitterionic – ion with both positive and negative charge attached to the same molecule with an overall neutral charge but can act as either a positive or a negative depending on pH.

flash foam – foam that develops immediately, may not have lasting power.

emulsifier – substance that stabilizes an emulsion by keeping both the water and oil phases mixed.

cloud point – point at which dissolved solids are no longer completely soluble, causing a solution to appear cloudy.

hydrophilic – has an affinity for water.

hydrophobic – repels water.

micelle – an aggregate of molecules that form in colloidal solutions.

pseudoplastic rheology – also known as sheer thinning. Viscosity will thin upon movement.

substantive – will bind to a substrate (hair) and not wash off with normal washing.

dent corn – a common variety of corn that has a ratio of about 76% amylopectin and 24% amylose. Used for making corn starches.

waxy corn – a variant of corn that contains 100% amylopectin. Used for making corn starches, not as common as dent corn.

amylopectin – a branched polysaccharide with α-1,4 and α-1,6 linkages. Makes up 76% of dent corn starch and 100% of waxy corn starch.

amylose – a linear polysaccharide with α-1,4 linkages. Makes up 24% of dent corn starch.

gelatinization temperature – the temperature at which a starch begins to swell.

antioxidant – substance that counteracts the damaging effects of oxidation.

sequestrant – form chelate compounds with metal ions often found in hard water. This allows for a shampoo to be rinsed easily from the hair without forming a layer of “scum” on the hair.

humectant – a substance that retains moisture.

critical micelle concentration (CMC) – concentration of surfactant above which micelles form and all additional surfactants added will spontaneously form micelles.

sebum – an oily secretion of the sebaceous gland that can be found on the scalp.

HAIR STYLING

Author
Charles Warren

a. Nonpressurized Styling Products

b. Pressurized Styling Products

The art of styling hair requires a broad spectrum of products to help achieve and maintain the desired coiffure. These products vary from those intended to simply hold hair in place (finishing products) to those intended to actually build a desired style (working products). A professional stylist would say that all styling is related to either lifting hair up or holding hair down. Styles can be achieved chemically by permanent waves or straighteners, mechanically by rollers, or thermally by irons or any combination of the former. In the development and maintenance of the desired configuration, a wide range of styling products may be used.

The styling product category is the largest and most confusing of all of the categories to the consumer. The formulator needs to understand what the product is to be used for in order to develop the best formula for the intended product. Once the targeted consumer and the desired functionality is understood, the formulator can develop the required formula and form to deliver the intended result in an aesthetically pleasing form.

In general, styling products can be separated into two categories: non-aerosolized styling products and pressurized aerosol styling products. Non-aerosolized styling products can be categorized into liquids, gels, nonpressurized sprays, and specialized (e.g., waxes, hairdressings) styling products. Pressurized aerosolized products can be categorized as fixatives (e.g., hairsprays/mousses) or specialty (e.g., shine sprays) products.

Because of the nature of styling products—the basic formulations and usage platforms—they are the most highly regulated category in hair care. The formulator needs to be aware of all of the regulatory requirements by category in order to develop functional, compliant formulations. The Volatile Organic Compound (VOC) regulations on styling products exist at the federal level (EPA) and at individual state levels, California being one of the strictest. Because the regulatory environment is dynamic and new interpretations arise on an almost daily basis, great diligence is required in formulating and even naming products in this category. The formulator must work closely with legal and regulatory advisors to avoid inadvertently developing a formula that will later be declared noncompliant and subject to punitive legal issues.

a. Nonpressurized Styling Products

Liquids and Gels

In general, both of these subcategories fulfill similar functions—to develop a style and then, once dry, maintain that desired configuration. Styling liquids are water-thin, aqueous, or hydro-alcoholic solutions of a holding, film-forming polymer (e.g., PVP and/or derivatives), modifiers to increase plasticity (i.e., flexibility) of dried film, and aesthetic modifiers (e.g., fragrance). They are generally applied to damp hair, worked through the hair, then dried after the desired configuration is achieved. They can be used in combination with brushing while blow-drying to achieve volume/fullness, which will be maintained as the film dries on the individual hairs.

Styling gels serve a similar function, but applied in a gel form. The gel itself is formed by the use of a polymeric material (e.g., carbomer) and provides a thicker coating to the individual hairs. Gels may be used to hold hair in a flat configuration or in conjunction with brushing and blow-drying to achieve volume or raise hair from the scalp.

When liquids or gels dry they form a film on the hairs and cause the hairs to hold together in a relatively rigid configuration. If combed or manipulated after drying, this film coating and the resultant "welding" of hairs together is disrupted and will no longer hold. This disruption can be negative if the desired configuration was achieved or positive if the desired configuration is less rigid and will be supplemented with other fixative products. Regardless, as the film is disrupted it breaks into small particles that can manifest themselves as flakes or dust. The formulator can incorporate materials to ameliorate this negative appearance, but must certainly be aware of the potential for this occurring.

Nonpressurized Aerosol Sprays

These sprays are hydro-alcoholic solutions of a hair-fixative polymer or polymers, film modifiers, and aesthetic materials. They are sprayed directly onto damp (working sprays) or dry (fixative) hair. They provide a modicum of coating to the individual hair fibers (used as working spray) or "spot welds" at the junction of individual hairs (used as fixative spray).

When used as a working product, these function in a similar fashion to liquids and gels, but allow lower levels of product to be applied. As a finishing product, these sprays dispense a fine coating of fixative polymer on the final coiffure to help maintain the desired configuration. Dispensing water or hydro-alcoholic solution onto dry hair will disrupt the hydrogen bonds of the hair and can cause the desired configuration to collapse or be disrupted. The formulator needs to be aware of how the product can disrupt a coiffure and can select a sprayer that, in conjunction with the degree of hold required (i.e., the amount of fixative polymer delivered to the hair), will ameliorate this collapse or disruption.

b. Pressurized Styling Products

Aerosol Hairsprays

Pressurized styling products (e.g., hairsprays and mousse) have been and are the largest section of the styling products universe and, combined with gels, comprise between 80–90% of the entire styling category.

Formulating pressurized hairsprays requires technical understanding of the basic formulas and mechanical understanding of the way that pressurized aerosols work and, specifically, how the formula, propellant, and spray button/valve system interact to deliver the desired outcome. In this particular subcategory, all of the parts make up the "formula," and changing any of the parts will have s significant impact on the final product. In addition, this category is highly impacted by the VOC regulations mentioned earlier.

The base formula for hairsprays is essentially an alcoholic or hydroalcoholic solution containing a polymeric resin or resins (fixatives), a neutralizing agent (if required by resin type), plasticizing agents to impact the stiffness/brittleness of the dried film, fragrance, and claims ingredients. The propellants used for hairsprays are propane, butane, isobutane, and in the world of VOC regulation, hydrofluorocarbon 152a.

The ratio of base formula to propellant (base-prop ratio) is important for product performance. In general, the lower the base-prop ratio, the finer and dryer the resulting spray.

In general, the volatile organic compounds in a pressurized aerosol hairspray are the alcohol (solvent for the base) and the hydrocarbon propellants. To achieve the requisite VOC maximum, the formulator would commonly use: a) a combination of alcohol, water, dimethylether (DME—a solvent/propellant that ameliorates propellant/base miscibility but is a VOC), and hydrocarbon; or, b) a combination of alcohol, hydrocarbon, and hydrofluorocarbon 152a. In the DME/water approach, the water, resins, neutralizing agents, and other miscellaneous ingredients are the non-VOC portion; the propellant, DME, and alcohol are the VOCs, which have a maximum level allowable. In the 152a approach, the resins, neutralizing agents, and other miscellaneous ingredients are the non-VOC portion; the propellant, 152a, and alcohol are the VOCs, which have a maximum level allowable. There are some special exemption formulations that have been used for compliance, but the two approaches indicated are the most common.

Water-containing hairsprays tend to be "wetter" when applied, and water can negatively impact coiffures, can cause corrosion in electro-tinplated steel cans and valves (commonly used for hairsprays), and can require special gaskets not negatively impacted by DME. The use of water in the hairspray can make the formula less expensive than the 152a approach. The 152a approach yields a finer, drier spray, does not impact the final coiffure, and is not corrosive to valves and cans. However, the 152a approach is significantly more expensive.

Mousse

Mousse styling products are used for a combination of styling and hair holding. In general, mousse formulations are an aqueous solution of holding resins (e.g., VP/VA copolymer), conditioners (e.g., polyquaternium-4, dimethicone copolyol), surfactant materials (e.g., polysorbate 60), aesthetic/claims ingredients (e.g., fragrance), and propellant (e.g., butane, propane, and isoubutane). When properly formulated, the propellant phase becomes dispersed in the liquid base phase such that when dispensed, the product immediately forms a thick foam in the hand, which can then be applied to wet or dry hair for styling. Some mousse formulations contain alcohol to assist the mixing of the water phase and the propellant phase.

Mousse formulations are generally used for a conditioning hold, with the ratio of holding resin and conditioners being varied to provide more or less of the desired property. These products are generally used as the preliminary styling product to create volume or create desired coiffure. They are then followed by a finishing spray to hold the configuration in place. They can be used alone to build and maintain style depending on the desired configuration or in conjunction with other styling forms such as gels or gums.

As are all pressurized styling products, mousse formulations are governed by VOC regulations. The levels of VOC allowed for mousse are substantially lower than that for aerosol hairsprays. The VOCs in mousse formulations are the propellant and alcohol, if included in the formula.

Pressurized Shine Sprays

Generally, pressurized shine sprays are an anhydrous solution of lightweight oils and lipoidal materials, fragrance, and propellant. These products are primarily used by consumers with relaxed, African-Caribbean hair to impart shine. Shine sprays are also regulated for VOC content, and the formulator must be aware of the categorization of the oils used before starting. In addition, the ultimate particle size of the dispensed spray must be closely monitored. Too fine a particle size can lead to inhalation of the oily particles, which can result in significant health issues. The formulator needs to check the current regulations.

SPECIALTY STYLING PRODUCTS

Author
Charles Warren

The category of specialty styling products is huge and grows on an almost daily basis. Products are developed to achieve styles and effects. These products usually come from the professional stylist arena and are the result of a creative stylist using an new or alternate material to achieve a particular "look" or style on a particular hair type.

Included in this category are waxes, hairdressings, silicone shine products, gums, etc. These products can all be used to impart a targeted effect on the hair. Waxes and gums are blends of waxes and other higher-molecular-weight fatty materials to impart stiffness to short hair or stiffness to small sections of a larger coiffure—small braids or sideburns for example. Hair dressings are blends of fatty materials or oil/water emulsions or microemulsions used to provide shine, immediate lubrication, and a modicum of control, especially on dry hair. Silicone shine treatments are blends of silicones used to lightly coat the hair and provide a glossy shine.

In general, the formulator needs to know the targeted consumer/hair type, the effect desired, the claims to be made, and the way the product will be used by the consumer to begin formulation work. A survey of the competitive products used for the same purpose will be helpful as a starting point.

PERMANENT WAVING

Author
Charles Warren

Permanent waves are two- or three-component systems applied to hair rolled on appropriate rods to achieve a specific curl or wave pattern that is durable ("permanent"). The first solution is either the waving lotion alone or a two-component system for creating the wave lotion. The waving lotion alone (cold wave) is an aqueous mixture of ammonium hydroxide (1–2% ammonia), thioglycolate (8–10% as thioglycolic acid), surfactant, and other water-soluble ingredients desired. (The pH of a traditional cold wave is 9–9.5.) Ammonium thioglycolate and monoethanolamine thioglycolate are the common forms of thioglycolate employed. It is the thioglycolate ion that is the reactive species. The two-component waving lotion involves an aqueous solution of ammonium hydroxide (1–3% ammonia) to which is added glyceryl monothioglycolate (GMT) immediately prior to application. Again, it is the thioglycolate that is the reactive species. In either case, the waving lotion is applied to the hair wrapped around rods of the appropriate size for the desired curl pattern. The waving lotion is allowed to process under a plastic cap (for the cold wave or some GMT waves) or with a cap under a hot dryer for acid GMT waves) until the desired curl pattern is achieved (determined by the operator unrolling a rod and reviewing a "test curl"). Once the pattern is acceptable, the waving solution is rinsed from the hair and the second component (neutralizer), an aqueous solution of hydrogen peroxide (2–2.5%) is applied to reform the cystine bonds in the new configuration. After five minutes, the neutralizer is rinsed and the rods are removed.

Permanent waves using bisulfate (ammonium or sodium) are also used. These function in a similar fashion to the thioglycolate waves, but have lower negative odor. They are slightly less aggressive on the hair than thioglycolate waves and are subject to a greater degree of reversion to the original hair configuration. Nonetheless, they can be effective on the right hair and with the right expectations.

Permanent waving is moderately damaging to hair due to the alkaline nature of the products and the fact that not all of the cystine bonds that are broken re-form, leaving the hair weaker than prior to the treatment.

PART 6.14

CONDITIONERS/TREATMENTS

Author
Charles Warren

Hair is continually being damaged by mechanical stresses (e.g., combing/brushing), thermal stresses (e.g., blow dryers), and chemical stresses (e.g., coloring/bleaching). As hair has no biological means of repairing itself, the damage is cumulative. Hair grows at a rate of 0.25 to 0.33 inches per month, so hair that is eight inches long (medium length) has undergone 2–2.5 years of cumulative damage. The additional mechanical stress of hair fibers rubbing back and forth across each other (fiber-fiber) interaction is an additional source of damage that is not usually even thought of.

Damaged hair becomes weaker, leads to breakage and fiber splitting, loses cuticle (the flattened outer protective layer of hair), and develops an overall negative surface charge. This negative charge results in "fly-away" hair, appearing frizzy and dull. Damage on the hairs' surface also interferes with the wicking of the natural oils (sebum) secreted at the hair roots, further exacerbating the negative appearance and lubrication of the individual fibers.

Conditioners and treatments serve to neutralize the negative charge on the hairs' surface, restore oil to the fibers' and leave the hair softer and shinier, at least on a temporary basis. Rinses, conditioners, and treatments generally serve the same functions, the difference being the amount and types of materials used. They are all usually oil-in-water emulsions (lipoidal ingredients suspended in a continuous phase of water, held together with emulsifiers). They usually contain a cationic (positively charged moiety) such as stearalkonium or cetrimonium chloride (quaternary ammonium compounds) and a blend of fatty alcohols, such as cetyl or stearyl alcohols. In addition, there are aesthetic ingredients such as fragrance and colors, microbiological preservatives and other conditioning/claims ingredients such as proteins, and vitamins.

Conditioners can be divided into the general categories of leave-in conditioners, rinses, moisturizing conditioners, volumizing conditioners, conditioning treatments, and specialty conditioners, such as oil or protein treatments. Again, there may be multiple names and types of conditioners, but they will usually fit into one of these categories.

The formulator needs to balance the ingredients to maintain a stable emulsion and deliver the end result claimed. Understanding the emulsion and the desired end result is usually a significant challenge and requires technical understanding as well as the ability to interpret all of the aesthetic requirements for the emulsion itself, the manufacture and dispensing of the emulsion, the feel of the product on the hands and hair as applied, and, most importantly, the final appearance and feel of the hair. Not enough conditioning will provide the hair with little benefit and too much conditioning can leave the hair looking/feeling greasy and weighed down. A poor emulsion will result in separation and instability, or if overemulsified, an unpleasant greasy and ineffective formula.

Leave-in conditioners are either water-thin aqueous solutions containing a cationic moiety (usually a cationic polymeric material) to neutralize charge and provide some conditioning to the hair fibers. They are low in lipoidal materials and usually dispensed via a spray directly on the hair or onto the hands and then worked through the hair.

Rinses are thin, rinse-out emulsions applied to the hair post-shampoo and contain lower percentages of cationic materials (quaternary ammonium salts), fatty alcohols, and ancillary or aesthetic ingredients. They provide a lower level of conditioning, desired by some consumers and effective in ameliorating the negative effects of relatively minor damage. As these are relatively thin emulsions, they can be problematic in maintaining stability over time and through extremes of heat and cold.

Moisturizing conditioners are emulsions containing higher levels of both cationic moieties (quaternary ammonium salts, cationic polymers) and lipoidal materials (fatty alcohols and oils). They are rinse-out, post-shampoo treatments and are dispensed into the hand and applied to the hair, left on for an interval, and then rinsed from the hair. They are generally thicker emulsions and have a creamy feel that is aesthetically pleasing to the consumer while being applied and worked through the hair, signaling efficacy while doing the actual conditioning of the hair. These conditioners are effective in neutralizing the negative charge, leaving residual oils on the hair surface and softening the hair fibers—the greater the degree of damage to the hair (and, thus, the porosity or ability for hair to absorb), the higher the degree of tolerance to lipoidal materials. For example, chemically relaxed (straightened) hair will tolerate and require higher levels of oils and conditioning materials than hair that is damaged by simple combing/ blow drying. The formulator needs to be aware of the targeted consumer/hair-type when developing a formula. What delivers an effective and aesthetically pleasing level of conditioning and hair-feel to one consumer will be viewed as oily/greasy to another.

Volumizing conditioners will provide conditioning benefits to finer/thinner hair at low levels and will have the added benefit of leaving behind materials (usually polymeric materials) that will attach to the hair electrostatically and thicken the hair, resulting in a fuller-appearing coiffure. These conditioners are generally trickier to formulate, as consumers with fine/thin hair are highly sensitive to materials perceived as weighing the hair down, leaving it looking flatter and appearing oily or greasy. This category of conditioner is probably the smallest of all of the categories.

Specialty conditioner treatments (e.g., oil or protein treatments) are rinse-out, post-shampoo treatments intended to be applied on an infrequent basis and are generally for a specific problem (e.g., severely damaged hair). In general, the formulas contain higher levels of specific ingredients (e.g., fatty materials), are applied and left on for extended periods (1–10 minutes), and may include the use of a plastic covering (cap) or a moist towel. Some specialty treatments require a shampoo step after the treatment to remove any excess oils or conditioning ingredients. Relaxed (straightened), bleached, or extremely fragile or dry hair are the targeted types for these products.

PART 6.15

HAIR COLORANTS AND PROTECTION

Author
Padmaja Prem, Ph.D
Vice President, Research & Development
Combe Incorporated, 1101 Westchester Avenue
White Plains, NY 10604

ABSTRACT

Most permanent hair-coloring technology is based on the 100+ year-old approach of oxidation of *p*-diamines and *p*-aminophenols by hydrogen peroxide at alkaline pH to form an active intermediate. These active intermediates then react inside the hair fiber with couplers that produce colored molecules of varying size depending on the nature of the primary intermediates and couplers. Being bigger, these color molecules are trapped inside the hair fiber, thus providing resistance to removal. Permanent hair color, however, is far from "permanent." Factors such as frequent washing, UV exposure, and heat styling are generally known to cause hair-color fading.

Additionally, hair-coloring process imparts oxidative damage to hair lipids and keratin and disrupts hair cuticle. When the cuticle is disrupted, it becomes fragmented and rough, resulting in less light reflection from the hair surface. The dramatic increase in the use of hair-coloring products and other chemical treatments requires specific products for the care and protection of color as well as the hair that underwent damage due to oxidation of lipids and proteins. Enhancing the protection of color, shine, vibrancy, and overall appearance and conditioning of color-treated hair requires products that are formulated differently from regular hair care products. Color- and shine-protecting products contain substances that smooth down the cuticle and increase light reflection.

This chapter describes the fundamentals of permanent hair coloring, the change in hair properties associated with hair coloring, and the factors that influence color fading, vibrancy, and shine. Further, it also covers formulation techniques to deliver long-lasting color, color vibrancy, and shine and remedies for protection of color-treated hair to preserved color vibrancy and shine. Beyond these approaches, the author has also provided a unique and critical review of selected ingredients and products in the market offering various benefits for color-treated hair.

The underlying reasons and remedies for hair-color protection described in this chapter provide important leads to ingredient-seekers and product formulators for color care and presents an opportunity for a myriad of novel products that consumers long for. The chapter is also unique in that it provides thoughtful, practical recommendations for developing better hair color and hair care products to address the needs of color-treated hair. This wisdom goes beyond the traditional approach of finding new ingredients or formulations to achieve the goals of beautiful hair that is shiny and vibrant. It is recommended that these approaches be incorporated in literature by product manufacturers as important information to consumers.

TABLE OF CONTENTS

6.15.1 INTRODUCTION

Hair-coloring products are a multibillion-dollar international industry composed of three types of products: temporary, semi-permanent, and permanent hair-color products. The majority of its growth (~70%) is derived from permanent hair-coloring products, which owe their popularity to their long-lasting effect, ease of application, natural look, versatility, and allowing virtually any color to be achieved.[1] This industry is poised for even greater growth in the future due to an increasingly aging, and thus graying, global population longing for a youthful appearance. Permanent coloring technology, which is also called lift and deposit technology, has the ability to lift the natural color of hair and deposit new color that lasts until the hair is replaced by new growth. Most permanent hair-coloring technology is based on the 100+ year-old approach of oxidation of colorless p-diamines and p-aminophenols by hydrogen peroxide at alkaline pH to form active intermediates. Permanent hair colorants are normally marketed in the form of a two-component kit comprising an alkaline composition of oxidation hair dyes in a liquid, gel, or cream vehicle and a developer composition that utilizes an oxidizing agent, usually hydrogen peroxide. The two compositions are mixed immediately prior to application to the hair. The alkaline pH of the resultant mixture causes the hair shaft to swell, allowing the dye precursors to penetrate into the cortex of the hair. These dye precursors are then oxidized and combine to form larger molecules. These larger molecules contain a significant level of conjugated double bonds, hence producing a colored product that is visible from the exterior of the hair. After an appropriate development time during which the composition resides on the hair, the mixture is rinsed from the hair. The color of the hair is then permanently altered.

Permanent hair color, however, is far from "permanent" due to color fading by factors such as frequent washing, light exposure, and other daily grooming habits such as heat styling. Permanent hair coloring changes hair structure due to removal of soluble lipids and oxidation of keratin protein and lipids. These changes in hair structure make colored hair to be more porous than virgin hair. As hair becomes more porous, it absorbs more color and it also removes more color on washing. The fading of permanent hair color due to frequent washing, daily grooming, and by environmental factors has become a common problem of color-treated hair and a source of frequent complaints by consumers.

Photo damage to the hair shaft contributes to dullness by altering the chemistry of the dyed hair through oxidative damage. UV exposure affects hair strength and elasticity and cause photo-oxidation, which triggers discoloration and fading in both natural and color-treated hair. Work by Ph. Maillan reports the use of a leave-on formulation with a polymeric organosiloxane sunscreen to protect the artificially colored hair. This polymeric filter was reported to be more effective than classic sunscreen ethylhexyl methoxycinnamate.

Luster or shine is another important feature of hair's appearance, and this visual effect is a key objective in the consumer hair care market. Thus, shine-protecting hair care products are worthwhile for the consumer with color-treated hair demanding youthful hair appearance. Color strength or color vibrancy is another important attribute for colored hair, but no parameter or test method has previously been developed to combine the two and enable quantified vibrancy claims. In relation, based on work by Lefaudeux et al., the authors define a new parameter for such claims, the hair-color vibrance factor (HCVF).

6.15.2 FUNDAMENTALS OF HAIR COLORING

Hair dyes can be divided mainly into three categories, each with a specific composition and action mechanism: temporary dyes (water-soluble dyes that withstand only one-time shampooing), semi-permanent dyes (which can withstand four to five shampooings), and permanent or oxidative dyes that needs reapplication only when new roots are shown. Temporary hair color works on the surface of hair to add sheer color and it typically only lasts one to two shampoos. When applied to prelightened or extremely porous hair, temporary hair color may penetrate further into the cortex and stain the hair shaft.

Semi-permanent hair color works on the surface of hair to deposit color, yet lasts longer than temporary hair color. Semi-permanent contains large and small color molecules that adhere to the outside of the hair, while some penetrate the cuticle layer, depending on the hair's porosity. Some color is removed with each shampoo, but color typically lasts from four to eight shampoos.

Oxidative hair dyes are the most popular hair-dye products. They may be further divided into three subcategories: permanent, demi-permanent, and auto-oxidative hair dyes. Permanent hair color contains ammonia and is mixed with developer, typically hydrogen peroxide, in various volumes in order to permanently change hair color. Depending upon the pH of the mixture and the strength of the developer, these systems have the capability to simultaneously lighten the hair's natural pigment and deposit color. The ammonia is an alkalizing agent that swells the hair fiber and opens the cuticle layer, allowing the color molecules and developer to penetrate into the cortex. Once inside, the developer lightens natural pigment and develops the color molecules so they remain permanently in the cortex. Permanent hair-color technologies' common uses include gray coverage, change of natural hair color, and lightening natural hair color. L'Oreal Excellence Crème hair color, Garnier Color Naturals Nourishing Permanent Hair Color Cream, Revlon ColorSilk, and Clairol Nice'n Easy are some examples of product in this category.

Demi-permanent formulas are ideal for enhancing, refreshing, or darkening hair color (either natural or previously colored). These formulas do not contain ammonia and use low-volume peroxide. Generally, they last up to six weeks, so they offer less commitment than permanent hair color. Because the developer is low strength, it is mild and the hair remains in optimal condition. Demi-permanents are also called "deposit-only permanent colors" as they do not lighten the hair, but only deposit color. Majority of the men's hair color in the market belongs to this class of dyes. Demi-permanent hair color is the fastest-growing color category in the industry because of its versatility. It is excellent for glazing or for refreshing previously tinted hair for added vibrancy and shine, and is essential for color correction. L'Oreal Healthy look crème gloss, Bigen Powder Hair Color, Just for Men Natural Hair Color, and Clairol Natural Instincts Hair Color are some examples of product in this category.

Auto-oxidative hair dyes involve the oxidation of dye precursors by oxygen in air without the use of an oxidant. This technology is based on precursors such as 1, 2, 4-trihydroxybenzene, 2,4-diaminophenol, 2-methoxy-p-phenylene diamine. Unlike, classic oxidative dyeing, hair is not lightened, so such systems are used to color gray hair or to change color from lighter to darker shades. Formulas containing these dyes involve no mixing, they are sold in one component and free of ammonia and hydrogen peroxide, and hence are milder than both demi-permanent and permanent hair-color products. Just for Men AutoStop hair color is an example of product in this category.

Concern over the safety of PPD and other hair-dye ingredients, the damage of hair due to oxidative coloring, and the demand for more convenient hair dyeing methods has fostered an increase in research in this area on new dyes and alternative hair-coloring technologies. Manufacturers have in recent decades embarked on intense research toward new dyes and precursors, as well as into alternative technologies for permanent hair dyeing. This research has been aimed not only at addressing potential toxicological issues but also technical weaknesses such as to mitigate hair damage, long-lasting color, no ammonia, no peroxide hair color, ease of application, and convenience.

6.15.3 FACTORS INFLUENCING COLOR FADING AND COLOR REMOVAL

Permanent hair-coloring products are formulated to provide excellent gray coverage, change existing hair color through removal of current hair color (lift) and deposit of new colors. Additionally, permanent hair-color products are formulated to give long-lasting and vibrant hair colors that provide overall youthful appearance. Several factors starting from formulation, product application, frequent washing, daily grooming habits, and environmental factors such as sun and pollution can accelerate color changes, color fading, vibrancy, and shine.

- **Color formulation and color application.**

When formulating hair-color products, several factors need to be taken into account in designing the appropriate vehicle. If color has not been given enough time to penetrate the hair shaft, color molecules will stay inside the cuticle layers and on the surface, allowing them to be washed away quickly. Most of fading appears after the first two washes, indicating that the color molecules settled on the outside of the hair shaft and had not penetrated deeply enough to be retained through washes. U.S. patent by Padmaja et al. teaches a two-step hair-color method, where the color precursors are applied in a first step that provides adequate time for effective penetration inside the hair fiber. In a second step, the hair is treated with hydrogen peroxide, so the reaction takes place inside the fiber and the dyes are trapped in the cortex, making them resistance to washing. The authors have shown more vibrant and longer-lasting color effect from this two-step system compared to conventional one-step hair coloring. In traditional permanent hair-coloring products as soon as the dye precursors are mixed with the developer, two competing factors come into play, the diffusion of dye precursors and peroxide into the fiber, the reaction of color precursor with peroxide outside the fiber. An optimal balance between the two factors contributes to overall color quality, long-lasting color, and color vibrancy.

- **Cuticle damage.**

The cuticle is the primary protection for the hair cortex where the majority of color molecules are housed. If friction or excessive chemical treatments damage the cuticle and strip away its protective fatty layer, the exposed cortex will chip away, and color molecules will escape during shampooing. Damaged hair is more porous and hydrophilic and hence absorbs more color during coloring and loses more color during washing. Protection of the cuticle with shampoos and conditioners that contain friction-reducing silicones helps reduce this type of color loss. Repair of hair damage using daily shampoos and conditioners containing protective polymers improves the state of the fiber and minimizes color loss due to the damage aspects of hair.

- **Rinsing with water.**

Fading due to water exposure is often related to a damaged cuticle. When the cuticle is overly compromised, water can more easily enter the cortex and some of the color molecules can be pulled out and washed away. Shampoos do not strip color. Studies show that water alone is responsible for the majority of color lost during shampooing.

- **Exposure to sunlight (UV and visible light).**

UV light is known to fade color in many substrates such as wood, cloth and paint. Hair is no different. UV radiation penetrates the hair and breaks down color molecules. The process happens with both natural and artificial pigments in the cortex and is the reason people develop highlights after spending long periods of time in the sun. UV protectants are added to some shampoos and styling products to help prevent hair color fade due to sunlight, although their efficacy is debated.

- **Some hair-color shades fade more quickly than others.**

Red shades tend to fade more than brown or black shades due to their relatively small molecule size, which can diffuse from the hair and wash away more quickly than other shades. UV exposure also breaks down the red tone more easily, while pure browns and blacks resist fading because their color molecules tend to be larger. Blonde shades have little color, so fading is less of a concern.

6.15.4 COLOR PROTECTION

Consumer demand for high-performance, vibrant, and fashion-oriented, yet natural-looking hair colorants continues to grow. To meet this trend, formulators must create high-impact products that provide lasting, natural-looking color as well as improved hair shine and conditioning effects. In recent years, the number of hair care products specifically designed to address such needs of color-treated hair is steadily increasing. The number of products claiming color protection continues to increase, and consumer product makers employ a variety of formulation strategies to address the needs of people who have color-treated hair. Rinse-off products such as shampoos and conditioners dominate the market and typically contain ingredients that emphasize the benefits of moisture retention, deposition of protective films on hair surface, and protection of color from sun fading using UV filters. Leave-on products, on the other hand, emphasize ingredients that serve to seal hair through deposition of polymers. Both formulation strategies address consumers who want to maintain the vitality of natural-looking hair following hair-color treatment. Naturally, consumers have a strong interest in adopting a hair care regimen that can extend the color vibrancy of hair, yet color fading and the loss of color vibrancy typically comes with everyday cleansing.

Studies by X et al. showed that color fading primarily occurs through physical removal of dyes by rinsing with water. These authors have investigated the physical and chemical factors that influence hair-color removal during the washing process by testing hair dye dissolution in water from dyed hair samples with variation of surfactant type, pH, and hair type. They have investigated a series of polymers with various functional groups and demonstrated that polymers with hydrophobically modified and cationic functionalities are the most effective in preventing hair-dye dissolution in water. A primary example of a polymer within this category is a cationic terpolymer of vinylpyrrolidone, dimethylaminopropyl methacrylamide, and methacryloylaminopropyl lauryldimonium chloride (INCI: Polyquaternium-55). Figure 1 shows the anti-fading test results of the four polymers in a leave-in treatment at 2% level using bleached hair tresses. The results demonstrate that Polyquaternium 55 (VP/DMAPA/C12-MAPTAC copolymer) leave-in treatment provides the highest color protection with 38% higher color improvement at the end of 10× washes over the control, and the effect is well perceivable by eye as shown in the picture.

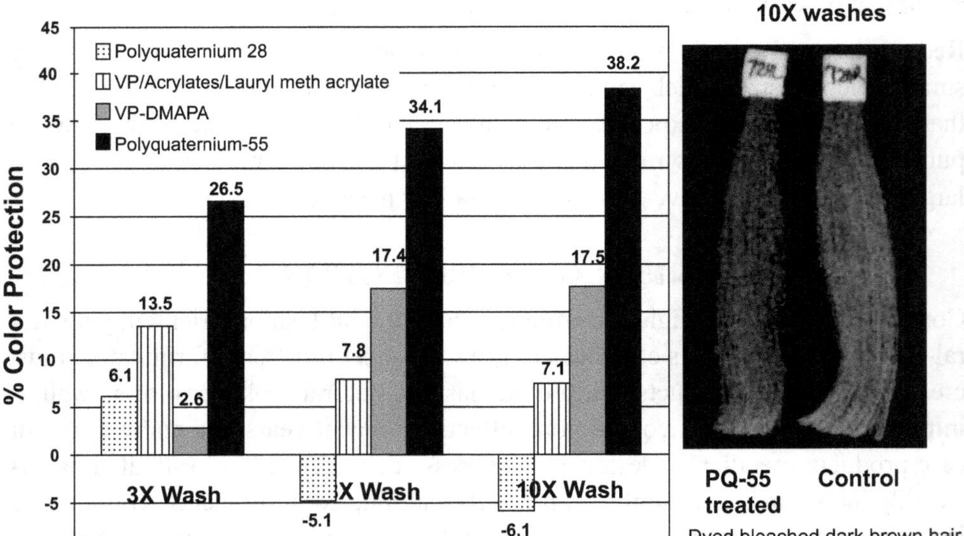

Figure 1. Pictures and percentages of color protection for dyed hair samples after 10× SLES washes and leave-in treatment of 2% of various polymers.

Both visual and instrumental measurement results indicate that Polyquaternium-55 provides a high level of color protection when formulated in a hair-color protection regimen with up to 50% color protection. Conditioning shampoos and conditioners with cationic surfactants and water proofing amino silicones can help combat the effects of water exposure.

Croda Inc. has commercialized a quaternized diester (ChromAveil) claimed to provide broad-spectrum sun protection to hair in rinse-off systems. It is a broad-spectrum UV filter that protected hair from color fading and hair integrity damage. Figure 2 below shows that hair treated with the diester shampoo protects the color from UV fading as evidenced by the lower value of Delta E, the total color change.

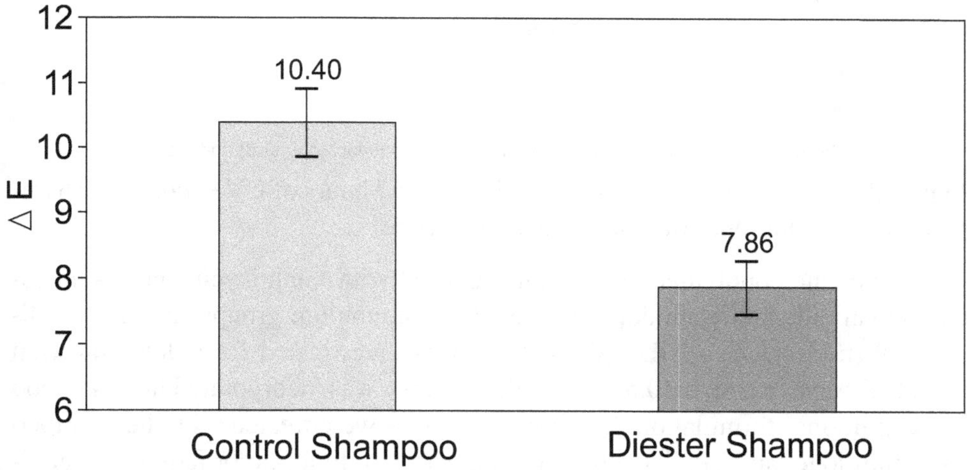

Figure 2. Total color change of medium brown-colored hair treated with different shampoos after 15 days of UV exposure

Silicones can help protect hair treated with permanent and nonpermanent colorants from discoloration and fading. Some color stays on the upper layers of cuticle and can be removed during washing. With its spreading behavior, silicone may help colorant further penetrate the hair cuticle for longer-lasting retention. By forming a water-insoluble film, the silicone may also help prevent color from washing out due to the hydrophobic nature of the silicone deposits on hair surface. Based on tests with several silicones, Figure 3 shows color retention properties for two silicones at 2% active level in a rinse-off conditioner. In this series of results, expressed by ΔE value, the silicones significantly reduced color loss compared to the control (the same rinse-off conditioner without silicone). The lower ΔE value for hair treated with the silicones indicates they help maintain color intensity and depth.

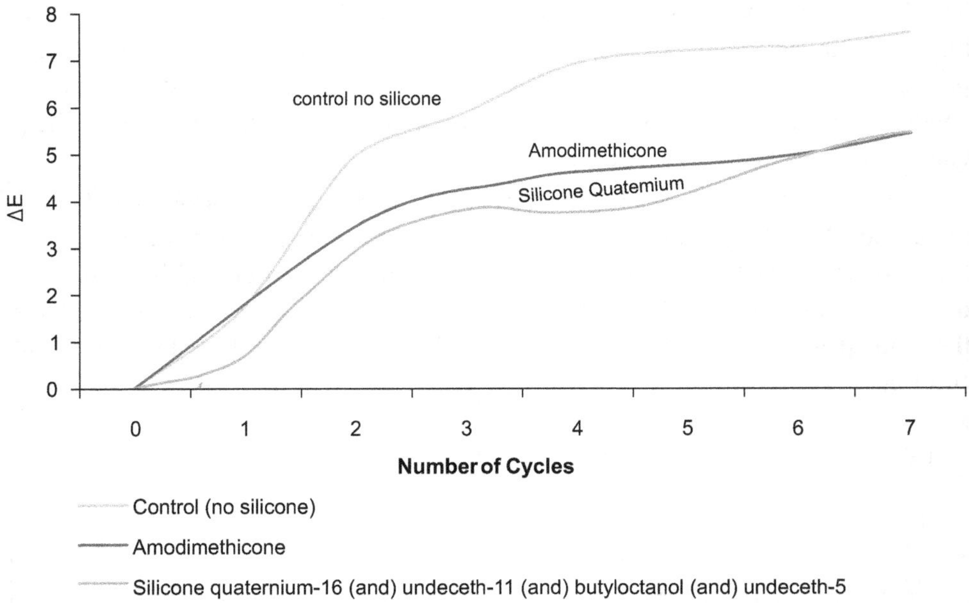

Figure 3. ΔE through seven cycles (each cycle = 7 hours of UV exposure + shampoo rinse + conditioner rinse at 2% active silicone)

A siloxane copolymer from Evonik grafted with methoxycinnamic acid ester and cationic alkoylamidopropyl dimethyl ammonium groups called Polysilicone-19 (trade name ABIL UV Quat 50) was investigated for color protection from UV. An active level (0.5–1%) of this silicone was incorporated in a shampoo and conditioner formulation. Colored hair tresses were treated with the shampoo and conditioner and irradiated by UV for a period of time. Color fading was compared to an untreated hair tress and other competitor ingredients. In a shampoo formulation at 0.5%, the silicone offered 50% reduced color fading and at 1.0% level from a conditioner application it offered 40% reduced color fading. The new silicone, Silicone Quaternium-22 microemulsion (trade name: ABIL® ME 45), offers significant color protection against washing. As a result, the combination of Silicone Quaternium-22 microemulsion and Polysilicone-19 in shampoos and conditioners can provide comprehensive color protection from UV and washing and premium hair-conditioning benefits with both visible and tangible benefits for consumers.

New color protection products include leave-on systems. Leave-on systems allow formulators to include functional ingredients like cationic film-forming polymers that bind with negatively charged amino acids on the surface of hair. These types of film-forming polymers can be found primarily in hair-styling gel and mousse formulations designed for hair hold, but they can also be used in personal care applications where a need exists to form a protective barrier on the hair cuticle. This protective barrier phenomenon can be strongly applied to products claiming hair-color protection. The film formed on the hair is believed to protect hair color from losing its vibrancy as a result of excess washing.

6.15.5 COLOR VIBRANCY AND SHINE

Human perception of color depends on the ability of our eyes and brains to detect and interpret the reflection of light on objects. When light shines on hair, part of it penetrates and is absorbed by the dye molecules, and part is reflected back. Shine-inducing shampoos and conditioners can be used on almost all hair types, creating the illusion of healthier hair. Darker hair tends to be shinier than lighter hair because it reflects light better, but as long as the cuticle and shaft are smooth, light is properly reflected off each individual strand. Hair shine is an important feature of hair appearance and this attractive visual effect is a key consumer objective in the hair care market. Hair-color intensity is another important attribute for colored hair.

Certain products and ingredients can enhance this effect. Conditioners are especially important when it comes to achieving shine because they replace natural oils and sebum that is lost further down the hair shaft. They penetrate, adding back lost moisture and giving the hair the ability to reflect light and therefore look shinier.

Consumers always want to have their colored hair appear bright and striking, or vibrant. Until now, neither a parameter nor a test method has been defined and developed to make such quantified "vibrancy" claims. Lefaudeus et al. have published principles for measuring hair luster (shine) using a Color Hair Visual Appearance Study System (SAMBA Hair system). SAMBA Hair System based on an innovative polarization camera SAMBA. They have observed that there are two bands on captured colored hair images: the "Shine" band (first reflection, no color) and the "Chroma" band (second reflection with color). The authors have defined an "Overlapping Coefficient" to describe overlapping degrees between "Shine" and "Chroma," the scalar product of the shine distribution and the chroma distribution. They have observed that the overlapping coefficient increases after specific cosmetic treatments and the treated hair demonstrated correspondingly shiner and richer color. Based on these observations and the established interaction mechanism between hair fiber and the light, a new parameter called "Hair Vibrancy Factor (HCVF)" is defined to describe shine and color intensity. Figure 4 shows the hair vibrancy factor measured on auburn-colored hair swatches after treatment with two hair-shine sprays using SAMBA.

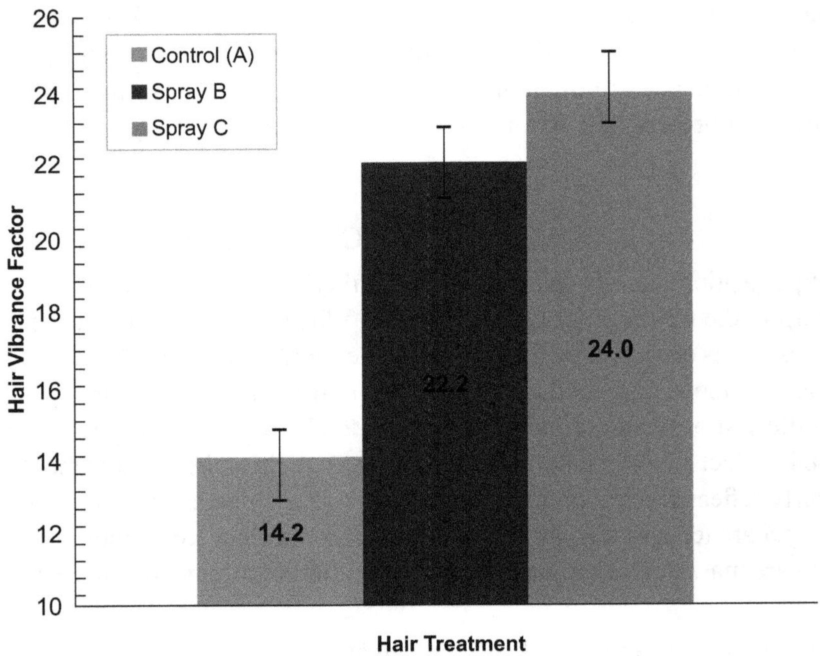

Figure 4. HCVF values of various hair samples measured using SAMBA

6.15.6 REMEDIES FOR COLOR PROTECTION, VIBRANCY, AND SHINE

The color-treated hair structure has a unique set of needs and characteristics. Dry hair that feels like straw and a dull, drab appearance are common complaints among those with color-treated hair. During oxidative hair coloring, the chemicals can also penetrate deep into color-treated hair and change the internal structure. Hair-strengthening proteins are attacked and porosity also increases, affecting hair's ability to hold the color molecules within the fiber. This leads to weaker hair that is more susceptible to hair-color fade. Red hair is especially susceptible to color fade, as the intense red pigments are the smallest and easily escape from a porous hair structure. Color-treated hair needs specialized care, so shampoos with gentle cleansing that protects the integrity of the color while still removing dirt, styling aids, and excess oils should be used. Damaged hair lacks moisture, so color-treated hair shampoos also infuse fresh hydration to help rejuvenate the hair's natural moisture. This grouping of products is further broken down into specialized formulas that provide additional capabilities, such as adding volume, protecting against UV damage, preserving color, enhancing color, augmenting highlights, and correcting tone.

Many color-safe shampoos and conditioners, particularly those that are geared toward a certain shade of hair color, will contain small bits of color and color enhancers to give your hair color a refreshed look after washing. They are wonderful for slowing the color-fading process. In addition to a good, color-safe shampoo and conditioner, you should select supporting daily products that contain sunscreens and light oils. Keep your hair thoroughly moisturized using conditioners that are specifically designed to address the needs of color-treated hair. Regular conditioning goes a long way toward preserving hair color and keeping the hair radiant.

Finally, use finishing products like hairsprays, spritzes, mousses, and gels sparingly. The alcohols used in these style-setting products are used to help your hair dry faster in your style, but can fade your hair color prematurely. Some have also reported that volumizing product lines, or those for fine hair, also fade new hair colors quickly because they allow a slight lifting of the cuticle layers to provide the illusion of increased hair-shaft thickness.

6.15.7 INGREDIENTS AND PRODUCTS FOR COLOR-TREATED HAIR

Ingredients for color protection, shine, and vibrancy include the well-established ones such as: silicones for color protection and shine, quaternary ammonium compounds for ease of combing, and conditioning and vegetable oils for shine. Formulating shampoos and conditioners with just 2% of Dow Corning's CE-8411 nonionic silicone emulsion provide color protection benefits, enhance hair shine, and help prevent hair breakage. Many ingredients are recently launched to address hair and scalp aging at the cellular level, improve follicle health, reduce hair loss, and offer antioxidant properties.

Natural vegetable oils provide nourishing conditioning and shine to hair. Coconut oil, being a triglyceride of lauric acid (principal fatty acid), has a high affinity for hair proteins and, because of its low molecular weight and straight linear chain, is able to penetrate inside the hair shaft.[21] Avocado and Jojoba oil are other oils for nourishing, conditioning, and shine benefits. Sunscreens are another category of ingredients now found in a variety of hair care products, including shampoos, conditioners, and hairsprays. They prevent breakdown of keratin due to sun exposure and also keep hair dye from fading in ultraviolet light. Ingredients like Crodasorb™ UV-HPP from Croda and PARSOL® SLX provide multiple benefits like prevention of color fading, strengthening hair, and enhancing gloss when delivered through hair color, or hair care products, especially leave-on sprays. Table 1 below lists some advanced functional hair care ingredients for color protection and shine popular in today's hair care market.

Table 1. Advanced hair care ingredients used for color protection and shine

Hair Care Ingredients	Benefits	Supplier
ABIL® UV Quat 50	Efficient protection of hair color against fading in sun light. Protection of fiber integrity against damage by V irradiation.	Evonik
Linseed Oil™	Linseed Oil provides hair-color protection and radiant shine to color-treated hair.	Textron
ChromAveil ®	Protects the hair from the damaging effects of sunlight. Gives color protection benefits to dyed hair from UVA and protects the mechanical properties of the hair from UVB.	Croda Inc.
Crodasorb™ UV-HPP	Polyester polyquaternized ingredient that is substantive to hair and protects against the damaging effects of UV-B radiation	Croda Inc.
Lustreplex®	Creates lustrous, healthy looking hair from anionic systems. Provides frizz control, shine, detangling, and conditioning benefits.	Croda Inc.
Dow Corning® CE-8411 Smooth Plus Emulsion	Repair colored, gray, and heat-damaged hair by restoring moisturized feel, shine, & alignment. Protects hair from further damage and color loss.	Dow Corning
Dow Corning® 5-7113 Silicone Quat Microemulsion	Restore smoothness, shine and Alignment. Prolong hair color. Protects hair from breakage.	Dow Corning
Coconut Oil	Provides conditioning, smoothness, and vibrant shine to color-treated hair.	Natural Sourcing
PARSOL® SLX	PARSOL® SLX is a silicone-based UV-B absorber delivers multiple benefits including prevention of color fading, gloss enhancement, and conditioning.	DSM

The hair care market is overloaded with products specifically designed to care for color-treated hair and protect the color from fading, so color can last longer. Redken has launched Color Extend, a collection of four products—shampoo, conditioner, treatment, and color protection—for complete care of color-treated hair. Shampoo for color-treated hair protects hair color from fading and provides UVA/UVB ray protection. Conditioner resurfaces the cuticle for a smooth, vibrant finish and helps with color retention; anti-fade protection maximizes color vibrancy and strengthens hair.

Protective treatment provides deep conditioning to leave hair manageable and vibrant. Specially formulated to provide stronger protection to extend life of hair color, this treatment for color-treated hair uses Fade Resist Complex with UVA & UVB filters to help lock in color and block out aggressors. Hair-color protection spray delivers anti-fade color protection and cuticle reinforcement to maintain color vibrancy and shine.

Pantene has recently launched a range of seven products for color-treated hair, Smooth Shampoo & Conditioner, Volume Shampoo & Conditioner, Color Seal Concentrate, two-minute Damage Rescue Treatment, and Instant Nourishing Shine Spray. The active formula in this shampoo helps to preserve the color for long-lasting brilliance. The active formula in this shampoo helps to preserve the color for long-lasting brilliance. This hair-moisturizing shampoo cleanses your hair while also infusing it with hydration. It features special moisturizers that build a layer around the hair fibers to protect hair from damage and color loss. Shampooing with the Pantene shampoo will add vibrancy and volume to color-treated hair.

6.15.8 CONCLUSIONS

Consumer demand for high-performance, vibrant and fashion-oriented, yet natural-locking hair colorants continues to grow. The global increase in hair-color products raises the need for color care products in the market. The number of hair care products specifically designed to address such needs of color-treated hair is steadily increasing and products claiming long-lasting color, shine, and color enhancement continue to increase. Rinse-off products such as shampoos and conditioners dominate the market and typically contain ingredients that emphasize the benefits of moisture retention, deposition of protective films on hair surface, and protection of color from sun fading using UV filters. Leave-on products, on the other hand, emphasize ingredients that serve to seal hair through deposition of polymers. Both formulation strategies address consumers who want to maintain the vitality of natural-looking hair following hair color. Despite the improvements made on color protection using specialized hair care products containing silicones, vegetable oils, and cationic polymers, a complete color protection is still far from reality. This is due to the fact that color loss, and loss in shine and vibrancy, are linked to hair damage and the majority of hair-color products in the market induce hair damage during the hair-coloring process. Over the years, hair-color product manufacturers have continually improved hair-color formulations to minimize hair damage. A complete damage-free hair color remains as a dream despite of the technological advancements. Regular use of color-treated hair care products significantly improves the appearance of color-treated hair, providing shine and vibrancy, and it prolongs the life color by 40–50%. This chapter provides an overview of the fundamentals of hair coloring, the factors influencing hair fading, and finally a compilation of some hair ingredients and color-protection products currently available in the market.

REFERENCES

Abil Quat. H.I. Leidreiter, U.Kortemeier, U.Maczkiewitz, M.Pascaly, Protection of Hair Fiber Appearance and Strength against UV-Damage, Proc of 23rd. IFSCC Congress (2004).

S. Herrwerth, I. Ulrich-Brehm, U. Kortemeier, P. Winter, M. Ferenz, B. Grüning, Silicone Quaternium-22: New Silicone Technology for Premium Hair Conditioning with Additional Benefits, SOFW J, 2009, 6, 11–18.

PART 6.16

REACTIVE HAIR PRODUCTS

Author
Charles Warren

TABLE OF CONTENTS

Reactive hair care products are those products that chemically react with or in the hair to provide a desired effect. These products are hair colors, bleaches, relaxers/straighteners, and permanent waves.

6.16.1 COLORS

Temporary Hair Colors

There are generally two types of products in this category: hair cosmetics and temporary stains.

Hair cosmetics are generally suspensions of colored pigments (e.g., iron oxides) and/or tinted glitter particles in an aqueous or hydroalcoholic solution containing holding resins (e.g., VP/VA copolymer). These formulas are applied directly to the hair and upon drying provide visual effects—"color" or "sparkle," depending on the formulation. The pigments/glitter are actually incorporated in the film on the hair and, therefore, can be easily removed by breaking the film and brushing the particulate out or by simply washing the hair to remove the film and the particulate.

"6 Wash" Colors

Temporary stains are actually mixtures of direct colors (i.e., the color molecules are the color they will remain) applied to the hair to stain the exterior (cuticle) with minimal penetration to the cortex. These "direct dyes" are usually applied in a shampoo or shampoo-like solution and can be simply washed in (color-enhancing shampoos) or applied and left on the hair for a period of time to achieve the depth and color desired. Color-enhancing shampoos provide minimal "gray" coverage and are used primarily to refresh existing color. Temporary colors (referred to as "6 Wash Colors") provide coverage to gray that is less than 10% of the whole hair volume and will remain on the hair for approximately six washes. Each washing or wetting of the hair will remove some of the stain, so care must be taken that the dyes are removed in a similar fashion so that the color remains as true as possible.

"Demi"-Permanent (non-ammoniacal, 12 wash colors)

Demi-permanent hair colors are two component colors. The first component, the color solution, is an aqueous mixtures of traditional hair-dye intermediates (e.g., paraphenylenediamine or PPD), monethanolamine (MEA), surfactants, and additives. The mixture of the dye intermediates is critical to the development of the desired colors and is very similar to the standard permanent hair-color mixtures. The MEA makes the solution slightly alkaline to assist with the color development when mixed with the developer.

The second component, the developer, is an aqueous solution of hydrogen peroxide (generally, 3–6%).

When mixed together, the MEA helps make the hydrogen peroxide more reactive with the dye intermediates to develop the highly colored polymerized color molecules that ultimately are the desired color. The MEA also serves to swell the hair and allow permeation of the developing color polymers into the subcuticular layers of the hair. Because the hydrogen peroxide is at a relatively low concentration and the MEA only slightly raises the pH (7–8), this coloring process results in little, if any, bleaching of the native hair color—thus, the "tone-on-tone" nomenclature for these type colors. Demi-permanent colors will not allow for a shade lighter than the starting shade. Demi-permanent colors will last for 12–20 shampoos and will provide coverage of gray hair that is less than 25–30% of the total hair volume.

Because demi-permanent hair colors function at lower pH and lower peroxide levels, there is relatively little damage to the hair. This category of hair color has seen the largest share of growth in the consumer market over the past 20 years.

Permanent Colors

Similar to the demi-permanent colors, the permanent color products are two component systems: the color solution and the developer solution.

The color solution is an aqueous mixture of reactive dye intermediates (e.g., PPD), ammonia, and additives. As in the demi-permanent colors, it is the mixture (quantities and types of intermediates) that yields the ultimate final color. The pH of this color solution is usually around 9, one of the significant differences between demi- and permanent colors.

The developer solution is an aqueous solution of hydrogen peroxide. The peroxide content of the developer solution can vary from 6% to 12%. There are some higher peroxide level developers, but those are predominantly only in the professional salon market and relatively few in number. Peroxides are also referred to by "volume" of oxygen delivered. For practical purposes, 6% = 20 volume, 9% = 30 volume, and 12% = 40 volume. In the retail market, 6% is the most common peroxide level.

When the two components are combined, the peroxide becomes extremely reactive and quickly initiates polymerization of the dye intermediates and, simultaneously, the bleaching of the native color. The high pH of the mixture swells the hair and allows the dye intermediates and peroxide to quickly penetrate throughout the hair shaft. The highly colored, polymerized dyes become too large to leave the hair and therefore replace the color of the hair. The higher the level of peroxide used will dictate the degree of bleaching that will be accomplished. Permanent hair coloring can lighten the hair significantly and can result in significant color change. These colors are durable and will usually last six weeks or through 24–30 wash cycles. By this time in the process, root growth has become the factor that usually requires the re-colorization process.

Permanent hair coloring is the most damaging of all of the additive coloring processes. This damage can be ameliorated by using a "conditioning" base, or a special conditioning treatment for post-coloring application.

6.16.2 BLEACHES

Bleaching is the process by which the native melanin in the hair is partially or completely destroyed, leaving the hair slightly to radically lighter than the starting point. Highlighting is the bleaching of selected portions of the hair to create a mixture of light and darker hair throughout the entire coiffure. Multiple techniques of application are used to create multiple effects, but the fundamental destruction of native melanin remains the same.

Bleaching can be accomplished by mixing an aqueous, ammonia (ph = 9–10), surfactant solution with 6%–12% hydrogen peroxide and monitoring the color removal until the desired shade is attained. Bleach powders, blends of highly reactive peroxydisulfates (sodium, potassium, and ammonium salts), can be mixed with peroxide to provide faster and more complete melanin destruction. Bleach oils, mixtures of lipoidal materials, and surfactants can also be employed to provide easier spreading throughout the hair and easier removal once the desired shade is attained.

Due to the high pH and high levels of peroxide (which not only destroys melanin, but can oxidize the inherent protein comprising hair), bleaching is one of the most damaging processes done on the hair. The hair is left in a weaker state and is therefore subject to more dryness and breakage than before the bleaching operation. Overbleaching, resulting from too high a level of bleaching or repeated bleach processing to the same hair, can and will result in breakage.

6.16.3 STRAIGHTENERS

Hair straightening has existed since the time of the ancient Egyptians. Extremely kinky, curly hair (e.g., Afro-Caribbean hair) or highly curly hair (e.g., European hair) can be very difficult to manage and style. Straighteners have been developed to release the natural curl of the hair and leave it more amenable to traditional styling.

Relaxers

The use of alkaline material to straighten curly/kinky hair has been documented from the time of the ancient Egyptian dynasties when women at court applied mud mixed with ash to the hair and left in place until the desired straightness was achieved. Today's relaxers are technically superior, but apply the same basic chemical principles.

The backbone of all human hair, the reason that hair has its configuration, tensile strength, elasticity, etc. is attributed primarily to the cystine (-S-S-) cross-linked bonds throughout the hair. Clearly to change the configuration of the hair, these bonds need to be altered. Highly alkaline conditions can convert the cystine linkages (-S-S-) to lanthionine linkages (-S-) while the hair is being mechanically placed into a new configuration.

As indicated, relaxing hair is both a chemical and mechanical process. The cystine bonds must be broken (chemical) and the hair must be placed and held in a new configuration (mechanical) until the new lanthionine bonds (chemical) are reformed, keeping the hair in its new configuration.

Sodium hydroxide (also known as lye) is one of the oldest alkaline agents used to straighten hair. At a concentration between 1.8% and 2.1%, sodium hydroxide–containing relaxers can effectively straighten hair to a level of manageability 15–20 minutes. The earliest versions of relaxers were simply lye (NaOH) mixed in with a thick animal fat (e.g., lard). Subsequent versions became more sophisticated, but still required a step called "basing," wherein a layer of non-lye-containing grease was placed as a protective barrier on the scalp and on the skin around the hairline. Modern relaxers do not require this "basing" step and are therefore referred to as "No-Base" relaxers.

The modern alkali relaxer is a mixture of an aqueous phase containing the alkali ingredient (sodium hydroxide, potassium hydroxide, or lithium hydroxide), propylene glycol, and other water-soluble ingredients and an oil-phase-containing petrolatum, mineral oil, and fatty alcohols held together in a slightly stable emulsion by an emulsifier. The oil phase is mixed and then the aqueous phase is added. The mixture is mixed hot until semi-emulsified and then cooled. As it cools the non-emulsified petrolatum thickens along with the emulsion and serves to physically hold the entire mixture together. The resultant mixture can best be described as a dual emulsion (part oil-in-water and part water-in-oil). This quasi-emulsion is by design so that when applied and worked through the hair, both oil and water containing the alkali will be released onto the hair to accomplish the chemical breakage of the cystine bonds. The thickness of the petrolatum helps hold the hair straight while the lanthionization process is completed and hair is chemically held in a new straighter configuration. When the desired straightness is attained the mixture is rinsed out and washed out with an acidic shampoo to neutralize any remaining alkali.

Alkali relaxation is damaging to the hair and is corrosive to skin if allowed to remain in contact for too long a period. Overrelaxation can result in immediate hair breakage or significant hair breakage over a short period after the process. Skin damage can result in mild edema or significant burning if contact time is prolonged. Once successfully completed, the hair requires conditioning and addition of significant levels of oil to remain soft, pliable, and have a pleasing appearance. Regrowth will still be kinky/curly and is usually the driving force for a new application (new growth only) in four to six weeks.

In the 1970s the modern consumer "no lye" relaxer was developed. These relaxers are two component relaxers. The relaxer crème is simply the oil phase (quasi-emulsified), similar to the alkali relaxer in which is suspended relatively insoluble calcium hydroxide particles. The activator is an aqueous solution of guanidine carbonate. When the two components are mixed immediately before application, guanidine hydroxide is formed, which chemically performs exactly like the alkali relaxers, creating the new lanthionine linkage in the new configuration. This process is slower than a straight alkali relaxer, as it takes time for the guanidine hydroxide to form and react with the cystine in the hair. This lower reactivity makes the relaxer less potentially damaging to the hair and scalp and is the main reason that most relaxers sold at the retail, use-at-home level are of this type. However, the potential safety issues are still there and hair breakage and skin damage are still possible. The opportunity to prevent these negative occurrences is greater with this type of relaxer. Thorough rinsing and shampoo with an acidic shampoo is still required. Guanidine hydroxide is unstable and will decompose in a matter of hours, so the mixed relaxer must be used immediately and disposed when process is complete.

Relaxers based on conventional reducing agents (thioglycolates and bisulfites) have been marketed. These relaxers are based on the reduction of the cystine bonds by the reducing substance, mechanical reconfiguration of hair, and subsequent reformation of the cystine bonds by the use of hydrogen peroxide (with thioglycolate) or alkaline shampoo (with bisulfate). The reducing agent is generally in an aqueous gel form, applied to the hair, combed straight and then placed under moderate heat. The reducing solution is then rinsed and followed with the neutralization step, an aqueous solution of hydrogen peroxide 2–3% or an alkaline shampoo (pH 8). These reducing relaxers are not as effective on kinky, curly hair and moderately effective on curly wavy hair.

The "Japanese" straightening system employs a reducing solution followed immediately by pressing the hair in a hot flat iron in thin sections. Peroxide neutralization follows. This system is highly effective but requires significant time and operator expertise.

The most recent relaxer/straightening system is the "Brazilian" or "Keratin" straightening system. This system is an aqueous solution of hydrolyzed keratin and a significant quantity of formaldehyde or formaldehyde precursor chemicals. When heat is applied via hot flat iron, the resultant formaldehyde cross-links the protein and holds it in the new, straighter configuration. While highly effective in straightening and retaining hair in straight configuration, formaldehyde has significant safety issues, especially in the gaseous form, created when the hot flat irons are used.

Blow Dry Lotions

Straightening lotions, creams, gels used with blow dryers are generally mixtures of high-molecular-weight silicones that allow the hair to be continually brushed while heat is applied via a blow dryer. This approach will straighten moderately curly hair, but the effect is temporary and highly susceptible to reversion of the hydrogen bonds from applied water or environmental humidity.

A SURVEY OF TEST METHODOLOGY USED IN EVALUATING THE DAMAGE, PROTECTION AND REPAIR OF HAIR

Authors
Ray Rigoletto Sr. Manager, Global R&D Applications Care Specialties: Hair Care; Home Care
Ashland, Inc.

Tim Gillece
Ashland, Inc.
1005 US Hwy No. 202/206 Bridgewater, NJ 08807

ABSTRACT

Human hair is continually exposed to various damaging factors that result in a negative impact on its cosmetic properties. Common sources of hair damage include daily use of shampoo detergents and normal grooming processes. In addition, there are more severe sources of damage. These consist of weathering from the UV-Visible components of sunlight, the action of chemically active hair products (such as oxidative hair dyes, hair relaxers, permanent waves), and the use of thermal styling appliances to create extreme hairstyles.

In order to understand the mechanism of the damaging process, as well as the actions of treatment compositions that protect or repair damaged hair, appropriate test methods need to be employed. These methods allow the study of hair from the macroscopic level (where whole hair attributes are assessed) to the determination of changes at the morphological and molecular levels. This chapter describes frequently used test methods for evaluating fiber damage and demonstrating the efficacy of protective or repair treatment systems.

TABLE OF CONTENTS

11.4.1 INTRODUCTION

"I am under a lot of stress" is a frequently heard complaint. Despite the advanced technology that tries to make our life easier, such as microwave ovens, dishwashers, voice-controlled devices, and the like, we still suffer from too much to do and trying to accomplish it all under a limited time frame. But, semantically speaking, are we actually under stress? Rather, it can be argued that we are being strained. Strain is an outside influence such as an ominous deadline that must be met and stress is our reaction to the applied strain. Some people are frazzled by life's complexities, whereas others can inherently adapt to more strain. Consequently, one's tolerance for internally felt stress is unique to factors such as the current psychological, biochemical, and social states of the individual. We can all relate to this on a human level; but in order to fully relate to the impact of stressors on hair it is imperative to gain an understanding of the physical relationship between stress and strain.

The relationship between stress and strain depends on whether force or distance is used to probe a material. If strain, or deformation of a material, is the mode of action, then stress in the system is the reactionary response. If stress, or force per unit area, is the mode of action, then the degree of strain is the measurable response. A simple model can demonstrate this easily. Take a rubber band and stretch it. The distance, or strain, applied to stretch the rubber changes the way the atoms in the solid are assembled. In reaction, the new physical configuration of the rubber band affects the resistance (i.e., stress response) to the applied deformation. Ultimately, at a critical strain, small irreversible fissures in the rubber begin to form, and applying further strain to the band induces stresses that ultimately cause a catastrophic break in the rubber.

During the course of explaining some of the test methods to determine the mechanical properties of hair, there will be stress-controlling devices that monitor changes in physical dimensions, and strain-controlling devices that measure the stress response of the deformed fiber; however, stress and strain do not have to be mechanical in nature. It is conceivable to expand the definition to include factors such as chemical, thermal, and environmental insult. In analogy, there are different limits to individuals tolerating a polluted city, or to resisting the sweltering heat, and ultraviolet radiation of the summer sun.

The subject of this chapter deals with human hair and the many factors that subject hair to stress. These include the various chemical and thermal treatments applied to hair in order to improve its cosmetic appearance, as well as environmental factors, especially UV radiation from the sun. The integrity and physicochemical state of the hair impacts the resilience of the fiber and its coinciding resistance to stress. Obviously, if the hair is compromised in some way, either chemically or structurally, it will not hold up to subsequent treatments.

An example of stress put upon hair by the strain of environmental conditions is the work done by Ratnapandian et al. where they studied the mechanical properties of hair after exposure to a controlled dose of solar radiation [1]. As reported by the authors (see **Table I**) the hair strength is compromised, as indicated by a positive percent loss in mechanical properties. The increase in the magnitudes of the turnover point (defined in **Table I**) and strain to break, as indicated by a negative percent loss values, actually represents hair weakening since they are due to the breakage of disulfide cross-links that consequently increase the mobility of the molecular chains. A full description of the mechanical properties of a hair fiber from the stress-strain curve and the molecular changes that occur at each stage can be found in Feughelman's treatise on the subject [2].

Table I: Percent loss of mechanical properties of hair with simulated solar radiation (300 hours; 70% RH). Data from Ratnapandian et al. [1].

Mechanical property from stress-strain curve	% Loss
Work to 20% extension	46.51
Stress at 20% strain	43.18
Initial modulus	46.69
Post yield modulus	60.63
Work to break	23.14
Stress to break	49.06
Turnover point*	- 36.54
Strain to break	- 43.14

* The intersection of the yield and post-yield part of the elongation curve; see **Figure 42b**.

In this experiment, the treatment of hair with a controlled time and intensity of solar radiation exposure is an example of straining the fiber, with weathering as the active agent. Also, the measuring device for evaluating the mechanical properties, which in this case is the tensile strength tester, is also a strain-controlling device since the rate of deformation imparted to the hair fiber is held constant.

In order to study the nature of hair damage from the multitude of strains and the consequent stressful factors that it is subjected to, as well as determining the efficacy of ingredients and ultimately products for protection and repair, appropriate test methods need to be employed. This is not a simple task. Hair has a very complex chemical makeup and morphology, and the imparted stresses and strains vary as a result of the type of cosmetic treatment being employed.

This chapter provides an explanation of the nature and utility of methods that are used in the assessment of hair damage, its protection, and repair. Methods are described in enough detail for the cosmetic chemist to utilize them appropriately and to make sound conclusions from the generated data. Sometimes an understanding of the damage mechanisms can be achieved with one method; however, it is prudent to use a combination of methodologies to build a case for proving product efficacy, especially with regard to claim substantiation. Throughout the course of explaining each method, an underlying theme is to keep in mind whether the stress-strain relationship is physical or chemical in nature. With regard to human hair, it will provide a reference for understanding the factors in the degradation of hair, its interaction and response to cosmetic ingredients, and the measurement of these effects with appropriate test methods.

11.4.2 THE NATURE OF HAIR DAMAGE

The major stresses that hair experiences are:

1. Shampoo fatigue—The distal ends of shoulder-length hair could be up to two years old and have gone through literally hundreds of shampoo cycles. Even if a mild shampoo had been used during the course of the lifetime of the hair, the surfactant slowly extracts the lipid of the hair as well as smaller-molecular-weight fractions of protein that are the result of other damaging treatments. This slow erosion of hair compromises its structural integrity over time.
2. Mechanical Damage—Combing or brushing of hair imparts shear stresses within the fiber. As a comb is pulled through a tress in the direction from root to tip, the bending of the hair fibers is also forced to propagate from root to tip. That is, it is a dynamic bend and not a static one. These shear stresses produce fine fractures within the interior of the cortex, which upon further combing, result in either a split end, or worse still, breakage. Compression, tensile, and torsional forces are also present from continual bending and add

to the stresses at work during combing and resultant fracture. The situation of fracture becomes magnified when hair is in the wet state. Hair that is wet is more extendable due to changes in hydrogen bonding between adjoining structural protein elements of the hair. Mechanical stress, such as towel drying or combing out a snag in the wet state, will also cause breakage.

3. Weathering—Sunlight affects hair in several ways. Light of shorter wavelengths and higher energy, designated as UVB, degrades disulfide bonds as well as structural components of the hair such as the lipids of the CMC. Once these are degraded, important hair attributes are compromised, resulting in a decrease in cosmetic effects, including shine and elasticity. The natural pigments of the hair, eumelanin and pheomelanin, defend against this by absorbing UV light and protecting the chemical components of the hair. Hair that is light in color, such as natural blonde or bleached fibers, does not have this natural defense and is more prone to damage.
4. Chemical processing—The chemistry of bleaching, oxidative hair dyeing, permanent waving, and relaxing have been well described in the literature; a recommended reference is by Robbins in *The Chemical and Physical Behavior of Human Hair* [3]. All of these chemical treatments have multiple damaging effects on the structural components of hair. When chemical bonds are broken, functional groups change their character and influence the cosmetic behavior of hair. One example is the removal of the lipid layer from the surface of hair, which is essential for important hair attributes. Another is the formation of cysteic acid groups, which makes hair more hydrophilic, and decreases hair characteristics such as detangling and hair manageability. Many other examples can be cited based on the varied chemical components of the hair.
5. Thermal Styling—Styling appliances configure hair through both mechanical manipulation and heat. Examples of these include curling irons and flat irons. It will be shown in this chapter that the excessive heat induced by these appliances tends to denature structural proteins in the cortex and cuticle of the hair. Although this treatment initially imparts attractive cosmetic effects, with continued use the hair becomes less manageable and suffers from a decrease in its cosmetic appeal. The result is that the consumer has to use intensive conditioning treatments to conceal the damage.
6. Thermal/mechanical (wet to dry styling)—After adding a styling gel or cream to damp hair, it is usually styled with a round brush and blow dryer. The subsequent insult is not only from the heat of the blow dryer, but also from the brushing process. Combing and brushing are damaging to dry hair, but when hair is wet, it is in a weakened state and is more prone to breakage during combing. If the styling product goes through a tack phase, brushing becomes very difficult and results in a large extent of breakage.

Damage imparted to hair can range from the molecular level, to the subassemblies of the fiber. The deterioration alters the complex structure of proteins in the microfibrils of the cortex and extends to macroscopic structures, including the cuticle and cortical cells. There are test methods appropriate for studying hair damage at each level. The ultimate level is observing changes in damage impacting whole hair attributes, where many fibers interact as an assembly. Cosmetically acceptable attributes from fiber interaction include, for example, curl definition, body, and shine; whereas the damage state exhibits a host of negative attributes including frizziness, poor comb through, and dullness.

Unfortunately, the state of hair is a bleak one since it cannot renew itself. As the dead fiber suffers more and more stress, there is a vicious downward trend until the fiber fractures and breaks. Since hair grows from the scalp, the hair's age increases along the fiber from root to tip so that the tips usually have the highest degree of damage. As hair is combed, the shear stresses imparted to the hair will be most destructive to the ends, with the result that the ends will fracture or produce split ends. Therefore, a fiber's ability to respond to multiple stresses depends on its current level of damage. Another factor is the morphology of hair. Since hair is a biological outgrowth of the expression of a person's genes, each individual then has a different hair type. In general, hair can be categorized by racial descent so that Asian hair is characterized by a larger diameter, and Caucasian hair is generally finer. Of course there is overlap of hair types between the races, but it can be concluded that morphological differences allow hair to be more or less hardy in its ability to handle the stress of damaging treatments. For example, during the use of a curling appliance, the thermostat has to be put on high to "curl-up" the larger diameter of Asian hair.

If hair was a living structure, then certain treatments may rejuvenate the broken structures so that hair can revert to its undamaged natural state, such as when it first emerges from the follicle. Unfortunately, this strategy cannot be employed and consumers resort to treatments that condition, protect, and what is more challenging, repair damaged hair so that they can continue with their usual styling behaviors. Some of these treatments are cosmetic and temporary in that the results from the treatment are usually washed away in a subsequent shampooing. Protective treatments help hair to take the insult of aggressive styling processes, such as hot flat ironing, so that damage is alleviated and the breakage of hair is postponed to a later date. But again, based on the dead nature of hair, its fate is sealed; ultimately there will come a day when the hair fiber will break.

Luckily, from a biological standpoint, there is hope. Each fiber is constantly renewing itself by generating new hair inside the follicle. Those follicles that are most active, those that are in the anagen phase, are producing keratin cells that mature in the follicular canal and then emerge from the scalp in its natural undamaged state, only to be cast into the world to suffer the stresses and strains of wear and tear.

11.4.3 SIMULATING DAMAGING HAIR TREATMENTS FOR STUDYING THE ALLEVIATING EFFECTS OF PROTECTIVE AND REPAIR INGREDIENTS

The manner in which hair is artificially damaged, and with respect to what has been described above, imparting a controlled strain on hair, depends on the particular objective of the experiment. Once the goal of the experiment has been established, then the scientist designs the experiment to maintain control of important variables. For example, some variables are held constant and one or more variables are purposely manipulated with the primary intent of determining effects.

a. Treatment Schedules

For each of the stresses that hair suffers from, a treatment can be designed to simulate the stress. These are usually performed on hair tresses of a particular configuration and hair type, such as fine or bleached fibers, for example. These treatments can be termed treatment regimen because the tress is purposely exposed to successive treatments that simulate what a consumer would do in real life. A simple example would be to wash and dry a hair tress with a shampoo to determine the damaging effects of the surfactant after multiple washes. Damage can be assessed periodically during the course of washing using, for example, a Scanning Electron Microscope to determine the state of the cuticle. Also, contact angle measurements with a tensiometer will indicate to what extent the protective lipid layer of the hair was extracted by the detergent of the shampoo. More complicated treatment regimens have been designed to study the effects of other strains on hair. Several examples from the literature will follow that have been utilized for assessing the effects of UV degradation by sunlight, thermal effects from appliances, color wash-fastness of permanently dyed hair from multiple washing cycles, and mechanical fatigue. These will serve as examples to demonstrate how to design a treatment regimen to study the effects of the key variables under study. These should not be considered as standard procedures, but as part of the experimental design to control and manipulate variables to determine effects.

1. Thermal Exposure

Hot flat irons that are used to produce a straight style can reach temperatures of up to 450°F. The styling procedure consists of taking about an inch-wide section of hair and applying the hot iron close to the root section and moving the iron from root to tip without hesitating. This procedure is continued until all of the hair on the head is treated. The thermal insult to hair can be done on hair tresses in order to run controlled experiments. A treatment regimen can consist of first washing and then treating the hair with a pretreatment to study its effect on alleviating the damage incurred to the hair from the hot ironing process. After the hair is dry, the hot flat iron is heated to a specified temperature. Then, in a controlled fashion, the iron is applied to the root section of the hair and moved down to the tip in a specified length of time. This is repeated a number of times to achieve a total time of heat exposure. Intermittent shampooing and re-treating with the experimental composition can be done as well. Measurements are taken initially, during the course of the treatment regimen, and then at it end. Alleviating damage of the hair due to the experimental composition can be determined by comparing results versus an appropriate control. A treatment regiment is illustrated in **Figure 1** that was utilized by Zhou et al. to study the thermal-protective effects of polymeric pretreatments and their alleviation of hair damage resulting from the hot ironing process. Methods utilized, which will be described in more detail in a subsequent section of this chapter, were Differential Scanning Calormetry (DSC), a specialized anti-breakage method, microscopic techniques, FTIR spectroscopic imaging, Dynamic Vapor Sorption (DVS), and thermal image analysis [4]. Results from this work indicated that several synthetically derived polymers were effective in thermal protection, especially those that were hydrophobically modified.

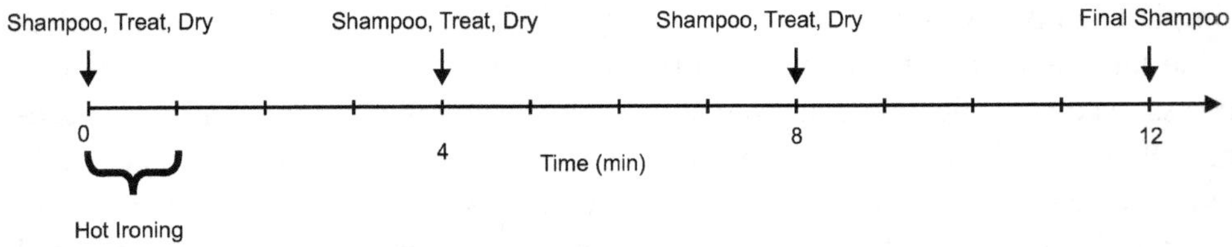

Figure 1: Treatment regimen used in the thermal insult of hair tress to study thermal damage and effects of protective pretreatments.

A similar treatment regimen was designed by McMullen and Jachowicz [5] in their efforts to study the effects on alleviating the damage to hair from curling irons. Again, the methodology consisted of exposing the hair to the heat from the curling irons for periods of time with intermittent shampooing and re-treating with the protective composition. However, in this case the mode of exposure of the curling iron was different than that of a flat iron in that the curling iron was clamped onto one section of the hair for a specific period of time. The window of exposure was then assessed to show the damaging effects of the heat as well as the alleviating effect of the pretreatment composition. This was accomplished by detecting a reduction in combing forces as tested through a mechanical combing device, and a reduction in the level of Tryptophan, an indicator of hair damage, by spectrofluorimetry.

There are many manually operated parts of the hot ironing process that are a source of variability in thermal treatment regimens. Maintaining a constant rate of descent of the hot iron from the root to the distal part of the tress is very difficult, especially if the polymer treatment on the hair creates a drag for the iron. The tension that the operator applies when pressing the plates of the iron against the bundle of fibers is a compound variable. As the operator uses more force to press the jaws of the iron against the fiber bundle, more force is applied to pull the iron down the tress to keep the rate of descent constant. This results in the fibers being stretched longitudinally. To control and monitor these variables, an automated apparatus was designed by Dussaud [6]. It consists of a tress mounted on the arm of a texture analyzer so that the rate of movement of the tress in relation to the hot flat iron is controlled. The two plates of the iron are brought into contact with the bundle of fibers and the tension is monitored by a force sensor. The stretching force is kept constant, as measured by the texture analyzer, by applying a certain contact force of the iron jaws against the hair. Hair temperature is monitored by the use of an infrared thermometer. Measurements by Dussaud after controlled thermal treatments with this automated apparatus included DSC, wet elasticity, and birefringence [6]. From this study, interesting conclusions on the permanent straightening of curly hair are described.

2. UV Exposure

References in the literature indicate that solar exposure degrades various components of the hair. These changes affect lipid components [7] and proteins [8]. Other aspects of the photodegradation process include understanding the role of melanin [9] in photoprotection, as well as other variables including moisture [1] content, and the degree of damage through processes such as bleaching, perming, and dyeing with an oxidative hair color [10].

A key piece of equipment requisite to performing a UV exposure study is a solar simulator. One could subject hair tresses to natural sunlight; however, variations in cloud cover, sun angle due to the time of day, as well as change of season, puts many obstacles into performing a controlled study. The solar simulator allows the experimenter to control important variables such as light intensity, wavelength, temperature, and humidity. The simulator consists of a light source such as a Xenon lamp, a filter that will subject the hair to a particular part of the electromagnetic spectrum, and a chamber that can control temperature and preferably humidity as well. The filter will allow simulation of normal daylight, or in more refined studies allow just certain bands of UV light to impinge on the hair such as UVA, UVB, or a combination of both.

As with thermal degradation, photodegradation studies also follow a treatment schedule. The experimenter will shampoo and pretreat the hair with a protective composition and then expose the hair for a certain length of time while keeping necessary variables, such as temperature, humidity, wavelength, and radiation intensity, held constant. The treatment and exposure cycles are usually repeated to represent the most practical consumer use conditions. In this way Locke studied the effect of a substantive UV photofilter by treating tresses with a protective composition and then putting the tresses into a sample holder that had an exposure window. Tresses were treated and exposed for eight hours. This was repeated for a total of 32 hours of exposure. Exposure consisted of placing tresses in a weatherometer that had the irradiation adjusted to simulate the same intensity of sunlight found during the day in Florida in April. Measurements were taken in the exposed and unexposed regions of the tress to determine and compare the degree of photodegradation and resultant protection by the UV photofilter. Measurements in reduction in combing and tryptophan degradation were conducted [11].

There are many references to help the experimenter with designing a protocol for study. One is by Signori where the author reviews the current understanding of the effects of ultraviolet and visible radiation on hair structure and options for photoprotection. Among some of her advice, she mentions that correlating the length and intensity of the simulated light to real-world conditions is an important factor to consider [12]. Also, many questions can be answered by referring to one of the manufacturers of the solar simulator [13].

3. Color Wash-fastness Techniques

Peroxide containing oxidative hair color is designed to "lift" the natural color of the hair and at the same time react dye intermediates inside of the hair. The intentions of this process are primarily for covering gray and/or changing one's natural color from brown, for example, to red. Although these products are termed permanent, a certain amount of fading takes place due to continuous cycles of washing and conditioning. Primarily, this is due to the surfactants used in these products that tend to slowly leach the water-soluble artificial pigment or dye out of the hair. This results in a change in both the intensity and hue of the hair, which is unacceptable for a consumer. Many products on the market consequently claim retention of the vibrancy of color with the use of protective ingredients.

To design a treatment regimen to test for color wash-fastness, hair tresses are typically first dyed and then cycled with a regimen of products. The regimen consists essentially of a shampoo, and may be followed by a conditioner and leave-in styling/conditioning products. Color measurements are then taken throughout the treatment cycle and measurements are compared to the initial state of the hair. Percent protection of the product in question is determined by comparing to appropriate controls. Such a treatment schedule was utilized to determine the color wash-fastness effect of a hydrophobically modified polymer in a treatment regimen of shampoo, conditioner, and leave-in treatment. In this case, bleached hair was dyed red, a color that is most prone to fading from shampooing, and cycled with a regimen of formulas both with and without the hydrophobic polymer. Results were substantiated with colorimetry measurements and image analysis. More sophisticated methods were used, such as water contact angle and FTIR spectroscopic imaging, to help propose a theoretical mechanism of action of the active ingredient [14].

4. Mechanical and Thermal/Mechanical Damage

Combing imparts mechanical strain to hair, i.e., hair gets stressed by the strain of combing. There are different components to this stress. **Figure 2** illustrates a hair tress being pulled through a comb that is being held stationary under a stereomicroscope. The various strain components are labeled and consist of shear stresses in the internal parts of the hair through dynamic bending, i.e. bending that is propagated from root to tip, longitudinal tension though extension, abrasion, impact loading, compression/expansion through bending, and torsional strain. As **Figure 2** illustrates, the combing process will include all of these strains. Specialized instruments have been designed and employed to isolate and test each component or combination of components of the multiple mechanical stresses that hair is subjected to during grooming to determine their effects on hair damage. The strength of hair, and in the case of cosmetic treatments, the alleviation of weakening of hair with its consequential breakage or reduction in cosmetic attributes, is quantified after a set regimen of specific strains. These strains can be designed to be in a longitudinal (tensile), radial (torsional), or tangential (bending) direction. Abrasion and impacting are other components that have been studied. One complicating factor is that other stresses, such as chemical, UV, and thermal exposure, tends to weaken the hair so that there is a greater propensity to break under mechanical strain. Many treatment schedules found in the literature, therefore, have as their regimen a combination of these stresses imparted to the hair. The application of these stresses as described in the literature will be described in the next section.

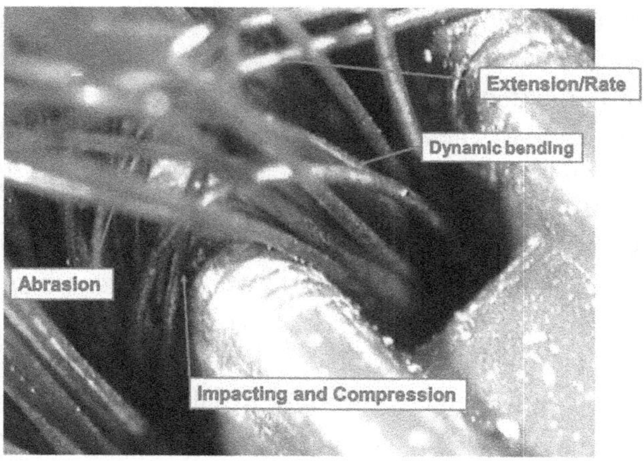

Figure 2: Mechanism of Hair Breakage-Various Stresses During Combing

11.4.4 INTRUMENTATION AND EXPERIMENTAL METHODS IN STUDYING THE DAMAGE AND PROTECTION OF HAIR

a. Physical-Chemical

1. Differential Scanning Calorimetry

Excessive thermal, chemical, weathering, and mechanical strains induce damage to the hair surface as well as the core of the fiber. Whereas surface analysis techniques, such as SEM, ToF-SIMS, and contact angle analysis, are all valuable in corroborating measurable stresses to the quality of the integument surface, thermoanalytical techniques, including Differential Scanning Calorimetry (DSC), may be used to probe the state of the subsurface fiber chemistry, such as the health of the cortical proteins.

The anatomy of a modern computer-controlled DSC instrument includes separate sample and reference holders, as well as vendor-specific cell closures, thermocouples, and gas purge inlets. The two principal types of DSCs are *heat-flow* and *heat-flux* instruments. Heat-flow instruments are based on the double-furnace design developed by Perkin-Elmer in the 1960s [15]. As a material passes through a thermal transition, the instrument uses local temperature readings and a feedback mechanism to ensure that the sample and reference pans are maintained at equivalent temperatures (i.e., $T_S=T_R$); hence, the amounts of power to the sample and reference furnaces are independent and are used to directly measure heat flow in or out of the sample. In heat-flux instruments, a single-furnace simultaneously heats both the reference and sample. Calibrations and temperature flow differences are then used to calculate heat flow during a thermal event (i.e., $T_S \neq T_R$).

In a DSC experiment, the impact of thermal energy on phase transitions, such as melting (T_m) or glass transition (T_g) events, is logged as a function of applied temperature. Heating a sample causes changes in the ability of the material to hold onto thermal energy—where the increase in kinetic energy is distributed to optimize the vibrational, rotational, and translational states of the molecules that define motion within the material. The ability of a material to hold heat, which is called its *heat capacity* (C_p), is subsequently used to monitor excess, or *differential*, heat flow. Depending on the category of the thermal event, excess heat flows to the sample, or from the sample, relative to the empty sample pan. Put another way, to maintain the sample and reference cells at equivalent temperatures in a heat-flow instrument, excess energy is either *added* to (endothermic) or *subtracted* from (exothermic) the sample pan. For example, heating a thermoplastic polymer from subambient to the decomposition temperature will display the T_g and T_m events as endothermic; whereas crystallization and some curing processes appear as exothermic peaks (see **Figure 3**).

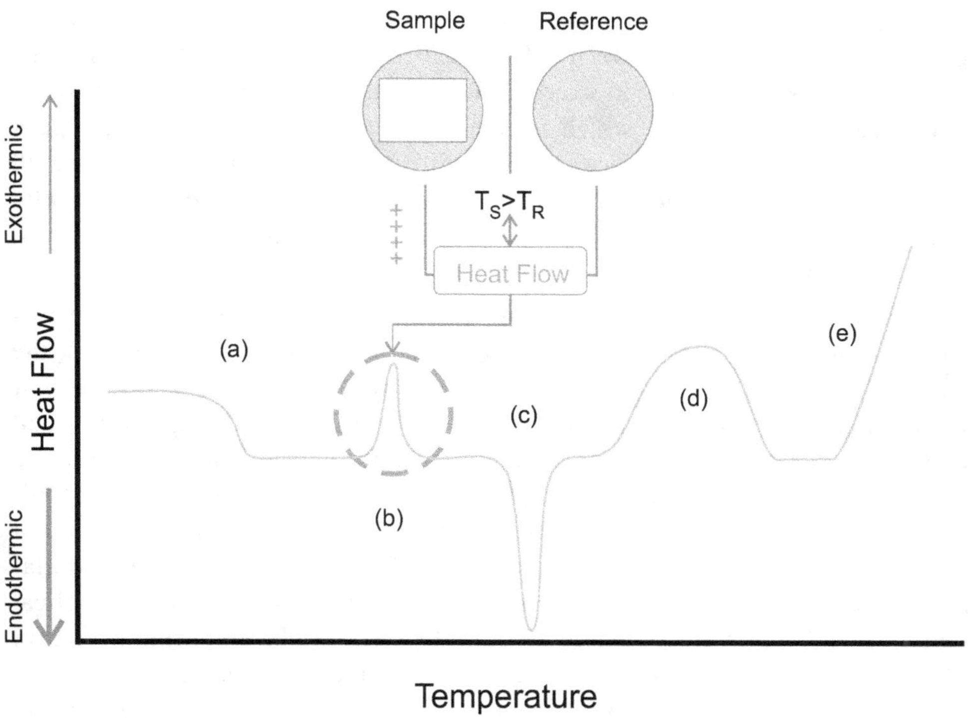

Figure 3: Peaks represent positive or negative heat flow (single-furnace). Characteristic DSC thermal transitions scanned from low to high temperature (exotherm points up): (a) glass transition temperature (T_g); (b) crystallization temperature (T_c); (c) melting temperature (T_m); (d) curing event; (e) thermal decomposition/oxidation (adapted from TA Instruments Thermal Analysis brochure, US).

In contrast to the aforementioned thermogram of a model synthetic thermoplastic, the human hair fiber is a very intricate composite and its intrinsic complexity typically adds intrigue to DSC data interpretation. Complexity aside, because applications of excessive heat, damaging chemicals, mechanical elongation, weathering strains, and combinations of each may alter the matrix cross-link density and/or irreversibly denature the secondary structure of the α-keratin to random coils and β-domains, DSC analyses of the endothermic denaturation temperature and enthalpy transitions are invaluable in quantifying the status of the stressed fiber cortex. That being said, consideration for the morphological complexity of a hair fiber is central in choosing whether to use "dry" or "wet" DSC methodology. In dry methodology, hair snippets are charged into a traditional, nonsealed aluminum DSC pan and water is evolved from the pan as samples are heated to decomposition. As a result, bookkeeping complexities arise as the denaturation (T_D) and decomposition peaks inconveniently overlap into a poorly resolved doublet (between 230 and 250°C). However, the doublet may be happily resolved by testing in excess water and taking advantage of the water-plasticization of the matrix, which conveniently shifts the hair denaturation peak (120–150°) clear of interference from the 250°C pyrolysis peak [16]. This result begs the question: Why does water plasticization—which is a property typically affiliated with amorphous materials—influence the magnitude of T_D for the crystalline α-helix?

The short answer is that water plasticity, in combination with prior chemical alterations, shifts the T_D of the α-helix due to viscoelastic changes in the morphological components of the *fiber composite*. The cortex of human hair is principally compartmentalized into macrofibrils, microfibrils, and the cell membrane complex. Various researchers have further postulated kinetic and physical models to both simplify and relate the fiber chemistry and morphology to water plasticity and/or thermally induced phase changes [16–27]. For example, in Feughelman's two-phase model (**Figure 4**) the intermediate filaments (IFs), or microfibrils, are composed of partially crystalline α-helical keratin bundles that are embedded in a highly cross-linked amorphous matrix [2, 17]. Typically, in most semi-crystalline polymeric materials, water interacts less with crystalline domains and more intrusively with amorphous, hydrophilic moieties; *however*, Wortmann suggests that, in human hair, water *absorbs* into the matrix and *adsorbs* to the periphery of the IFs equally well, meaning that water distributes within the cortex "quasi-homogeneously [18]." Therefore, as *isolated* IFs in hard keratins are soft and pliable when extended in water, it is clear that the surrounding matrix, which is also covalently bound to the IFs, plays a large part in the rigidity of hard keratins [16, 19]. Consequently, the two-phase model conveys that the magnitude of T_D (i.e., thermal stability) for α-keratin is kinetically controlled by the cystine-based crosslink density and the viscosity of the nonhelical *amorphous matrix*, whereas the energy to denature (ΔH_D) correlates with the structural rigidity of the *α-helices* in the IFs [20, 21]. In an augmented interpretation of the two-phase model, Istrate uses a variety of technical arguments to weigh the limitations of the Feughelman model. Instead, a third physical phase is introduced that links chemical changes (i.e., rate limiting S-S scission) in the nonhelical terminal domains of keratin filaments to the thermal stability of the IFs [22]. In a final example, Greenberg et al. studied hard keratins from various sources and concluded that an important function of the matrix is to keep the IFs in a semi-dehydrated state—suggesting that an intact matrix is key to maintaining the mechanical strength and stability of the IFs [19].

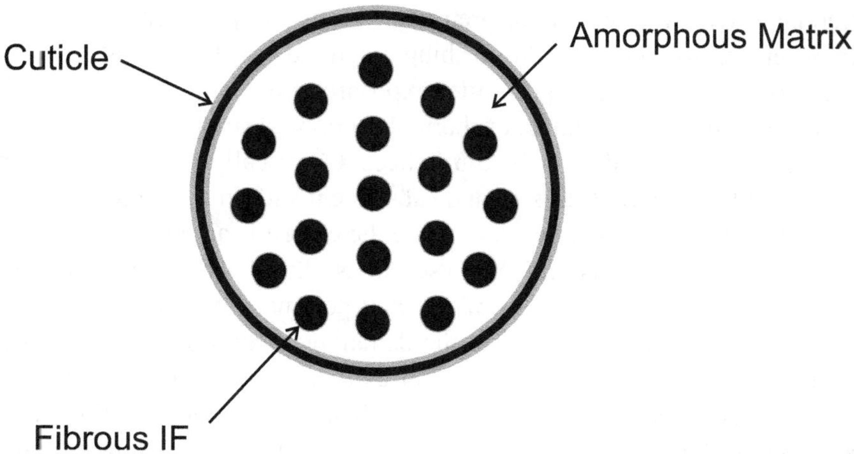

Figure 4: Diagram of a transverse section of hair fiber showing the traditional Feughelman (two-phase) morphological model where the composite fibrous intermediate filament(s) phase is immersed within a highly cross-linked amorphous phase.

As an illustration for the utility of DSC in evaluating cortical damage, **Figure 5** shows the impact of hot flat ironing on virgin and polymer-treated fiber assemblies. The overlay was produced by following the methodology of Wortmann and Deutz [21]. Polymer-treated hair samples were prepared by applying model formulations to hair tresses. The tresses, including a freshly prepared virgin tress, were first blow-dried and next thermally treated with a timed regimen utilizing a high-temperature commercial flat-iron [4]. The virgin and thermally treated hair tresses were sectioned into small snippets and equilibrated at 60% RH overnight to normalize hydration history. Five to ten milligrams of the equilibrated snippets were subsequently charged into stainless-steel, pressure-resistant, large-volume DSC capsules, and 50 µL of water was added to each capsule. After sealing each pan, the hair snippets were hydrated overnight prior to charging into the DSC autosampler. In terms of the robustness/precision of the method, fastidious attention to the preparation protocol is critical to developing data worthy of inter-study (i.e., historical) comparisons. Specifically, art and tedium are intrinsic to the preparation of snippets, and variables such as water quality, heating rate, and application of all pretreatments must be precisely controlled.

Now that the hard part is done, it's time to let the machine earn its keep. Depending on the thermal history, *hydrated hair fibers* characteristically denature between 110 and 150°C; hence, DSC investigations are accomplished by heating samples at 2–5°C/min over the 60–185°C temperature range. For example, thermograms *a* and *e* (**Figure 5**) depict the resultant outcomes of high-pressure DSC scans for wet, untreated virgin, and wet, thermally treated virgin hair snippets, respectively; and curves *b-d* and the trends in **Table 2** show the effects of various commercially available polymeric pretreatments on the preservation of the secondary α-keratin structure. The diminishing magnitudes of the T_D and ΔH_D, which is the area of the endothermic peak after exposure of the hair tresses to the rigors hot flat-ironing, reflect the impact of thermally imposed strains on the integrity of the amorphous matrix and embedded α-helices. Chemically speaking, it has been suggested that the imparted stresses and subsequent shift in T_D are related to a decrease in the matrix crosslink density, where the culprit is an increase in the number of thermally-induced disulfide bond scissions [22, 6]. Additionally, relative to flat-ironed virgin hair, the addition of selected polymeric treatments (e.g., *b* and *c*) to virgin fibers appears to mitigate the damaging effects of excessive thermal insult. Thus, for example, although the precise efficacy mechanism of "thermoprotective additives" is complex and currently debatable, the trends in **Figure 5** and **Table 2** suggest that treatment *b* is more successful than treatment *d* in hindering the irreversible progression of thermally induced α-keratin denaturation.

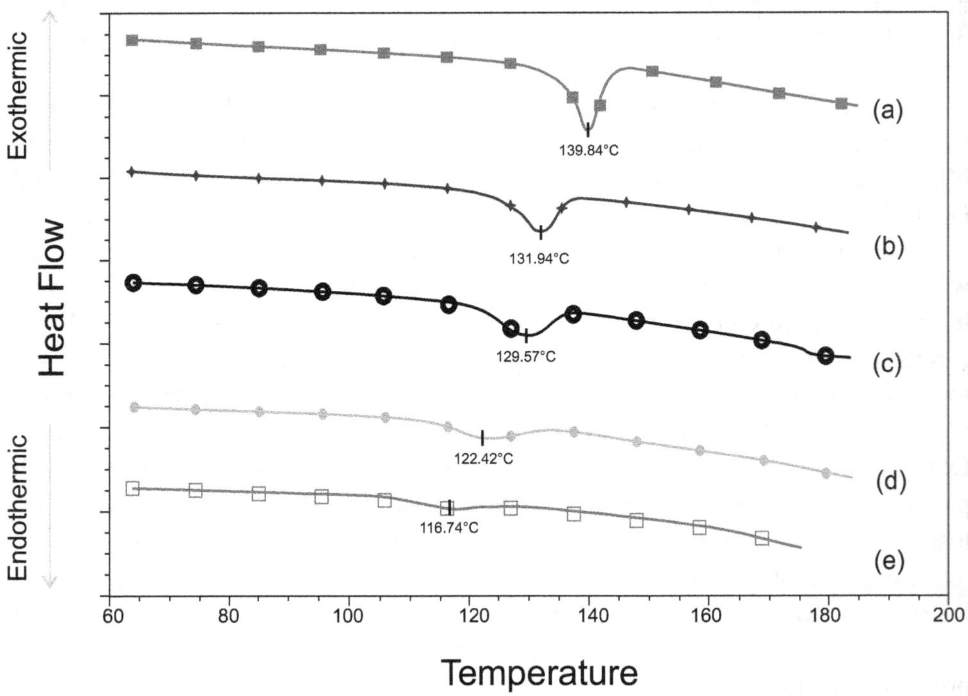

Figure 5: Effect of thermal styling treatment (232°C) on the α-helix melting temperature and associated enthalpy change (offset on *y*-axis for clarity). (a) Profile of untreated virgin hair; (b-c) flat-ironed hair/cationic polymer composites; (d) flat-ironed hair/non-ionic polymer composite; (e) flat-ironed virgin hair. Shifts in the peak minima from higher to lower temperature and decreased peak areas indicate presence of thermomechanically induced cortex damage (courtesy of D. Koelmel, Ashland Specialty Ingredients, US).

Table 2: Effects of thermal treatment on the denaturation temperature and denaturation enthalpy of European Dark Brown Hair

Sample Description	Shift in TD (°C)	ΔHD Loss (%)
Virgin	—	—
Flat-ironed + B-treated	8	22
Flat-ironed + C-treated	10	12
Flat-ironed + D-treated	17	53
Flat-ironed Virgin	23	81

Although thermal damage has been exemplified in portraying the merit of DSC methodology in measuring stresses in the fiber cortex, the influence of chemical [6, 17, 20, 22–26] and weathering strains [27], which also inflict damage to native cortical protein conformations, can also be discerned by DSC analyses. In extension, because the tensile mechanical properties of hair fibers are tied to the structural integrity of the cortex, thermal analysis enables a measurable connection between protein structure, bulk fiber performance, and the inception of novel keratin-preserving prototypes.

2. Surface Tension, Wetting, and Contact Angle Analysis

Interactions of a liquid and hair at the interface may be used to probe the physical and chemical states of the hair surface. The physicochemical state of the hair typically varies with hair length as weathering, cosmetic treatments, aging, and genetic strains induce measurable stresses on the fiber's perimeter [28]. Depending on the extent, type, and location of damage, chemically unique segments of the F-layer, epicuticle, A-layer, exocuticle, endocuticle, cell membrane complex (CMC), and exposed cortex may all contribute to the measurable fiber-fluid interface. For instance, water is a very polar liquid and its wetting interaction with the hair surface depends on the summation of the accessible chemistry of the interface—explicitly, undamaged virgin hair fibers are lipophilic, whereas damaged fibers are on average more hydrophilic. Consequently, depending on the state of the hair, certain fluids tend to spread across the hair with film-like behavior, whereas others will bead on the surface, or form patchy domains on the hair's heterogeneous landscape. Hence, the efficacy and performance of hair-damage repair treatments are affected by the current condition of the fiber, as well as the surface activity of the applied treatment formulation. Specifically, any treatment that lowers the tendency of the applied fluid to form cohesive and spherical droplets will increase the likelihood of that fluid wetting the hair surface. When done carefully, comparative measurements of the contact angle between the applied fluid and different substrates facilitate a description of comparative wetting behavior.

Insights into the likelihood of a fluid spreading across a surface may be gleaned by the parameters of the Gibbs equation (Eq. 1). Ignoring the intimidating squiggles of calculus, one only needs to focus on a couple of variables to see that *surface tension* (γ) is key to wetting a surface—and, via a mental extrapolation, that *wetting* is described by the magnitude of the *contact angle* of a fluid at the solid-liquid interface. The Gibbs equation relates the extent of adsorption of one phase (e.g., water) onto another (e.g., hair fiber) and suggests that a system that reduces the surface tension (γ), such as a surfactant, will have the propensity to be adsorbed onto a surface,

$$\mathbf{\Gamma}_i = - 1/RT\ (\partial\gamma/\partial \ln \mathbf{a}_i)_{T,P} \quad (1)$$

where Γ_i is the surface concentration of the spreading fluid, a_i is the concentration of the adsorbing phase, T is the absolute temperature, and R is the gas constant.

Hence, prior to discussing the importance of contact angle in quantifying wetting processes on hair, it is useful to introduce surface tension, which, by dimensional analysis arguments, is equivalent to the *surface free energy*. As depicted in **Figure 6**, the atoms at the surface of a liquid are in a different environment than those in the bulk. Bulk molecules interact with neighboring molecules equally; however, the molecules at the surface of a liquid may only interact with neighboring surface molecules and with adjacent subsurface molecules. The net result of the asymmetry in attractive forces is that interfacial molecules are pulled inward until molecular collisions with bulk molecules arrest their contraction [29]. The surface is now analogous to a tight skin covering the bulk fluid, and the tight skin of the contracted interface requires energy to penetrate it or to extend its area. Thus, surface tension (or surface free energy, *G*), which has units of N/m (or J/m^2), is defined as the force (or work) applied parallel to the surface of the fluid divided by the length (or area) over which it acts,

$$\gamma = F/l, \text{ or } \gamma = (\partial G/\partial A)_{T,P,n} \quad (2)$$

where, in either form, Equation 2 infers that it requires energy (ΔG) to extend the surface (ΔA) and to bring molecules from the lower energy bulk to the stretched, higher-energy interface. Another way to view the surface ensemble is to envision that parameters affecting hydrogen-bond packing influence the cohesiveness and consequently tension of the interface. Conventionally speaking, the term "surface tension" is typically applied to forces at the liquid-vapor interface; because elastic forces confound and dominate the energy needed to expand the surface of a solid, measurements at the liquid-*solid* and vapor-*solid* interfaces are typically described by *surface free energy*.

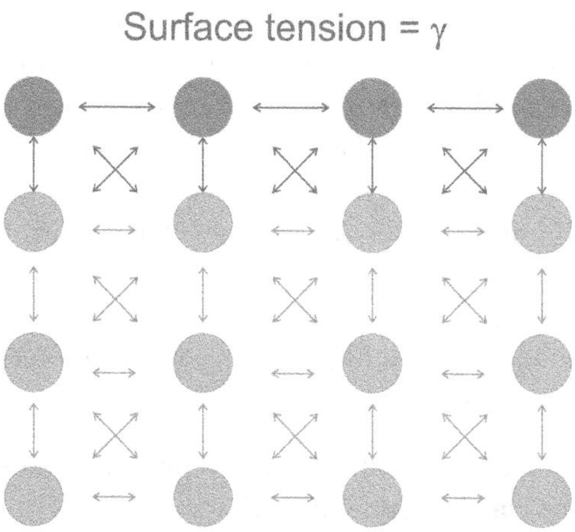

Figure 6: Model of an air-condensed phase interface. ○ =interfacial molecules. ● =bulk molecules. The interfacial molecules are not solvated equally and are in a higher energy state than those in the bulk fluid.

Surface tension measurements are typically accomplished with a *surface tensiometer* and Wilhelmy Plate or du Noüy ring methods [30]. In surface tensiometry, the high-energy and pristine surface of the plate or ring is inserted into the solution to form a meniscus. As the probe is slowly removed, a microbalance follows the maximum force needed to overcome the wetting force, which is proportional to γ (or σ in **Figure 7**).

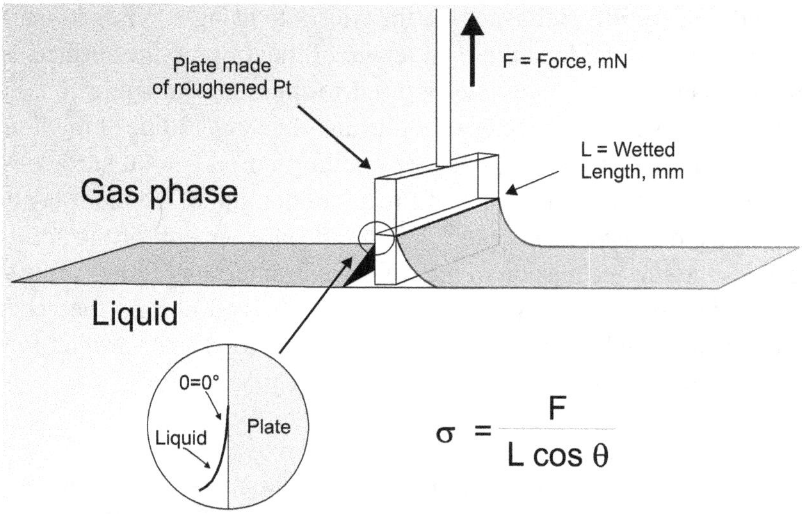

Figure 7: Wilhelmy plate method for determining surface tension. L=wetted perimeter; F=force exerted on microbalance; σ=γ=surface tension; θ=contact angle. θ is typically zero and, hence, cos 0 = 1 (courtesy of Krüss GmbH).

Wetting is an intuitive term and refers to the process of a liquid displacing a gas to make intimate contact with the surface of a solid. When interacting with a solid, poorly wetting liquids tend to bead, while exceptionally wetting liquids spread evenly across the exposed surface. The process of wetting a surface is related to the molecular interactions between the liquid and the solid. For example, if the liquid-liquid attractions within the droplet are stronger than the molecular attractions at the liquid-solid interface, the liquid will exhibit *cohesive* properties and will tend to bead at the surface of the solid. Conversely, if the molecules of the liquid and solid interact strongly, the liquid will counter *adhesively* by stretching its volume uniformly across the interface (**Table 3**).

Table 3: Description of cohesive and adhesive properties and relation to contact angle [courtesy of ramé-hart Instrument Co.]

Contact Angle	**Wetting Description**	**Solid-Liquid Interaction**	**Liquid-Liquid Interaction**
0°	Complete	Strong	Weak
60°	High	Strong	Weak
90°	Moderate	Weak	Weak
120°	Low	Weak	Strong
180°	None	Weak	Strong

The *static contact angle* of a fluid on a solid is typically measured with a modern Drop Shape Analyzer (DSA). In a DSA experiment, a *sessile drop* (i.e., liquid drop on solid) is carefully deposited on the substrate using a syringe. A mounted video camera is then used to capture an image of the drop on the surface, and accompanying image analysis software is used to measure the angle (i.e., contact angle) between the solid-liquid interface line and the tangent line at the liquid-gas interface. **Figure 8** shows a water drop at equilibrium on a solid surface—a hair fiber. The equilibrium contact angle is the result of the sum of the interplay of three surface tensions, or *surface energies*: γ_{sl} is the surface tension of the solid-liquid interface, γ_{sv} is the surface tension of the solid-vapor interface, and γ_{lv} is the surface tension of the liquid-vapor interface. By definition, at equilibrium the vector sum of the three tensions, which sums along the parallel of the fiber-droplet interface, must be zero, and rearranging produces the *Young equation* (Eq. 3).

$$\cos \theta = (\gamma_{sv} - \gamma_{sl}) / \gamma_{lv} \tag{3}$$

As indicated in **Table 3**, at $\theta > 90°$ the solid-liquid interface is at higher energy than the solid-air interface. In this instance, the vapor preferentially wets the surface and the liquid beads (i.e., minimal wetting). At $\theta = 0°$ (i.e., $\cos \theta = 1$) there is perfect wettability and, due to deviation from equilibrium, the Young equation no longer holds true [31, 32].

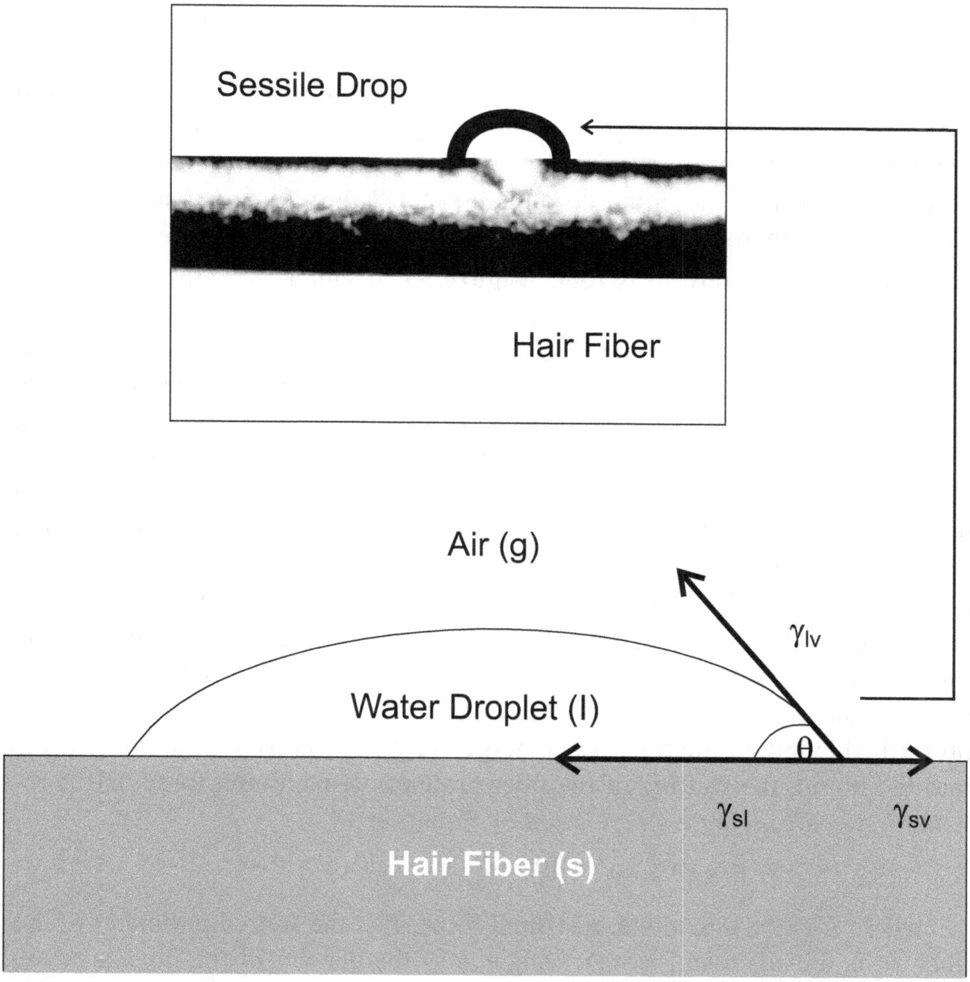

Figure 8: Top: 100 pL static water drop on surface of hair fiber (courtesy of Krüss GmbH). Bottom: Model of the interaction of liquid-vapor (γ_{lv}), solid-liquid (γ_{sl}), and solid-vapor (γ_{sv}) interfacial tensions.

The advantage of the sessile drop method is that multiple measurements on the sample surface may be used to gauge surface energy heterogeneity. That is, if measurements are done carefully, the variation between contact angle measurements will be indicative of the wetting variability as well as the gradation in surface topology as a function of x-y space. However, to make things interesting, by definition the static drop and associated Young equation apply to smooth and homogeneous surfaces; because a hair fiber is naturally porous, has variations in sebum and integral fatty acids, and has a jagged cuticular structure with natural and damage-dependent chemical and morphological inhomogeneity, good sense must be implemented when characterizing the meaning of the data and/or applying them to surface-free energy models. Further, DSA experiments are sensitive to droplet rearrangements (i.e., lateral motion), humidity, static electricity, volatility and/or sorption of the liquid—especially if applying low-volume droplet sizes to hair fibers. Hence, in the literature the use of the liquid drop method for determining contact angles on hair fibers is rather sparse.

Prior to recent advances (e.g., **Figure** 7) in video technology and drop volume [33] control, the application of DSA to the rough and chemically heterogeneous surface of hair rendered contact angle measurements difficult and unreliable [34]. Hence, historically speaking, the prevalent method in the literature for measuring the contact angle of a fluid at the interface with a single fiber is based on *force tensiometry* and the single-fiber Wilhelmy balance method. The Wilhelmy technique is considered a *dynamic contact angle* method because, unlike the sessile drop approach, the phase boundaries and shape of the meniscus are in perceivable motion as the fiber is advanced or receded from the fluid. In the application of the Wilhelmy method to hair, a small section of the hair fiber is affixed to a thin wire hook and suspended from the microbalance. The mass of the fiber is tared, and a moveable stage containing the fluid, such as high-purity water, is subsequently raised or (lowered) until a prescribed length of the fiber is submerged (e.g., 2–5 mm). As the fiber moves into the liquid, the wetting of the fiber produces a maximum force that is related to the *advancing contact angle* by Equation 4,

$$F = \gamma P \cdot \cos\theta_{a,r} + W - \rho g y A, \tag{4}$$

where F is the maximum measured force, P is the wetted perimeter of the fiber, θ_a is the advancing contact angle, ρ is the density of the fluid, g is the gravitational constant, y is the immersion depth, W is the weight of the fiber, and A is the cross-sectional area of the hair fiber [34]. The second and third terms of Eq. 4 are ignored because the fiber mass is initially tared, and because the buoyancy of a human hair is negligible. Subsequent retraction of the fiber from the fluid stretches the meniscus along the wetted fiber surface, and the maximum force produced is related to the *receding contact angle* (θ_r) by Eq. 4. **Figure 9** depicts the Wilhelmy balance model and **Figure 10** shows a force versus distance profile for a typical experiment. As with DSA, force tensiometry is sensitive to extraneous vibration, temperature fluctuations, and surface contamination. Also, for the Wilhelmy methodology, the wetting perimeter (**Figure 11**), the direction of scales (**Figure 10** inset), and the rate of introduction or removal of the fiber from the interface affect equilibration processes and must be carefully controlled [35].

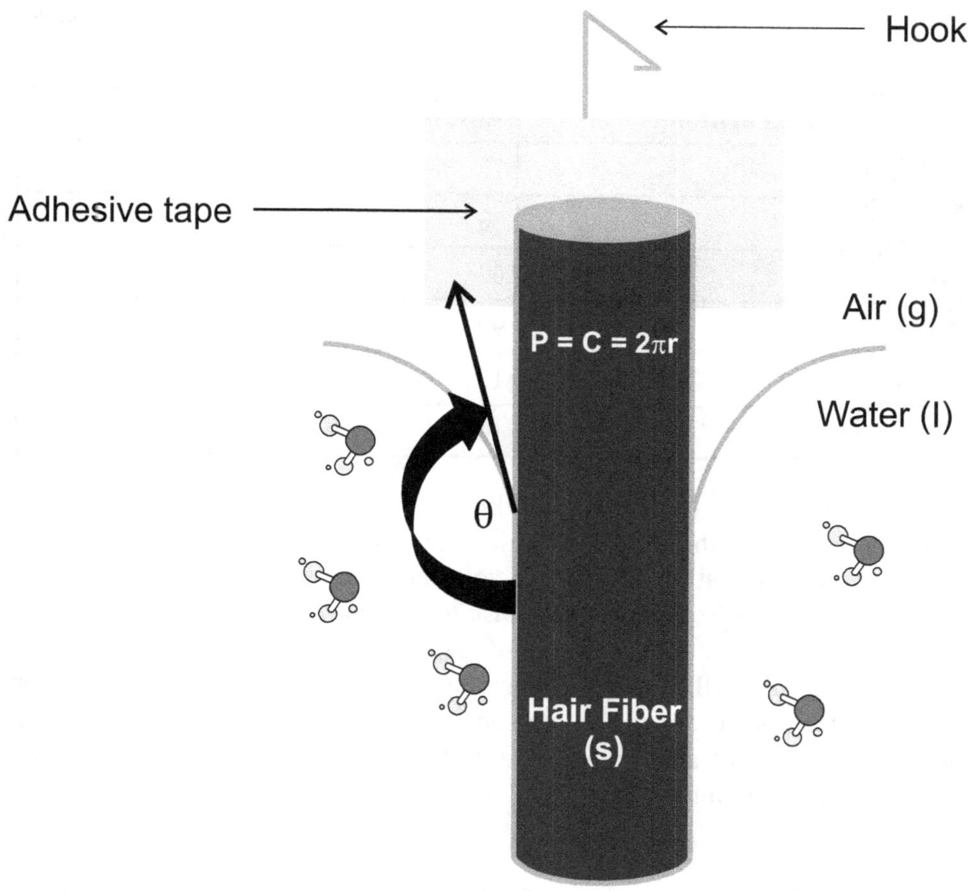

Figure 9: Diagram of dynamic contact analysis on hair using Wilhelmy methodology. Contact angle analysis is reduced from Eq. 7 to cos θ= F/γP, where *P* is the wetted perimeter of the solid, *θ* is the advancing or receding contact angle, and *F* is the wetting force corrected for buoyancy and fiber mass. *P* is approximately 2*π*r for a hair fiber.

Kamath et al. [36] employed the Wilhelmy balance technique to study the effects of weathering, chemical, and mechanical insults on the water wettability of the fiber surface. The extent of daily mechanical strains and natural weathering processes (i.e., UV damage) was inferred by sectioning 10-inch-long fibers and next measuring the wetting forces as a function of root-to-tip distance. **Table 4** suggests that daily UV and grooming processes introduce cuticular stresses that augment the hydrophilicity of a hair fiber as a function of time, or hair length. Hair that emerges from the scalp (zone 6) shows nonwettability properties, while zones 3–6, which are closer to the tip, show wettability traits similar to those seen in bleached fibers [34].

Table 4: Effect of root-to-tip distance on the magnitude of the advancing contact angle [38]

Tip	Fiber Partition	Advancing contact angle (θa)
	1	72
	2	73
	3	67
	4	99
	5	101
Root	6	103

Using Wilhelmy techniques, Molina et al. [37] studied the impact of chemical strains on the physicochemical properties of the integument. They evaluated the application of alkaline solutions with and without 0.6% H_2O_2 and compared to untreated hair. Because hydrogen peroxide is known to oxidize cystine to cysteic acid residues, the assumption is that this influences the hydrophilicity as well as the number of ionizable moieties on the cuticular surface. Attempts were made to augment wetting trends by characterizing the *physical* (dispersive) and *chemical* (acid-base) contributions to the work of adhesion across the interface,

$$W_{SL} = W_{SL}^{LW} + W_{SL}^{AB}, \tag{5}$$

where W_{SL} is the equilibrium work of adhesion, W_{SL}^{LW} is the Lifshitz-van der Waals (i.e., dispersive or hydrophobic) component, and W_{SL}^{AB} is the contribution of acid-base interactions between the liquid and solid. W_{SL}^{AB} may subsequently be solved for by applying Equation 6 to the empirical data [37],

$$W_{SL}^{AB} = \lambda_L(1 + \cos\theta) - 2(\lambda_L^{LW} \cdot \lambda_S^{LW})^{1/2}, \tag{6}$$

where λ_L is the surface tension of the dry solid, λL_{LW} is the dispersive component of the surface tension for the liquid, and λS_{LW} is the dispersive component of the surface tension for the dry solid. Not surprisingly, the results confirmed that untreated hair is less wettable than alkaline-treated and/or peroxide treated fibers. Further, by controlling the aqueous pH during tensiometry measurements, it was shown that alkaline-treated fibers have an increase of ~2 times increase in W_{SL}^{AB}, and oxidized fibers have an increase of 3–4 times increase in W_{SL}^{AB} relative to untreated fibers—confirming that alkaline and/or oxidative treatment increases the number of hydrophilic and ionizable functionalities on the hair surface.

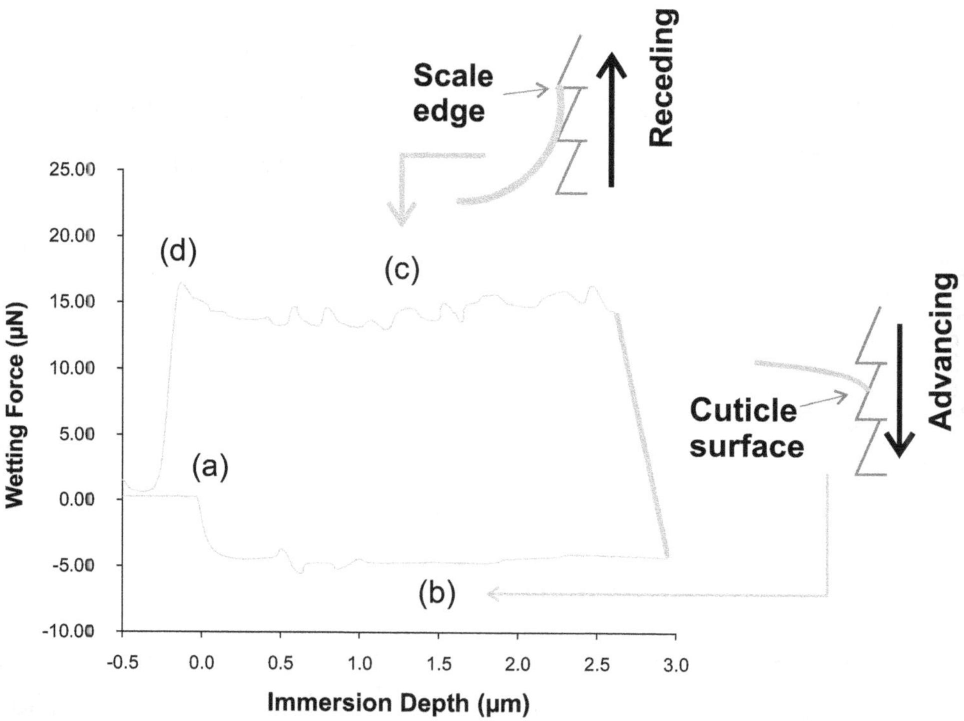

Figure 10: Wetting force as a function of immersion depth for a virgin hair fiber. The fibers are typically mounted in the against-scale direction. (a) Fiber penetrating the liquid interface; (b) fiber advancing into liquid surface; (c) fiber receding from interface; (d) meniscus breaks from fiber. The insets depict one reason for contact angle hysteresis (θ_a-θ_r). During advancing of fiber into liquid, the meniscus interacts with cuticle surface; in the receding step, the meniscus strongly adheres to scale edges [34, 36, 37, 39].

Using Zisman's approach [38] to find the *critical surface tension* (λ_C), where plotting cos(θ) versus λ_{lv} with test liquids and extrapolating to θ=0 to find λ_C, Kamath [37] detailed the λ_C wetting argument into dispersive and polar terms,

$$\lambda_C = \lambda^d{}_S + \lambda^p{}_S, \tag{7}$$

where λ_C is the critical surface tension, and λ_{dS}=24 mN/m and λ_{pS}=4 mN/m are the polar and dispersive components for untreated hair, respectively. The low-magnitude dispersive component reflects the dominating *average* hydrophobic nature of virgin hair, and also intimates that very high surface tension fluids will bead on the pristine hair surface. However, intuitively, the ensuing chemical effects of oxidation significantly increase λ_C and $\lambda^p{}_S$ – and, therefore, increase the likelihood of additional homogenous chemisorption interactions between higher surface tension conditioners, such as water-soluble cationic polymers, and the modified higher-energy surface.

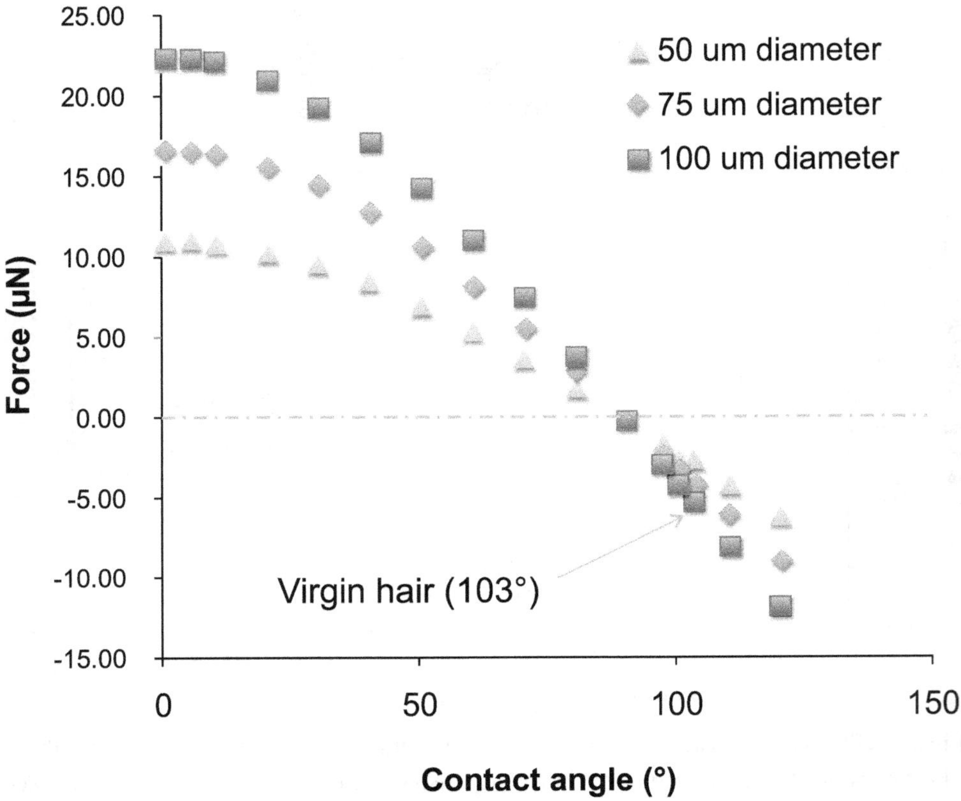

Figure 11: Consequence of the magnitude of the wetting perimeter on the profile of the force curve (see Eq. 4). Nonwetting solids are less dependent on fiber diameter. Virgin hair has a negative wetting force, and θ_A is approximately 103° [34, 36, 37].

Kamath et al. [35], and also Lodge and Bushan [34], studied the wetting properties of virgin, chemically treated, and subsequently conditioned, hair tresses. Lodge observed a statistically significant (p=0.05) reduction in the dynamic contact angle (Wilhelmy balance) with permanent waving (70±7°) and with the application of conditioner (88±9°) to virgin hair (103±4°); however, application of commercial conditioner to permed hair (79±1°) caused an increase in the contact angle, relative to the permed hair. To explain the trends, both Kamath and Lodge speculated that the state of the fiber may dictate how the conditioning surfactant associates with the hair. For example, on damaged hair, the cationic groups will electrostatically bind more strongly to the copious cysteic acid moieties and the lower-energy alkyl chains of the surfactant will be directed towards the surface (i.e., higher contact angle, decreased wetting). Yet, on application of cationic conditioner to virgin hair, with a presumably intact F-layer, the hydrophobic alkyl chains of the surfactant may physisorb with the bound lipids and the higher-energy cationic moieties will be exposed to the surface (i.e., lower contact angle, increased wetting).

Lodge [34] also rationalized that contact angle hysteresis ($H = \theta_a - \theta_r$) could be used to study the location of the deposition of conditioners on a hair fiber. Relative to the permed-fiber curve, very little contact angle hysteresis was seen for the bleached-and-treated fiber. This indicated that the conditioner deposited significantly on the cuticle edges, producing a larger θ_r than expected because the intrinsic hydrophilicity of the scales was "hidden." This result was corroborated by Dupres et al. [40, 41], who used noncontact AFM to examine the *microscopic* heterogeneity of wetting behavior for a range of solvents on hair fibers—including silicone oil (21 mN/m), decane (23 mN/m), and squalane (31 mN/m). Results indicated that only silicone oil wets the hair surface completely; however, the cuticle edges, which are proteinaceous and more hydrophilic than the cuticular surface, were wet homogenously by the oils (**Figure 12**). Using critical surface tension arguments, this clearly suggests that the cuticle edges have a higher λ_C than the cuticle surface, and that the hydrophobic oils have λ less than the λ_C of the cuticle edge.

Trends in surface tension, wetting, and contact angle trends are valuable tools for following the deleterious effects of chemical, mechanical, thermal, and weathering strains on the integrity of the cuticle. Due to chemical and surface heterogeneity, hair fibers are a challenging substrate for both static and dynamic contact angle measurements. Advances in DSA technology have rendered small-volume, sessile-drop DSA measurements on single fibers feasible, although the surface heterogeneity of hair renders challenges to evaluating instrument precision. Due to an abundance of examples in the literature, the Wilhelmy balance method is still the established method for measuring the wettability of single fibers. By employing surface energy models to contact angle results, it is possible to gain insight into the chemical modifications of the surface and to accordingly develop treatments to ameliorate the compromised wetting properties of damaged hair.

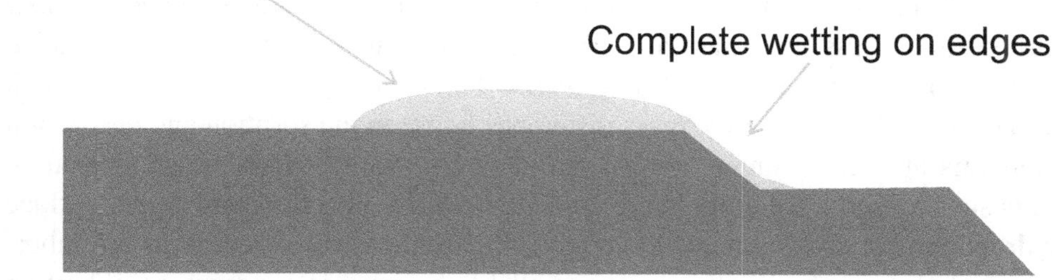

Figure 12: Preferential wetting of virgin hair by squalane. Squalane spreads uniformly across the relatively polar cuticle edge, whereas sparse wetting is visible on the hydrophobic cuticle surface.

3. *Dynamic Vapor Sorption (DVS)*

Prior to the advent of commercialized Dynamic Vapor Sorption (DVS) technology, the interaction of relative humidity (RH) with a sample was principally studied by exposing pre-dried samples to isothermal air over a series of saturated salt solutions (42). Samples were then periodically removed from the desiccators and weighed to study sorption kinetics and to obtain the equilibrium sorption isotherm. Understandably, the methodology was both tedious and time consuming due to the lack of automation. Furthermore, it was more difficult to accurately monitor the rate of sorption and to strictly control the environment of the samples within the cumbersome desiccators—including temperature, dry gas type, sorbent vapor type, vacuum, and the logistics of transferring highly hygroscopic materials between the desiccator and balance.

In general, modern DVS analysis is a fully automated, gravimetric technique used to monitor the interaction of a gaseous probe molecule (e.g., water, cyclohexane) with a substrate of interest (e.g., polymer film, hair). The relative vapor pressure (i.e., RH for water vapor) is accurately controlled by streaming a mixture of dry (e.g., nitrogen, air) and vapor-saturated gases in correct proportions using mass flow controllers. The mass changes of the sample are monitored with an ultra-sensitive microbalance, and changes in the chemistry of the sample can be simultaneously followed with NIR spectroscopy, Raman spectroscopy, and/or optical microscopy. Depending on the instrument model, one or several very small samples (< 30 mg) can be dried at 0% RH, pre-heated to high temperatures (e.g., 100–300°C), pre-humidified, cooled or heated, exposed to stepped or oscillating humidity, or influenced by reduced pressures—all automated and all *in situ*. Because all aforementioned processes can be programmed into the DVS control software using sequences, and without altering the position or controlled environment of the sample, both equilibrium and kinetics trials may be used to fully differentiate comparative sorption processes. During water vapor DVS analysis, which is the method typically used in the literature to study interactions with hair fibers, the relative humidity in the sample compartment is varied stepwise with time and changes in mass are continuously monitored. A subsequent plot of the *equilibrium* sorbed vapor mass (i.e., mass regain) against the relative humidity at a controlled temperature is termed a *sorption isotherm*. The resulting *hysteresis* plots, which are generated by plotting the mass difference between the sorption and desorption isotherms at each isohume, are insightful in contrasting characteristic substrate traits such as equilibrium moisture content, bound versus unbound water, surface hydrophobicity, and porosity. Although fully equilibrated experiments are inherently time consuming for porous or swellable biomaterials, proper equilibration between the *adsorbent* (substrate) and *adsorbate* (vapor) facilitates the determination of accurate equilibrium moisture contents and diffusion coefficients. In addition, application of comparative isotherm data to theoretical sorption models may be used, albeit controversially (43), to visualize the allocation of *adsorbed* and *absorbed* vapor at the surface and within, respectively, a porous substrate—such as a hair fiber.

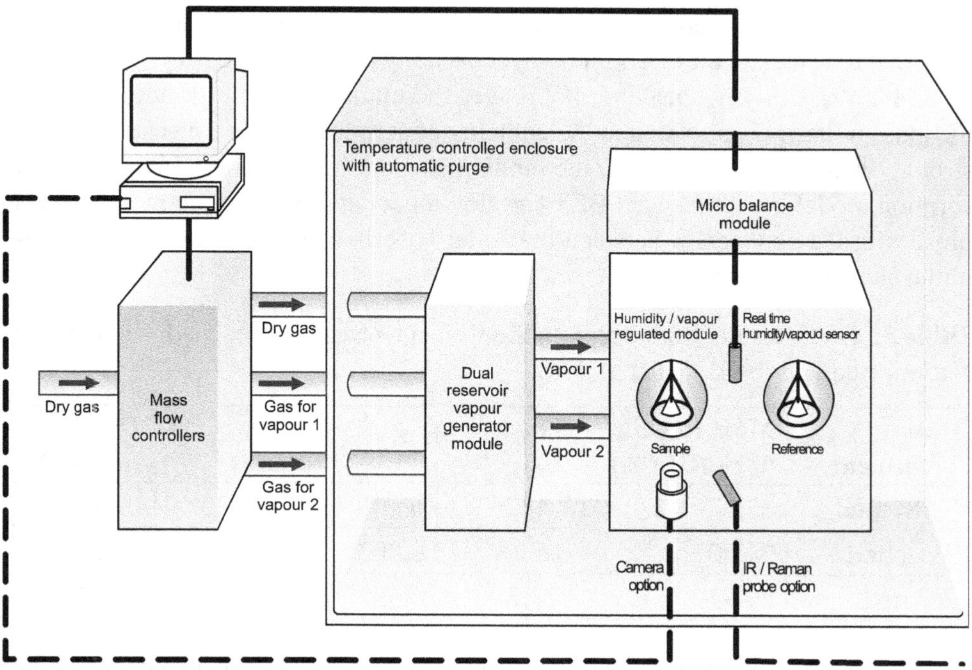

Figure 13: Modern DVS Instrumentation (courtesy of Surface Measurement Systems, UK).

Hair fibers are hygroscopic, yet an undamaged hair fiber with endogenous sebum and intact integral fatty acids has a low surface tension and effectively repels water (44). Although contradictory, the net result is that hair has a penchant for slowly absorbing and slowly desorbing water vapor, as indicated by its characteristic sigmoidal DVS isotherm and noted hysteresis between the sorption and desorption steps. The hysteresis lag and the exothermic heats of sorption suggest that once water negotiates a path through the cuticle and into the cortex (i.e., *absorbed* water) it is tightly held by the hydrophilic peptide residues within the fiber (45). As absorbed water induces radial swelling of the fiber and affects the free volume and mobility of α-keratin, any treatment that affects hair's water transport processes will induce transient changes in properties such as dye mobility and mechanical strength (46). Hence, DVS analysis is a tool to forecast the impact of weathering and the efficacy of protective or repair remedies on the quality and health of a keratinous fiber.

Bleaching and perming are processes that impart chemical strains to the hair. Bleaching is a harsh oxidizing process, whereas perming involves the reduction of disulfide bonds followed by an oxidative process to reform the bonds in a newly styled position. Barba et al. (47) contrasted the water transport processes of untreated, bleached, and permed natural red hair using DVS. Subsequent fitting of the sorption data to the Guggenheim, Andersen, and De Boer (GAB) sorption model was used to calculate the GAB monolayer capacity (W_m) and GAB energy constant (C_g) (48, 49). Loosely speaking, W_m relates the number of vapor-binding sites to the mass of hair; C_g is related to the enthalpy of sorption, and is a measure of how strongly water vapor adheres to the binding sites in the hair fiber (50). The GAB sorption model is an enhanced BET sorption model and has been shown to give a physics-based connection between the water absorbed and the number of hydrophilic sites on the substrate (51).

Table 5: DVS Results from Sorption Studies on Untreated, Bleached, and Permed Natural Red Hair by Barba et al. (46)

Hair Treatment	**Max. Regain, 95% RH (%)**	***Wm* (%)**	***Cg***	**t_T (min)**	**D_A (min-1)**
Untreated	25.87	7.487	6.706	3204.22	0.0163
Bleached	24.60	6.630	6.803	2895.12	0.0203
Permed	29.97	7.518	6.597	3297.16	0.0175

The authors rationalized the results in **Table 5** by noting that oxidative degradation mechanisms corrupt the surface and the way hair naturally intermingles with water; therefore, although perming significantly increased the maximum regain, bleaching is considered to have the most detrimental effects on hair by rendering the fibers more permeable to water. Bleaching lessens *Wm*, increases the apparent diffusion rate (D_A) of sorption/desorption, and decreases the amount of time it takes for the sample to reach equilibrium mass (t_T); however, neither treatment significantly affects *Cg*. In a 2009 report by the same research group, bleach-damaged hair was subsequently treated with isolated wool intermediate-filament peptides and proteins. Relative to bleached fibers, the DVS results, including improvements in D_A, t_T, and *Wm* data, all suggest that the keratin treatments reestablish the original water-management properties of the untreated virgin hair (52).

High-temperature flat ironing introduces deleterious structure and chemical effects that alter the water management properties of the hair—including cuticle cell lifting; thermal softening; and the formation of deep holes, cracks, and fractures of the cuticle structure caused by protein denaturation and the rapid expansion of water vapor within the fiber structure (53, 54). Moreover, protein denaturation and changes in lipid structures may significantly affect the accessibility of water-binding residues. Hence, as conduits to water-vapor sorption may be closely tied to physicochemical damage of the hair fiber, DVS analysis is a logical asset for studying the efficacy of remedies for diminishing thermal damage.

Following the work of Zhou et al. (4), tresses of virgin European dark brown hair were washed with 10% SLES, then blow-dried to remove dampness, and subsequently hot flat-ironed (232°C) for 12 seconds. The process was repeated three times over a 12-minute period. If a protective treatment was applied, the treatment was added after washing, and prior to the blow-drying step. To minimize the experimental cycle time, the chosen method revolved around time constraints and comparative vapor penetration kinetics (i.e., samples were nearly equilibrated). Rather than introducing edge effects (**Figure 14**) to the sorption processes, the sample preparation consisted of carefully wrapping 20–30 strands of hair fibers into a loose coil (**Figure 14**) and loading them into the DVS apparatus (55). All DVS experiments were performed at 25°C and used the following procedure:

1. Preconditioning: Prior to drying of the loops, samples were exposed to 95% RH for 1 hour to minimize the variations in "humidity history" (56).
2. Initial drying: The loops were dried at 25°C and 0% RH for 12 hours.
3. Absorption curve: The humidity was ramped from 0% to 90% in 10% RH steps. Each sorption step was 4 hours in duration.
4. Desorption step: The humidity was ramped from 90% to 0% in 10% RH steps. Each sorption step was 4 hours in duration.

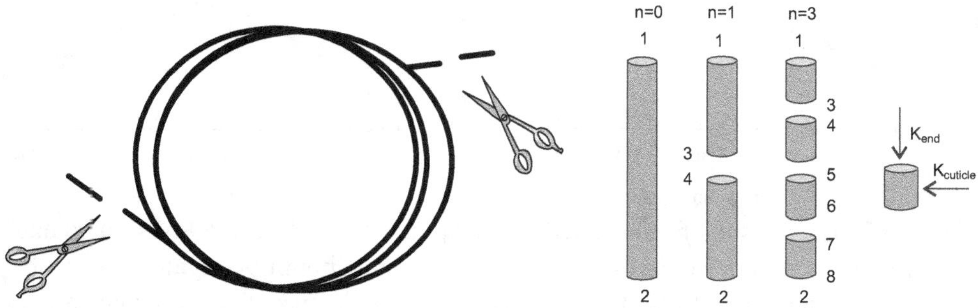

Figure 14: Formation of DVS hair loop and the potential implication of edge effects. Coiled fiber bundles were used instead of chopped hair segments to model "real-life" cuticle-permeation kinetics.

Figure 15 shows the DVS isotherm and D_A overlays for the unheated, heated and untreated, and Polyquaternium-55 (PQ-55) treated and heated hair tresses (PQ-55, **Figure 16**). Note that the maximum water vapor regain trend is unheated > PQ-55 treated and heated > heated and untreated (Fig. 3a). This suggests that the PQ-55 treated and heated composite sustained less thermomechanically imposed damage to the microstructures involved in water binding than did the heated and untreated tress. **Figure 15b** echoes the same trends seen in the isotherm overlay and implies that, in the desorption process (upper portion of diffusion curve), water diffuses most quickly from the heated and untreated hair at moderate humidity levels (40–80% RH). With the aid of supplementary empirical evidence, the authors speculated that changes in the water-management properties of the damaged heated and untreated fibers were due to combined surface and cortex damage. First, the hydrophobic boundary mediating the transport of water vapor to the cortex was compromised through the introduction of cracks, holes, and the formation of micropores in the cuticula. Further, on a molecular scale, degradation of protein moieties and conformational changes in the keratin structure, such as α-keratins denaturing to β- or to other unfolded forms, may have reduced the number of water-binding sites within the cortex.

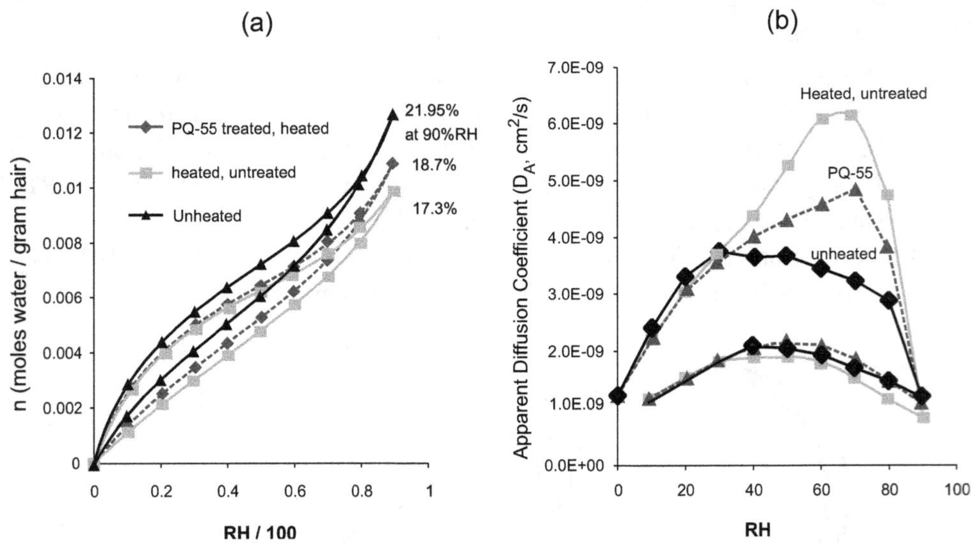

Figure 15: DVS results for unheated, heated and untreated, and PQ-55 treated and heated hair fibers; (a) isotherm overlay depicting maximum % regain values; (b) overlay of D_A showing effect of thermal treatment on kinetics of water management.

Whereas untreated and heated samples were irreversibly damaged by thermal insult, the PQ-55 heated and treated fibers exhibited less protein degradation and denaturation and, for this reason, retained structural elements critical for effective hydrogen-bond stabilization of the α-keratin helices. The resilience in physicochemical structure resulted in the preservation of natural water sorption processes—which were deemed important for the preservation of moisture retention, moisture restoration, and subsequent thermal protection properties (4).

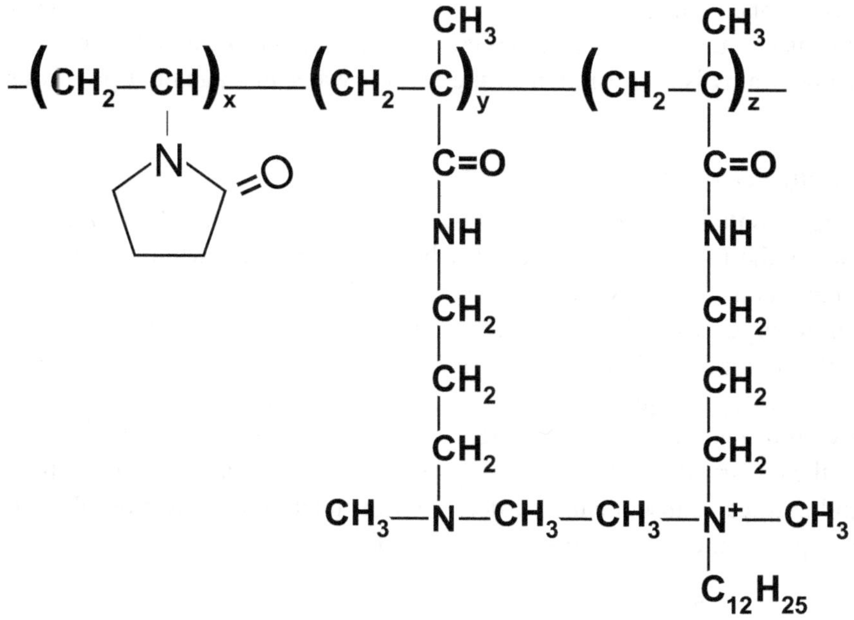

Figure 16: Repeating unit structure for Polyquaternium-55

Keis et al. (57) used DVS to study the retention of moisture after the application of oil films to surfactant-washed hair. The results indicate that the moisture regains for the coconut, sunflower, and mineral oils were 23.7%, 22.5%, and 22.1%, where the maximum regain (R_{max}) is a function of the dried hair mass (M_D) and the equilibrium mass of the fibers (M_v) at 95% RH:

$$R_{max} = Mv / M_D * 100 \tag{8}$$

At low humidity levels, calculated hysteresis plots demonstrate that oil increases the retention of water, which is suggested to be an effect similar to moisturization of the hair. The authors proposed a diffusion barrier mechanism wherein the pathway for permeation of water vapor into the hair is primarily through the endocuticle and the Cell Membrane Complex (CMC). The oils are thought to accumulate at the cuticle edges before subsequently penetrating into the endocuticle, CMC, and possibly the cortical envelope: thereby slowing the rate of sorption and lowering R_{max} (relative to virgin hair, where R_{max} = 27.4%).

By means of empirical pathways, many researchers have speculated on the mechanisms of applied oxidative and/or thermal damage and the resulting stresses subsequently acquired by the maltreatment of hair's chemistry and microstructure (4, 5, 22, 53, 54, 59–65, 66). Others have made efforts to critically speculate on how and why effective barrier oils and polymeric additives function in thermal protection applications (5, 58, 67). Although the complete damage and protection mechanisms are not fully understood, it is clear that a glaring symptom of applied weathering strains is a corruption in the natural water management processes of hair.

4. Streaming Potential

Streaming Potential, or *Dynamic Electrokinetic and Permeability Analysis* (DEPA), incorporates the measurement of electrochemical properties while a flowing test solution interacts with the surface of a planar or fibrous sample. It has been used to study the adsorption and desorption of various ingredients on hair [68, 69, 70]. The empirical data for a single DEPA experiment includes the streaming potential (E), conductivity (κ), pH, liquid flow rate, and temperature—all measured as a function of flow volume and time. The zeta potential, ζ, which is an important parameter for gauging the electrostatic attraction or repulsion between an applied rinse-off treatment and hair, can subsequently be derived as a function of time from the DEPA data by applying the Smoluchowski equation (Eq. 9),

$$\zeta = 4\pi\eta\kappa E / P\varepsilon, \tag{9}$$

where P is the drive pressure applied to the flowing liquid, and η and ε are the viscosity and dielectric constant of the streaming polyelectrolyte solution, respectively.

In a DEPA experiment designed to discern the consequences of oxidative damage, the hair sample is wetted in dilute electrolyte solution, chopped into small, compressible pieces (4–6 mm), and then placed in a special flow cell that houses two perforated silver chloride electrodes (**Figure 17**). Dilute electrolyte solution (5×10^{-5} M KCl) is next pulsed through the cell (30 s on, 30 s rest) five times to properly equilibrate the sample [68]. Following equilibration, the dilute KCl test solution is pulsed unidirectionally through the fiber plug for 75 minutes while monitoring the E, κ, flow rate, and ζ. The more highly damaged sample (as assessed by the alkaline solubility test [70]) showed a higher initial solution conductivity and a longer decay to a constant conductivity plateau than the less-damaged tress. Both samples showed a negative decay in ζ and E as a function of rinsing time. Jachowicz et al. suggested that the observed variations in the electrochemical properties of the bleached samples, relative to the untreated control, were more than likely related to residual bleaching components leaching from the hair.

DEPA provides detailed information about the electrokinetical properties of the fluid-fiber interface. By developing a detailed understanding of the dynamics of interactions with the damaged-hair plug, including the kinetics of rinse-out, E, ζ, and κ data may be used to better design intelligent treatments to ameliorate fiber damage.

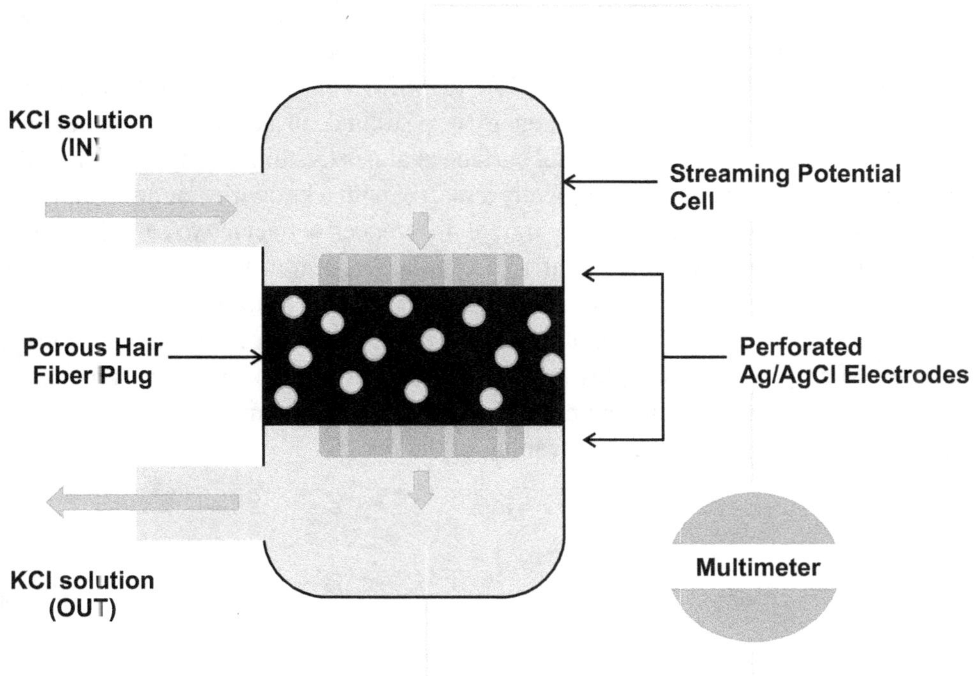

Figure 17: Schematic of Streaming Potential Cell showing perforated Ag/AgCl electrodes surrounding the compressed hair fiber plug (Adapted from Dynamic Electrokinetic Analyzer manual, Better Cosmetics LLC, US).

5. Time-of-Flight Secondary Ion Mass Spectrometry (ToF-SIMS)

Time-of-Flight Secondary Ion Mass Spectrometry (ToF-SIMS) uses a pulsed, finely focused ion beam to bombard the surface of a substrate and release secondary atomic and molecular ions. The desorbed organic or inorganic ions are subsequently accelerated to a Time-of-Flight (ToF) analyzer where their arrival times are correlated with mass (**Figure 18**).

In its simplest mode, ToF-SIMS provides a mass spectrum of the region of interest. However, by rastering the primary ion beam across the surface, two-dimensional images are generated to view the spatial distribution of specific chemical moieties as a function of x-y space. For each pixel in the image, an entire mass spectrum is subsequently obtained, ranging from 1 to approximately 10 kDa. Further, depth profiles are obtained by using a sputter beam technique, where surface layers are removed from an area prior to acquiring images of newly exposed subsurface monolayers (**Figure 19**).

An advantage of ToF-SIMS is that concatenation of images facilitates imaging of fairly large samples (e.g., 9 cm × 9 cm). Further, as the lateral resolution for a surface can be as low as 60 nm [71], ToF-SIMS enables an excellent understanding of the true chemical heterogeneity of a studied surface. A disadvantage is that although ToF-SIMS is a powerful surface analysis technique, quantification of analytes is not straightforward. Typically a matrix with a known amount of analyte must be used as a reference, or comparative differences between two samples may be determined by referencing an internal standard common to both sample matrixes (e.g., protein moiety on the surface of hair). Further, because x-y scanning only examines the first few monolayers of the sample surface, proper care must be taken when preparing samples for ToF-SIMS analysis. For example, touching hair fibers with unwashed fingers may introduce sebum contamination to the fiber surface, thereby confounding the meaning of the results.

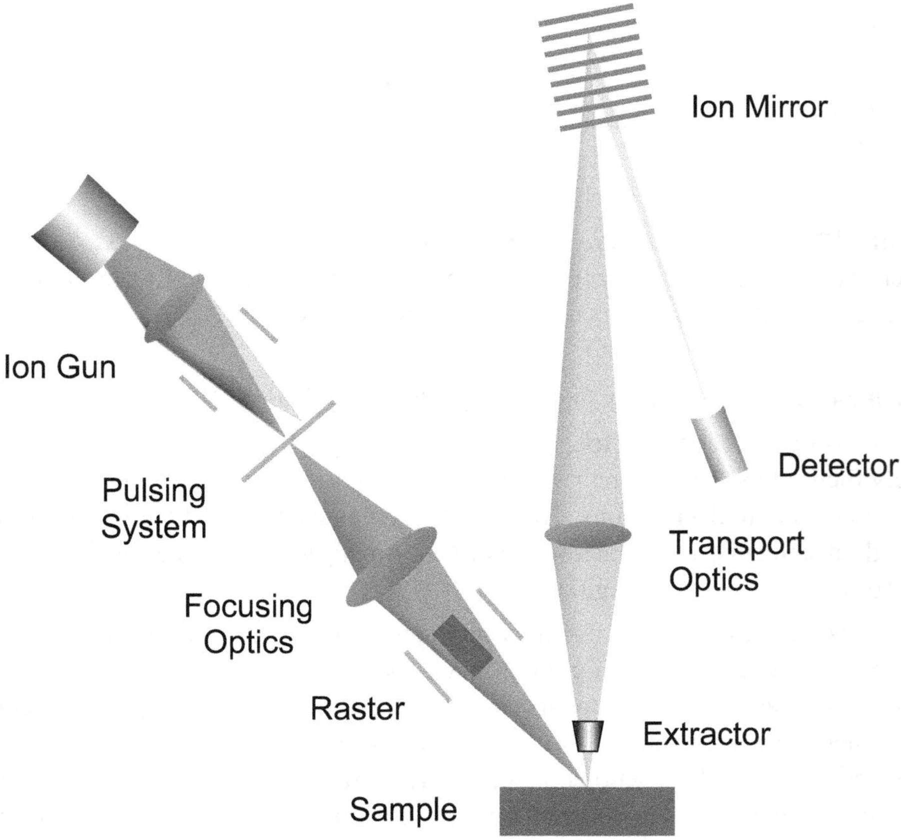

Figure 18: ToF-SIMS schematic: A pulsed primary ion beam (orange) is focused on the sample and secondary ions (blue) are desorbed from the surface, focused, and counted by the detector as a function of time (courtesy of ION-TOF GmbH, DE).

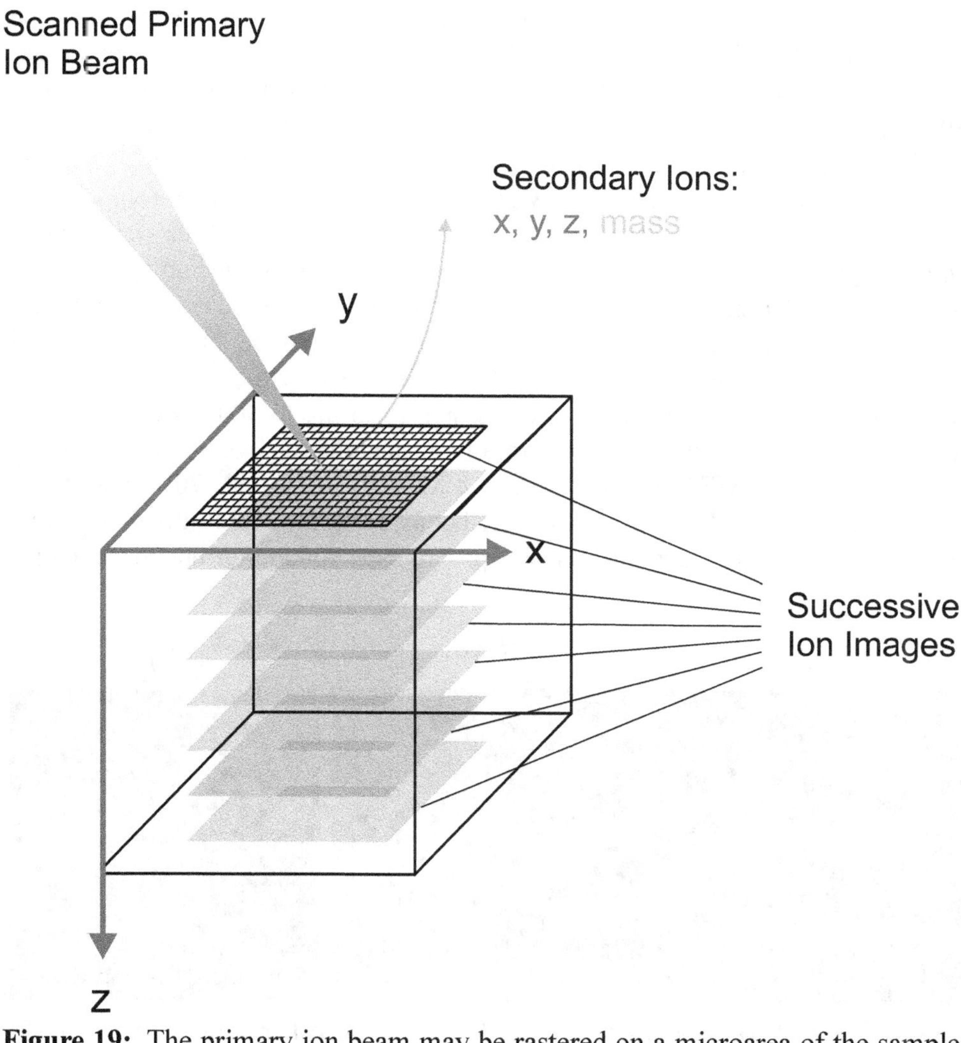

Figure 19: The primary ion beam may be rastered on a microarea of the sample to generate a 2-D image. By using a sputter beam to remove successive surface layers, a depth profile of the substrate (3-D) may be generated to view the layers of substrate below the surface monolayer (courtesy of ION-TOF GmbH, DE).

In the literature, ToF-SIMS has been applied to characterization of the detailed chemical structure of the hair surface (e.g., **Figure 20**). Surface and cross-sectional analyses have been used to evaluate a wide range of fiber applications, including evaluation of surfactant deposition [72], conditioning pretreatments [73, 74], oil penetration [75], dye distribution [76], and elemental distribution [77].

Clear examples of applying ToF-SIMS methodology to studying the weathering and chemical strains of the hair's native hydrophobic barrier include the work of Okamoto et al. [78, 79, 80]. The investigators utilized ToF-SIMS to follow the depletion of 18-MEA as a function of hair length, bleaching, and UV exposure. In the initial work [78], hair fibers were collected from a Japanese woman, aged 30, with no history of cosmetic chemical treatments, such as bleaching, permanent waving, or coloring. Some of the pristine hair fibers were subsequently bleached with H_2O_2, and others were treated with UV light (3500 $\mu W/cm^2$) for various exposure times (48–480 hrs). For each studied fiber, a 75 × 75 μm area was scanned and changes in the negative ion spectrum intensity signals, including 18-MEA *thioester*-bound (m/z 341) and 18-MEA *ester*-bound (m/z 325) surface lipids, were monitored. Relative to an internal peak from fiber protein, the results showed that ~80% of the thioester-bound 18-MEA and ~40% of the ester-bound MEA were removed in one bleaching cycle. Further, exposure to 400 hrs of UV radiation (~2–3 months of summer exposure) diminished the relative intensity ratios of thioester-bound 18-MEA and ester-bound 18-MEA by ~85% and ~70%, respectively. Hence, the researchers concluded ester-bound 18-MEA is presumably less susceptible to chemical oxidation and UV exposure than its thioester-bound analogue.

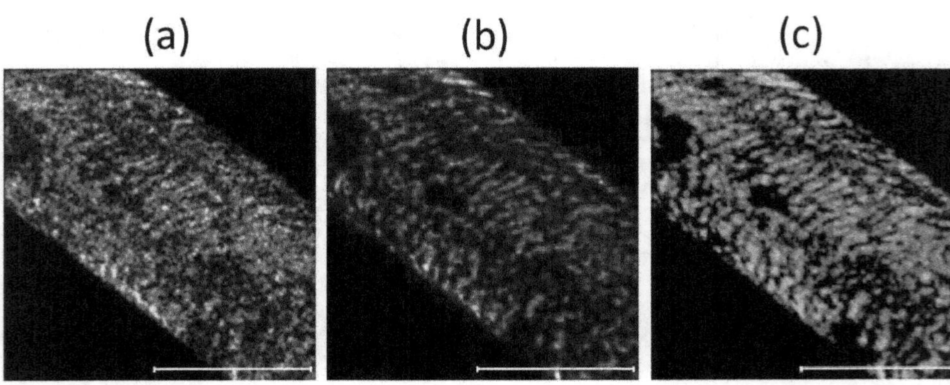

Figure 20: 2-D ToF-SIMS images of (a) CNO^- moiety, from surface protein, (b) $(\text{lauryl sulfate})^-$ from shampoo residue, (c) and $(\text{18-MEA})^-$ distributions on the fiber surface. Pixels with lighter colors represent larger ion counts (courtesy of Physical Electronics Inc., U.S.).

In addition to employing ToF-SIMS to investigate the impact of weathering and chemical insults on 18-MEA depletion, subsequent work by Okamoto et al. [79] discussed resultant changes in surface wettability and potential treatments to mend damage. Hair samples from Japanese women, aged 20–30, with varying exposure to hair-coloring treatments, were analyzed by ToF-SIMS and dynamic contact angle analysis to correlate 18-MEA damage with hydrophobicity data. The results inferred that the 18-MEA thioester content was drastically modified by coloring treatments, especially for exposure to >1 treatments per year. Further, as the ratio of 18-MEA to fiber protein decreased to <1, the dynamic contact angle dropped from ~100° to ~57°. For reference, the ratio of 18-MEA to fiber protein for *untreated hair* decreased to <1 at a hair length of >40 cm from the root—where the authors suggested that cumulative solar weathering, grooming, and daily shampooing affected the F-layer quality. Finally, ToF-SIMS was used to study formulations of 18-MEA combined with cationic surfactants. Both ToF-SIMS and contact angle measurements showed that the treatments replenished the hydrophobic integrity of the damaged surface, as evidenced in the recovery of the dynamic contact angle (from 65° to ~90°) and the uniform distribution of 18-MEA/surfactant complex on the hair surface.

Although intermolecular interactions within the surface limit the molecular weight of *intact* emission ions, recent technological advances in ToF-SIMS primary ion beam sources, depth profiling, and analyzer technology have increased the applicability of the technique to more complex matrixes, such as biopolymers [81, 82] or biocomposites. In conclusion, ToF-SIMS imaging offers insights into the spatially resolved chemical modifications imparted by applied physicochemical insult; subsequent coupling of ToF-SIMS imaging with data from other performance measurement techniques, such as optical, wetting, or mechanical data, enables a feasible route to designing damage repair treatments.

6. X-Ray Photoelectron Spectroscopy (XPS)

XPS, which is also known as Electron Spectroscopy for Chemical Analysis (ESCA), is a technique employed for the qualitative and quantitative analysis of surface elements within the first 1–10 nm of a solid, such as a hair fiber. The sample is irradiated with photons from a beam of monochromatic X-rays while a hemispherical energy analyzer simultaneously monitors the number and kinetic energy of the emitted electrons [83]. The kinetic energy of the emitted electrons is then normalized into element-specific binding energies (Eq. 10) that can be used to identify and quantify surface elements (± 0.1–1.0 atom-%). As the adjoining chemical environment affects the binding energy of a surface element, XPS may be used to compile information regarding the chemical state of an atom [84]. In addition to resolving the elemental composition of spots as small as 10 μm, XPS may be applied to larger areas comprising a few square millimeters. Further, by combining XPS with ion-induced sputtering, it is feasible to describe the elemental composition as a function of penetration depth.

$$\text{Binding energy} \approx \text{X-ray energy} - \text{Kinetic energy of emitted electron} \quad (10)$$

In combination with SEM, Beard et al. [84] studied the application of surface specific XPS to spectroscopically discern the effects of bleaching and subsequent conditioning on the surface chemistry of hair fibers. The impact of pH and the addition of surfactant on the efficacy of the bleaching process were also investigated.

Because XPS is not suitable for detecting atoms with atomic numbers less than 3, the measurable untreated hair surface is primarily composed of carbon (C), oxygen (O), nitrogen (N), sulfur (S), silicon (Si), and calcium (Ca). C, O, N, and S are components of the surface protein, and the fatty "overlayer" is principally composed of C and O (e.g., 18-MEA). Ca and Si are noted as minor "natural constituents of hair," with Ca levels supplemented by tap water [21, 85].

Bleaching treatment systems for the study included (A) 3% hydrogen peroxide, (B) 3% hydrogen peroxide, sodium bisulfate activator, pH=9, and (C) 3% hydrogen peroxide, sodium bisulfate activator, pH=9, 0.25% SLS. Each treatment was applied to a hair tress for 0, 30, or 45 minutes prior to rinsing. To examine the effect of the rinse-off conditioning treatments on bleached hair, the aforementioned bleached swatches were subsequently treated with a 10% conditioning dispersion (including 2.8% diester quaternary amine, 0.9% dimethicone, 0.7% glyceryl stearate, 0.8% stearamidopropyl dimethylamine, 2.7% fatty alcohols) for 60 seconds and then washed with warm water prior to XPS and SEM analyses. XPS (Al k_α X-ray source) was then used to monitor the surface composition of the bleached tresses, focusing on the C, N, S, and O counts; additionally, fluctuations in the content of Si and Ca were followed for the conditioned samples.

The investigators used the photoelectron transitions from sulfur to monitor changes in the disulfide and sulfonate surface concentrations as a function of the formulation and bleaching time. The data, which are summarized in **Figure 21**, indicate that time, pH, and the presence of surfactant affect the kinetics of oxidation, as indicated by comparative changes in the levels of cysteic acid. The authors rationalized that SLS reduces the induction time for effective oxidation via effective wetting of the formulation with the hair surface; in addition, it was surmised that surfactant facilitates more effective rinsing of the hydrocarbon overlayer during the 30-second rinsing step. Arguments were similarly presented for trends in changes of the C, O, and N chemical states. Clearly, alkaline bleaching removes the protective covalent lipid and subsequently exposes more of the hydrophilic protein surface to the oxidative effects of H_2O_2.

Finally, relative to the bleached sample, XPS analysis of the conditioned tress showed dramatic increases in Si and O, but a decrease in protein-specific N, and the absence of Cl^-. Further, high-resolution XPS was used to confirm the presence of deposited diester quaternary amine. Examining the data, the authors concluded that the conditioner is not deposited homogeneously on the surface, as evidenced by the existence of Ca and N, which are components of the fiber. Additionally, the dimethicone is more than likely associated with the hydrophobic tails of the ester quat, rather than the proteinaceous surface. Conversely, the Cl^- counterion is absent because it is released when the N^+ of the ester quat directly associates with the anionic sulfonic functionalities of the oxidized protein surface.

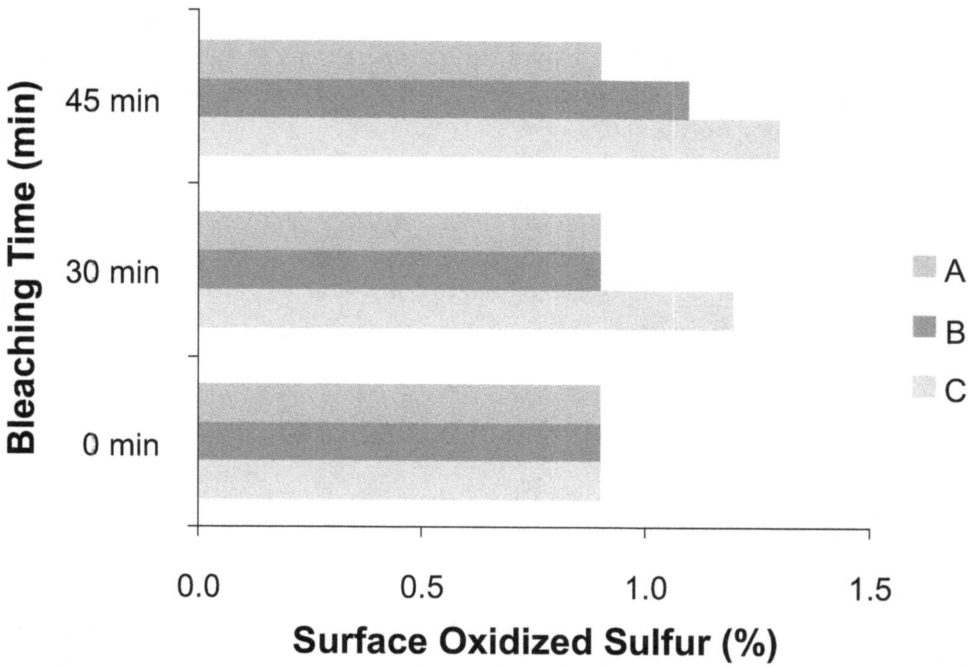

Figure 21: Total oxidized surface sulfur content (cysteic acid) by XPS for (A) bleached hair, (B) bleached hair, pH=9, (C) bleached hair, pH=9, SLS. Comparing *B* and *C* at 30 min., note that the addition of SLS eliminates the inherent induction period for surface oxidation (adapted from Beard et al. [83]).

In summary, XPS enables the direct spectroscopic measurement of deleterious changes in the hair's proteinaceous surface. Correlation of XPS data with data from other techniques, such as SEM, contact angle analysis, AFM, and ToF-SIMS, facilitates a robust description of the chemically damaged fiber surface while offering a means to match the modified surface chemistry with a properly targeted remedy.

7. Inverse Gas Chromatography (IGC)

Inverse Gas Chromatography (IGC) is a dynamic sorption method used to measure the thermodynamic properties of surfaces. Contrary to traditional gas chromatography, as the name of the technique aptly implies, the analyte is not probed by a known stationary phase. Instead, the analyte is represented as the stationary phase in the custom GC column and helium is used to sweep volatile probes through the solid sample (e.g., hair fibers) to a chromatographic detector, such as a flame ionization detector (FID). Depending on the available surface physicochemistry of the sample in the column, the probe vapors will elute at different retention times (see **Figure 22**). The retention times are subsequently converted to net retention volumes (V_N), and the V_N values are then used to derive the total surface free energy for the sample—where the total surface energy is a summation of *dispersive* (e.g., van der Waals) and *specific* (e.g., hydrogen bonding, polar, acid-base) surface energy components (86).

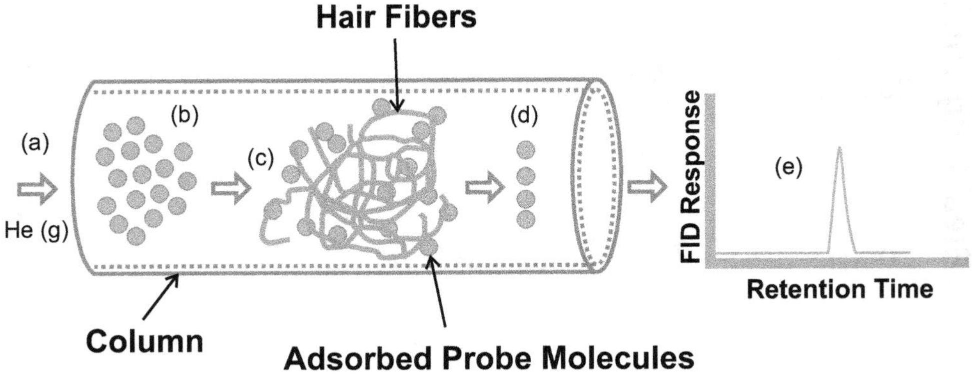

Figure 22: Diagram of an IGC experiment showing the interaction of probe vapor with intact hair fibers that have been packed into a custom-sized chromatography column. (a,b) Helium carrier gas and vapor pulse introduced to the column head; (c,d) retention time of the probe molecules delayed by fiber-probe interactions; (e) model chromatogram showing single peak of vapor probe as detected by the FID (adapted from SEA brochure, Surface Measurement Systems, UK).

Further, surface energy heterogeneity may be determined by pulsing precise amounts of the probes that interact with the substrate (87). Surface energy heterogeneity is essentially a map of the probe-sample surface energy distribution as a function of surface coverage. That is, at very low probe gas volumes, or at infinite dilution, probe-probe interactions are minimized and only a small high-energy fraction of the sample surface interacts with the probe gas; however, at higher volumes of probe vapor (i.e., BET region), perhaps all of the active sites on the surface will interact with the probe gas (88, 89). Contrastingly, if a pulsed volume of adsorbate vapor that is equimolar to the spectrum of active sites on the analyte surface is introduced, then the resulting total surface free energy value will be composed of an average of all interactions between the surface and vapor—as is the case in a traditional surface tensiometry measurement done on a single hair fiber (e.g., Wilhelmy balance method).

The cortex of a healthy strand of hair is protected by a very sophisticated 4–5 μm thick cuticular structure. In virgin hair, the protective sheath emerges from the scalp approximately ten cuticle sheets thick (90); however, as mechanical, thermal, ultraviolet radiation, and chemical insults apply daily strains to the exposed shaft of the complex composite, the damaged sacrificial surface gradually weathers and sheds to spawn a fresh, new surface (91). Consequently, one could argue that most virgin hair samples have been exposed to surfactants (chemicals), a brush or comb (mechanical), and sunlight (UV radiation), and as a result should have varying degrees of history-dependent chemical and morphological micro-heterogeneity at the cuticular surface (**Figure 23**).

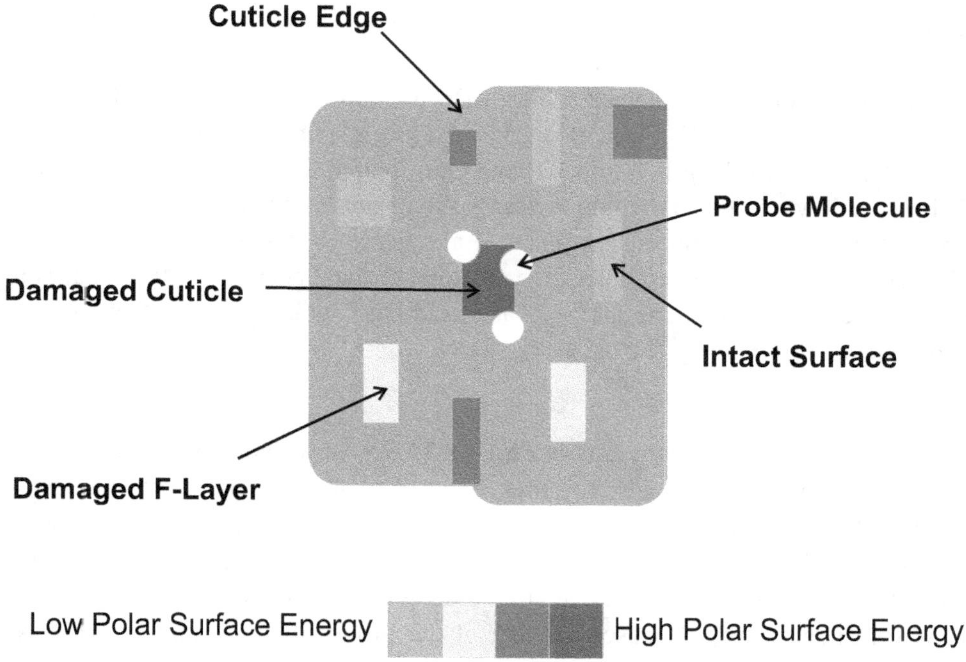

Figure 23: Depiction of model probe-surface interaction as a function of the fiber's x-y surface. Cuticle edges and damaged cells have higher specific (e.g., acid-base, polar) surface energy than the untainted, hydrophobic cuticle surface; hence, small volumes, or small coverages, of polar probe vapors will first interact with high-energy polar sites prior to adsorbing to lower-energy lipophilic locations on the cuticular surface.

Because established methods to calculate the surface energy of fiber surfaces, such as contact angle goniometry or Wilhelmy-based dynamic tensiometry, place relatively large droplets of a liquid onto the surface of the hair fiber(s), these methods inherently produce single-point averages that oppress the realistic distribution of energy sites beneath the voluminously applied droplet (87). In addition, as Young's equation applies to contact angle measurements on smooth and homogeneous surfaces, bulk solvent absorption and roughening of the fiber surface by mechanical, chemical, and aging processes [92] affect the fundamental meaning of the data. In contrast, by varying and strictly controlling the introduction of small volumes of gas/vapor probe molecules, IGC probes the nooks and crannies of the available fiber surface a bit at a time to produce surface energy distribution maps that better describe the breadth of available adsorption sites on the fiber surface.

To better scrutinize the use of IGC in examining damaged hair surfaces, a series of tresses was exposed to a range of mechanical, thermal, environmental, and chemical strains. **Table 6** describes the hair tress preparation details for IGC experiments that were performed on untreated virgin, as well as mechanically, thermally, and chemically strained European Brown hair tresses. Each nontrimmed, full-length hair sample (1.5–2.0 g) was packed into a silanized glass chromatography column (30 cm length, 4 mm ID) and equilibrated for one hour at 25°C/30% RH with a flow of 10 sccm helium carrier gas to normalize the level of physisorbed water. Samples were subsequently run at a series of surface coverages with *n*-alkanes and polar probes to determine the total surface energy (γ_S^{Tot}), which is a sum of the dispersive (nonpolar, γ_S^{D}) and acid-base (polar, γ_S^{AB}) surface energy components, respectively (Eq. 11).

$$\gamma_S^{Tot} = \gamma_S^{D} + \gamma_S^{AB} \tag{11}$$

The initial, low-coverage data in **Figures 24–25** show that pulsing, rather than flooding, the hair samples with limiting moles of *n*-alkane or polar probes results in a treatment-dependent distribution of surface coverages. Introducing incrementally small volumes of probe gas ensures that the full range of the spectrum of surface energies is accurately represented. In contrast, flooding the column with larger volumes of probe vapor causes binding of the probes to high- and low-energy adsorption sites alike; consequently, the coverage data indicate that controlling the extent of the interfacial contact surface ensures that important adsorption contributions from the lower-density, highest-energy adsorption sites of the exposed hair surface are not lost in the statistics.

Table 6: Details of treated European Dark Brown hair tresses later examined by IGC

Sample	**Sample Details**
Flat-ironed, wet	The tress was equilibrated for 30 min in tap water; the excess water was gently removed followed by immediate exposure to five 12 s sweeps with a 190 °C flat iron; subsequently washed with 3% SLS.
Virgin	The tress was washed with a relatively mild 0.3% SLS solution.

Sample	Sample Details
Heavily abraded	The tress was spread evenly on lab bench (1–2 fibers thick) and was scraped from root to tip 100 times on each side with a stainless-steel razor blade; subsequently washed with 3% SLS.
Bleached	The tress was exposed for 30 minutes to a commercial bleaching formulation followed by 3% SLS wash.
Permed	The tress treated with a 2-step home-perming formulation (ammonium thioglycolate) for 1 hr followed by 3–4 min tap water rinse; in step 2, the tress was neutralized with hydrogen peroxide and treated with conditioner (Quaternium-52); tress subsequently washed with 3% SLS.

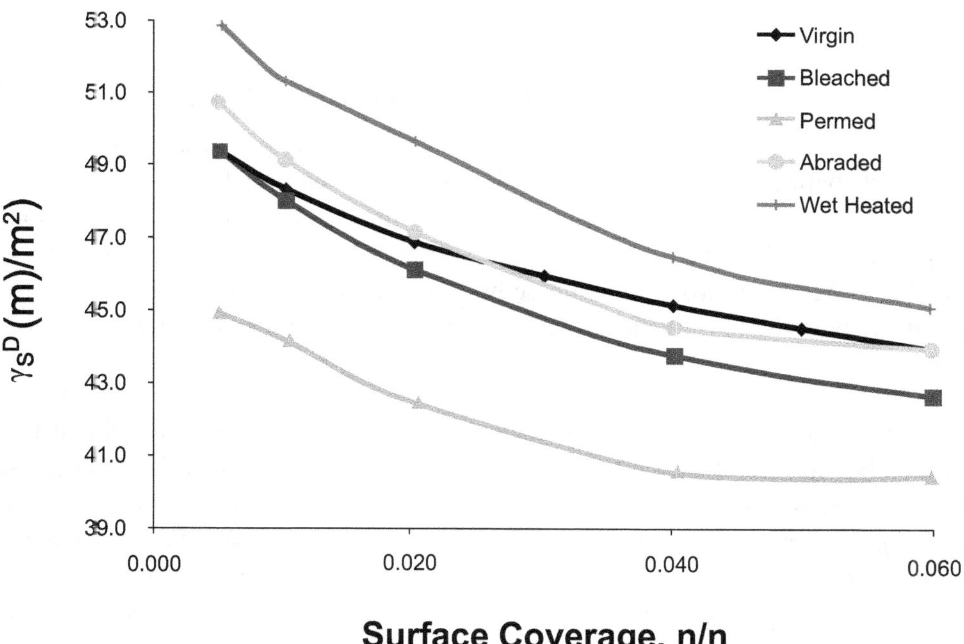

Figure 24: Dispersive surface energy profiles overlay for virgin, bleached, permed/conditioned, abraded, and flat-ironed wet hair fiber bundles. Pulsing discrete volumes of nonpolar probes into the column controls the fraction of probe-covered surface, where 100% coverage = 1.00 (i.e., $n = n_m$), where n_m = number of moles of probe to completely cover the sample surface. Results were produced with the iGC Surface Energy Analyzer (Surface Measurement Systems, UK).

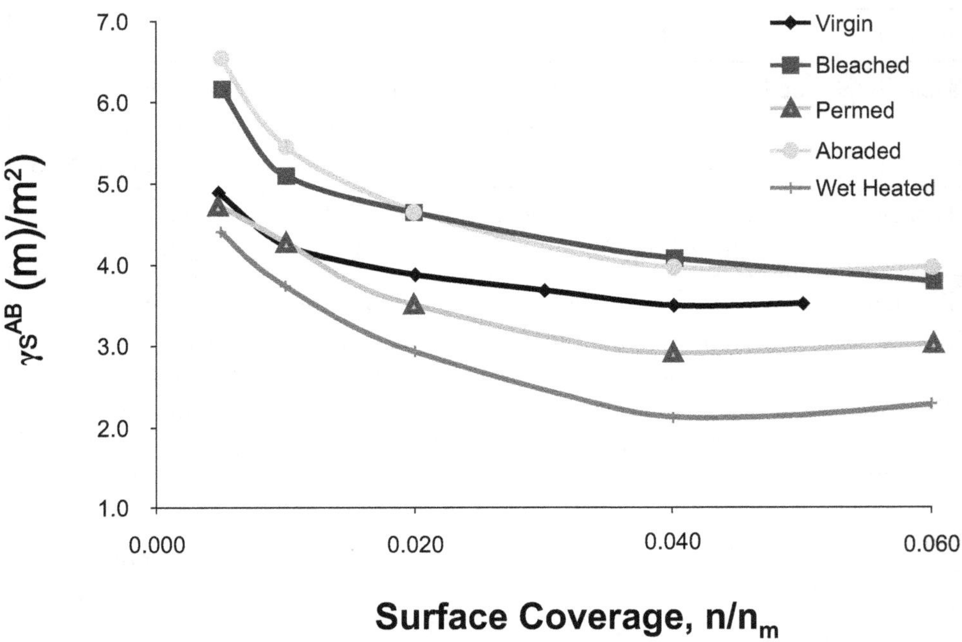

Figure 25: Specific (acid-base) surface energy profiles overlay for virgin, bleached, permed/conditioned, abraded, and flat-ironed wet hair fiber bundles. Pulsing discrete volumes of polar probes into the column controls the fraction of probe-covered surface, where 100% coverage = 1.00 (i.e., $n = n_m$), where n_m = number of moles of probe to completely cover the sample surface. Results were produced with the iGC Surface Energy Analyzer (Surface Measurement Systems, UK).

Before speculating on the relationship between fiber damage and the chemistry of the fiber surface, it's useful to gain a visual perspective for the relationship between dispersion, specific, and the total surface energy of the hair surface (refer to Eq. 11). The heterogeneity profile in **Figure 26** shows an overlay of the aforementioned surface free energy distributions for the bleached hair assembly—where the surface energy distributions estimate the percentage of active surface sites at a particular surface energy. Note that the dispersion and acid-base components are shown relative to the total surface energy and suggest that the γ_S^{Tot} distribution more resembles γ_S^{D} rather than γ_S^{AB}. Hence, the contributions to γ_S^{Tot} by induced temporary and complementary shifts in electron density dominate the energetics of the vapor-solid interface.

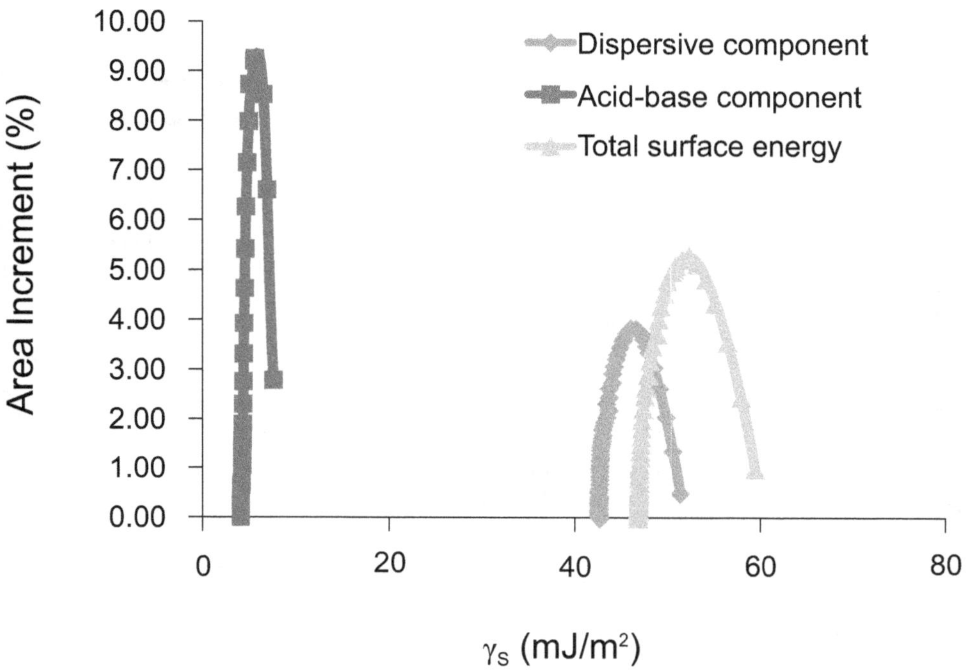

Figure 26: Dispersive, acid-base, and total surface energy distributions for the bleached hair sample. Results were produced with an iGC Surface Energy Analyzer (Surface Measurement Systems, UK).

The trends in the dispersive and acid-base energy profile/distributions in **Figures 24–28** clearly suggest that abrading, bleaching, perming/conditioning, thermal abuse, and associated grooming and SLS washing processes modify the accessible surface chemistry of the respective cuticles. Heavy abrading likely removes layers of cuticle cells and exposes inordinate levels of subsurface protein, including those in the endocuticle and, perhaps, grants limited access to the fiber cortex [90]. Lengthy bleaching with alkaline hydrogen peroxide causes oxidative cleavage of thioester-bound fatty acids and surface cystine, thereby generating higher levels of cysteic acid on the cuticle and exposed endocuticle [93, 94]. Along with many side reactions [95], permanent waving decreases cystine levels and increases cysteic acid and thiolate anion levels [96]. Further, perming may affect the quality of cystine cross-linking in endocuticle bridging structures, leading to higher protein solubility and subsequent cuticle cell delamination [97]. Heating wet hair above the boiling temperature of water can generate internal pressures from steam rapidly escaping from the matrix, CMC, and cuticles, leading to changes in protein and lipid composition/conformation, and to the production of fragments, lifted cuticles, cracks, and holes in the cuticular surface [98, 99, 100]. Further, the ensuing SLS washing and rinsing steps (see **Table 6**) assuredly strips remaining free surface lipids from the fibers [101, 95].

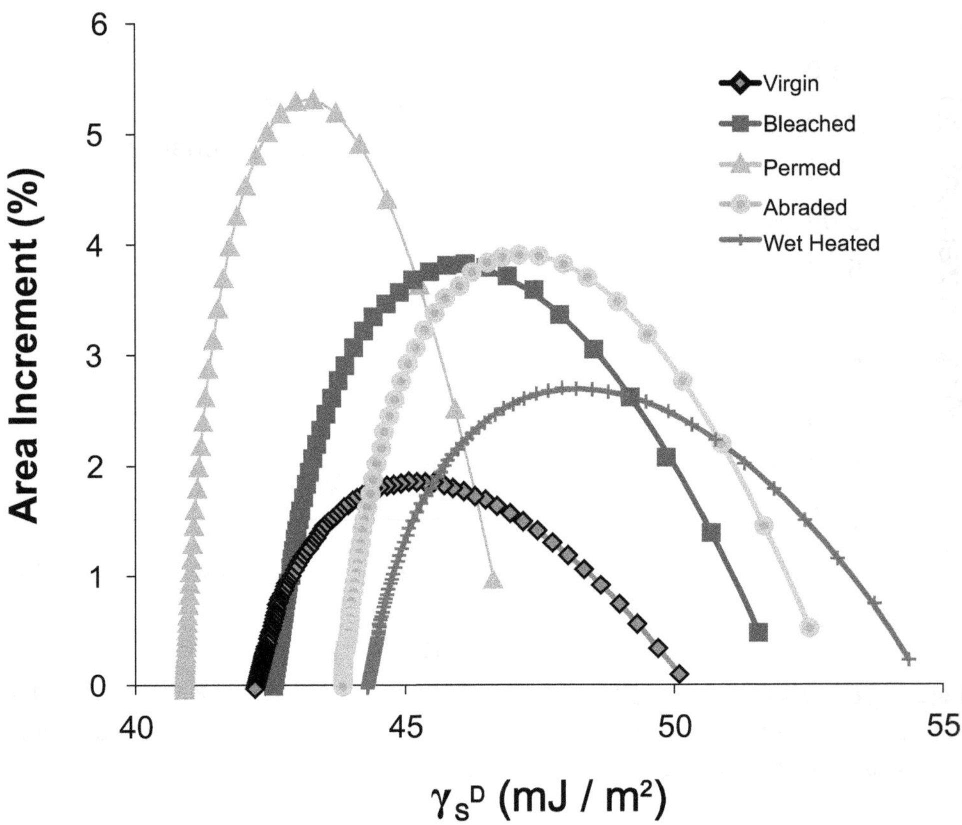

Figure 27: Dispersive surface energy distribution overlay for virgin, bleached, permed/conditioned, abraded, and flat-ironed wet hair samples. Results were produced with an iGC Surface Energy Analyzer (Surface Measurement Systems, UK).

The IGC experiments ranked the γ_S^D *surface heterogeneity*, which is gauged from the breadth (i.e., highest γ_S^D - lowest γ_S^D) in each dispersive surface energy profile in the overlay (**Figure 24**), as follows: wet flat-ironed > abraded ≈ **virgin** > bleached > permed. The γ_S^D *peak maxima* trends, which are captured from the maxima in the surface energy distributions (**Figure 27**), ranked as follows: wet flat-ironed (54.33 mJ/m²) > abraded (52.52 mJ/m²) > bleached (51.51 mJ/m²) > **virgin** (50.07 mJ/m²) > permed (46.68 mJ/m²). The results suggest that the heterogeneity in dispersive surface energy on the fiber surface is increased, relative to virgin assemblies, by wet flat-ironing and heavily abrading processes; whereas the damaging consequences of oxidative bleaching and chemical perming/conditioning appear to modify the surfaces more homogeneously. Additionally, the frequency maxima trends specify that the applied thermal and mechanical processes resulted in the largest γ_S^D peak maxima—indicating that the applied non-chemical strains impart surface stresses that increase the interaction between nonpolar probes and the highest energy sites on the fiber surface. Although changes in surface chemistry are no doubt involved, treatments involving heat, abrasion, perming, and bleaching may add uniform submicron-level surface roughness to the cuticle surface; hence, it is likely that the number of active adsorption sites increased accordingly. Interestingly, bleaching and the lengthy perming process produced the narrowest γ_S^D heterogeneity and lowest γ_S^D peak maxima. Why? Both treatments diminish the interaction of the nonpolar fractions of the surface with dispersion probes. Oxidation increases the number of cysteic acid residues and possibly results in some loss of surface-bound lipids. Perming should also result in increases in cysteic acid surface moieties. However, the γ_S^D trends may be more complex for the perming-conditioning process, as the pH of the combined acidic neutralization and conditioning step may affect the ensuing binding conformation and deposition pattern of quaternary surfactant on the hair surface. More explicitly, at low pH the adsorption mechanism of cationic surfactant may be hydrophobically, rather than electrostatically, driven; therefore, the lower γ_S^D may be due to hair damage as well as the additive influence of accessible polar groups on the deposited cationic surfactant [102].

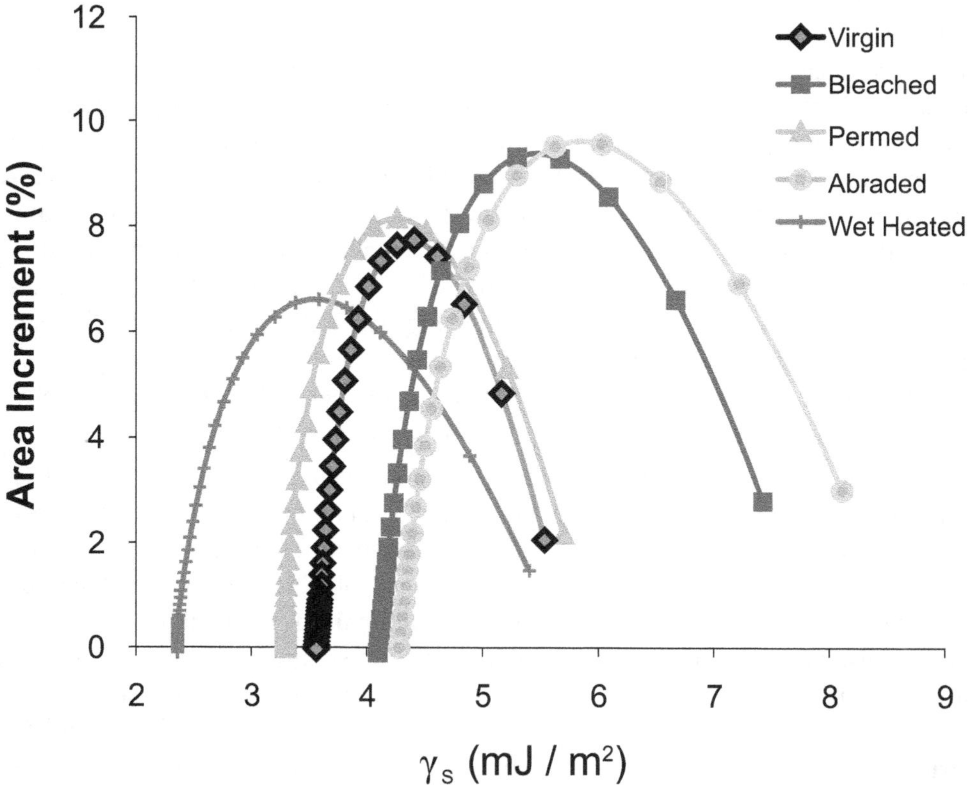

Figure 28: Polar (acid-base) surface energy distribution overlay for virgin, bleached, permed/conditioned, abraded, and flat-ironed wet hair samples. Results were produced with the iGC Surface Energy Analyzer (Surface Measurement Systems, UK).

Figure 28 depicts the specific (i.e., polar, acid-base) surface energy distributions for the five hair samples. The γ_S^{AB} *heterogeneity* ranked in the order: abraded ≈ wet flat-ironed > permed > **virgin** ≈ bleached; whereas the trend in γ_S^{AB} *peak maxima* positioned in the following way: abraded (8.10 mJ/m^2) > bleached (7.42 mJ/m^2) > permed (5.68 mJ/m^2) ≈ **virgin** (5.53 mJ/m^2) ≈ wet flat-ironed (5.39 mJ/m^2). The virgin and bleached samples had the narrowest γ_S^{AB} distribution profiles, indicating that the surfaces had the narrowest allotment of polar sites on their respective surfaces. Because the polar sites on healthy virgin hair are mainly at the cuticle edges and aged fiber tips, and oxidation generates widespread cysteic acid on a bleached hair surface, one can surmise that the γ_S^{AB} distributions should be well defined. In comparison, abraded and wet flat-ironed samples have damaged and missing cuticles, including an augmentation in the available surface area, as well as exposed cuticular and cortical proteins. Therefore, one would expect to see larger breadth in γ_S^{AB} surface energy heterogeneity. The γ_S^{AB} maxima rankings imply that the abraded and bleached samples have elevated fractions of accessible higher energy γ_S^{AB} adsorption sites—indicating that these fibers possess higher fractions of acid-base interactions with the polar probes (e.g., more probe-protein interactions). The data for the wet flat-ironed sample infers that heating the tress may have melted and redistributed the lipids on the fiber surface, thus preventing considerable changes in the number of accessible protein-polar probe interactions. In combination with the observation that the treated assembly was shiny and healthy-looking, the virgin-like γ_S^{AB} data for the permed sample suggest that the conditioning step may have masked some of the chemical damage provoked by the perm treatment. Further evidence is evident in the γ_S^{AB} to γ_S^{Tot} ratio, which is indicative of trends in fractional surface polarity, or surface wettability. **Figure 29** shows that the abraded and bleached samples have the highest fraction of acid-base surface free energy component; whereas the wet flat-ironed, UV-treated, and permed/conditioned samples appear to maintain similar hydrophobicity to that of untreated virgin hair.

In conclusion, IGC has proven useful in gaining insight into changes caused by the damaging effects of environmental, chemical, and thermal strains on the fiber surface. Parameters such as surface energies and enthalpies, surface heterogeneity, and acid-base interactions can be measured at controlled temperature and humidity. As evidenced by the impact of mechanical, thermal, environmental, and chemical strains, as well as the impact of a conditioning step in the perming process, appreciating the interactions between known vapor probes and the hair surface enables an improved understanding of externally induced stresses within the surface structure. Moreover, with the assistance of complimentary surface analytical techniques, such as SEM and IR imaging, IGC may enable a deeper and fundamental understanding of important hair care properties, such as the principles of adhesion, deposition, conditioning, and structure repair.

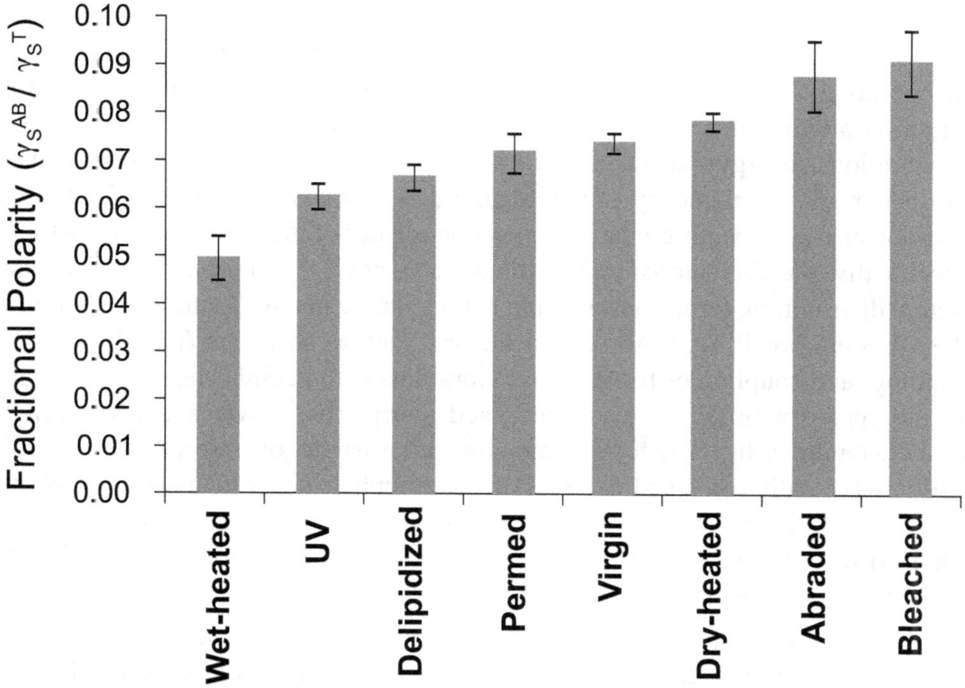

Figure 29: Fractional polarity ($\gamma_S^{AB}/\gamma_S^{Tot}$) comparisons for thermally, environmentally, chemically, and mechanically strained European Dark Brown hair fiber assemblies. The error bars indicate slight variation in polarity as a function of surface coverage. Results were produced with the iGC Surface Energy Analyzer and SEA Analysis software (Surface Measurement Systems, UK).

b. Spectroscopic

1. Infrared Imaging (IR imaging)

Infrared (IR) light is radiation that resides between the visible and microwave regions of the electromagnetic continuum. The IR spectrum is arbitrarily divided into the near, mid, and far infrared spectral regions. The wavelength (λ) of near IR (0.8–3.0 μm) is closest to red visible light, whereas the wavelength range of far IR (30–300 μm) is nearest to the microwave region. Since mid IR (3.0–300 μm) has applicability to functional group analysis, it has arguably been the spectroscopic region of choice for chemical investigators.

Not all bonds are active to IR energy. The ability of a particular bond to absorb IR radiation (i.e., IR active) depends on the presence of a net change in dipole moment as the interatomic distance of the bond fluctuates. If a bond is IR active, the imposed IR radiation couples, or resonates, with the electrical field of the vibrating charge, and the absorbed radiation is subsequently transformed into larger-amplitude bond oscillations (excited state) that have increased rotational-vibrational energy. Fortunately, each functional group has an unambiguous, intrinsic resonant frequency as the magnitude of the discrete, or quantized, absorption energy depends on the native characteristics of the vibrating bond. More specifically, the characteristic absorption frequency for a bond is related to its spatial distribution, force constant, and to the relative masses of the atoms within the vibrating bond [103]. Additional factors, such as solvation (e.g., hydrogen bonding) and coupling of fundamental vibrations with neighboring fundamental vibrations (or with higher overtones), add interpretive power and complexity to the technique. In IR spectroscopy, absorption bands, or absorption frequencies, are typically conveyed in terms of wavenumbers ($\bar{v}$), which are in units of cm^{-1} (i.e., λ^{-1}). Note that the term "absorption frequency" is synonymously interchanged with "wavenumber" because the two magnitudes are both proportional to the imposed IR energy.

A modern FT-IR instrument uses an interferometer to produce a superimposed interference spectrum called an interferogram that contains a complete description of all of the IR frequencies produced by the IR source. The produced interferogram is then passed through the sample, which subsequently absorbs IR energy corresponding to the specific resonant frequencies of its IR active functional groups. The transmitted (or reflected) beam finally passes to the detector. The resulting interferogram is subsequently digitized and sent to the computer for Fast Fourier Transform (FFT) analysis, which basically converts the interferogram, which is in the time domain, to a frequency-based spectrum that can be interpreted by the scientist.

IR Imaging is an extension of FT-IR spectroscopy, and was initially developed to automate the surface composition of larger samples. The system consists of an automated, high-precision x-y stage that sequentially rasters the focus of the IR microscope from spot to spot on the sample. At each position on the surface, complete FT-IR scans are collected. The powerful, nondestructive technique produces high-resolution images that visually illustrate the 2-D distribution of chemistry as a function of x-y sample space [4, 105, 106, 107]. A schematic of the process is portrayed in **Figure 30**.

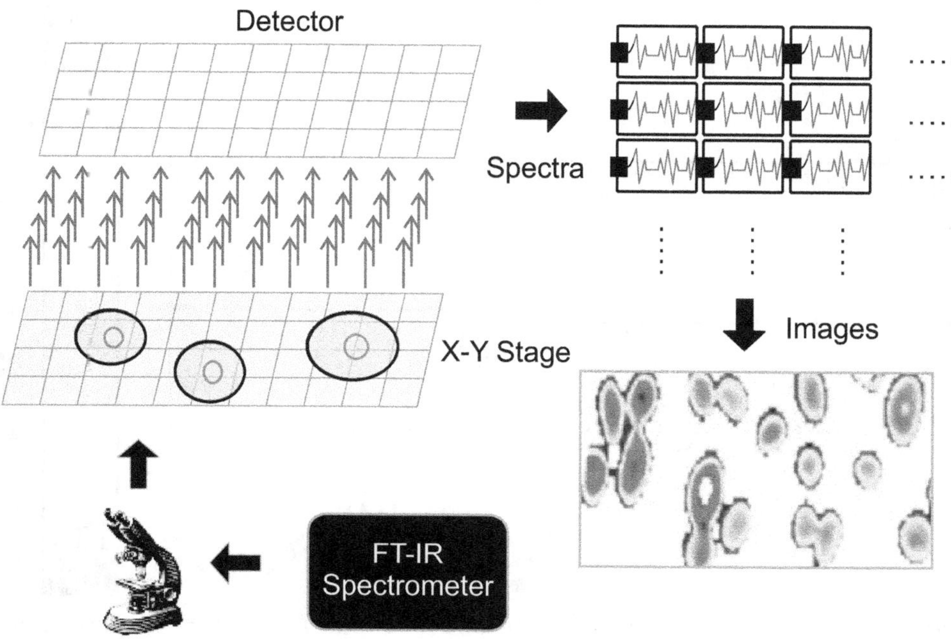

Figure 30: Schematic portraying the assembly of spatially resolved, high-resolution IR images. The spectrometer produces mid-IR radiation that is focused through the optical microscope. The automated stage rasters the sample to reposition the focus of the spectrometer (IR beam) to the new x-y space. The resulting interferograms are generated and processed by the software (FFT) to FT Images for further analysis. Each pixel in the image represents a 6.25 μm spot (Courtesy of Y. Zhou, ASI, Wayne, NJ).

Zhou et al. (4) applied IR Imaging to hot flat-ironed hair tresses to investigate the impact of excessive heat on European dark brown hair. Prior to flat-ironing, tresses *B* and *D* (**Figure 31**) were treated with polymer (0.5 g w/w of 1% solution) and then blow-dried. Subsequently, all four tresses were hot flat-ironed (232°C) with the same treatment protocol: 12 minutes total thermal insult, using 12 s exposure periods and intermittent 10% SLS washing cycles. Small bundles of the tresses were then microtomed to produce very thin 4–5 μm thick cross-sections that were collected on CaF_2 windows for conducting FT-IR image analyses. An MCT linear diode array detector and optical microscope equipped with a high-precision XY sample stage were used for the image mapping process. The individual scans were analyzed and concatenated to produce images (**Figure 31**).

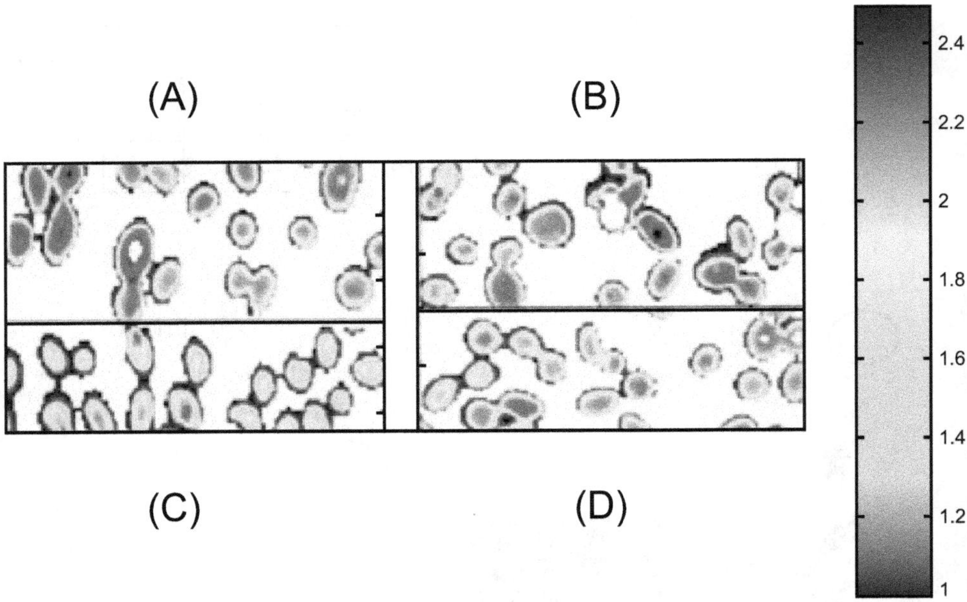

Figure 31: –CH asymmetric stretching band (2960 cm^{-1}) from $-CH_3$ terminal residues of fiber protein, with a minor contribution from the hair lipids. The trends indicate changes in the protein and lipid concentration due to thermal insult, especially for cross-section *C*; where A=Untreated virgin, B=cationic polymer treated virgin; C=thermally treated virgin, and D=pseudo-quat treated virgin fiber cross-sections (courtesy of G. Zhang, ASI, Wayne, NJ).

Each pixel on the image represents the results of a separate scan and corresponds to a specific 6.25 μm × 6.25 μm x-y area coordinate on the sample surface. More specifically, the pixels correspond to the relative concentration of terminal CH_3 residues in the fiber protein (with a minor contribution from the integral lipid), which absorb mid-IR energy at 2960 cm^{-1}. The intensity bar, on the right of **Figure 31**, is used to visually gauge the relative surface concentrations of the chemical species—where more red represents higher levels of intact protein/lipid, and more blue represents a change, truncation, or absence of the species described by the 2960 cm^{-1} asymmetric C-H stretching frequency. As indicated by the marked decrease in the band, the results suggest that the pretreated and thermally exposed fibers (**Figures 31B and 31D**), which were pretreated with quaternized and pseudo-quaternized styling polymers, respectively, fared better in the excessive heat than the untreated hair assembly (**Figure 31C**). The investigators developed similar spectroscopic trends to visualize fiber-protein damage at the molecular level, including changes in α-helix cortical hydrogen bonding, which affected the quality and sustainability of the secondary structure (e.g., irreversible α-helix conversion to β-sheet).

IR Imaging is an indispensible tool for viewing molecular changes to materials such as keratinous substrates. By coupling the technique with other analytical tools, such as DSC, DVS, and sensorial appeal, it may be possible to directly relate claims and performance attributes to trends and variations in the molecular structure.

2. Spectrofluorimetry

The physical basis of fluorescence that makes up the basis of spectrofluorimetry, also known as fluorescence spectroscopy, entails the electronic state of a molecule where a photon is first absorbed by the molecule, which elevates an electron from a ground to a more excited state. This initial phase is termed excitation and has a characteristic wavelength for a particular molecule. Photons are then emitted by the molecule when the excited electron drops down to lower energy levels; this is termed its emission spectrum. The spectrofluorimeter utilizes this physical phenomenon to identify and quantify the amount of the fluorophore present in a system. There are certain amino acids that make up the protein of hair that will fluoresce when they are exposed to a certain wavelength of light. One such compound is tryptophan which, being a heterocyclic amino acid, has an emission spectrum when excited by a certain wavelength of light. Since tryptophan is part of the structure of the various types of proteins of hair, its quantification can be used as an indicator of the level of damage to the structure of these proteins so that conclusions can be made as to the effects of stressful treatments such as UV light and thermal styling as well as the alleviation of this damage through cosmetic pretreatments.

The fundamental research performed by Chandra and Jachowicz formed the basis of using the degradation of tryptophan in hair as a marker of hair photodamage [108]. Their initial experiment consisted of taking sections of hair from a person that had hair previously oxidized by the sun. They exposed the undamaged root section and sunbleached tip sections of the hair to light that had a wavelength of 295 nm, resulting in a strong emission at approximately 340 nm. Thinking that tryptophan was responsible for this response, they subjected L-tryptophan powder and the undamaged brown hair to the same excitation wavelength. The same emission spectrum was produced, proving that they were indeed measuring the amount of tryptophan in the hair of the subject. To further explore this phenomenon, they irradiated hair in a controlled fashion and found that the degree of tryptophan degradation was directly correlated to the time of irradiation. Later, McMullen and Jachowicz performed experiments showing the utility of quantifying tryptophan degradation as applied to the thermal degradation of hair. Controlled experiments using specified treatment regimens with the heat from a hot curling iron indicated that the hair suffered degradation of tryptophan that could be quantified spectrofluorimetrically [109].

Those molecules that are part of the chemical makeup of hair that are considered chromophores will exhibit fluorescence when exposed to a particular wavelength of light. The amino acid tryptophan is one such compound. This heterocyclic compound is illustrated in **Figure 32** with its associated excitation and emission wavelengths. The intensity of the decrease in the emission of tryptophan is an indicator for hair photo or thermal degradation. Typical equations utilized for calculating percent protection from a photofilter or pretreatment to thermal exposure follow (Eqs. 12, 13, and 14).

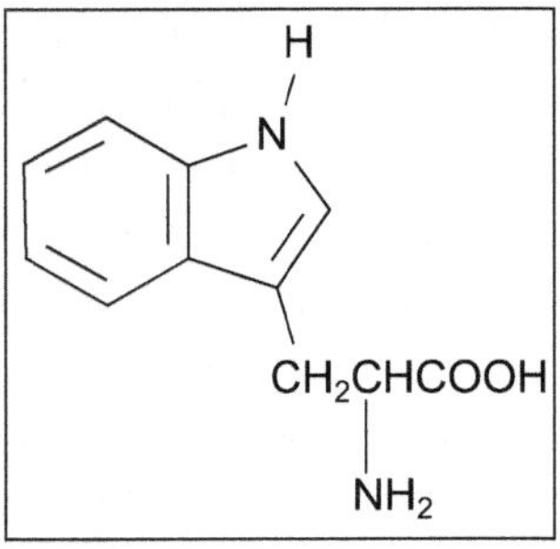

Tryptophan
Excitation: 290 nm
Emission: 336 nm

Figure 32: Heterocyclic structure of tryptophan

$$\text{Ratio of tryptophan intensity} = \frac{\text{Emission intensity at 336 nm of experimental}}{\text{Emission intensity at 336 nm of reference}} \tag{12}$$

The fluorescence emission intensity for an unheated and untreated hair tress is also included in this study as a reference response factor to standardize the tryptophan emission intensity of the experimental hair tresses.

% Degradation is calculated as follows:

$$\left(\frac{\text{ratio tryptophan intensity before treatment - ratio tryptophan intensity after treatment}}{\text{ratio trytophan intensity before treatment}}\right)100\% \tag{13}$$

% Protection is calculated as:

$$\left(\frac{\%\ \text{degradation of control} - \%\ \text{degradation of experimental}}{\%\ \text{degradation of control}}\right)\times 100\% \tag{14}$$

Figures 33 and 34 provide examples of fluorescent spectrums of hair tresses. They consist of with and without protective polymer pretreatments, and before and after exposure to 12 minutes of hot flat-ironing. The spectrum before exposure is indicated by the blue line in **Figures 33 and 34**. The initial amount of tryptophan is measured at the emission peak at 336 nm. After exposure both tresses suffer tryptophan loss as indicated by the lower red spectrum; however, there is also a decrease in the amount of tryptophan lost in the tress with the polymer pretreatment. Percent protection can then be calculated by the difference in degradation from control versus experimental.

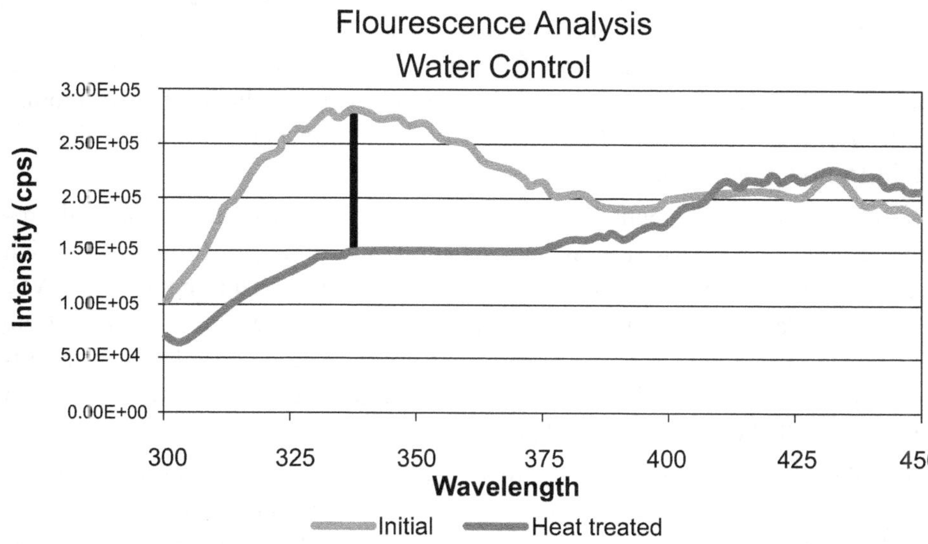

Figure 33: Fluorescent spectrum of control tress before and after thermal exposure

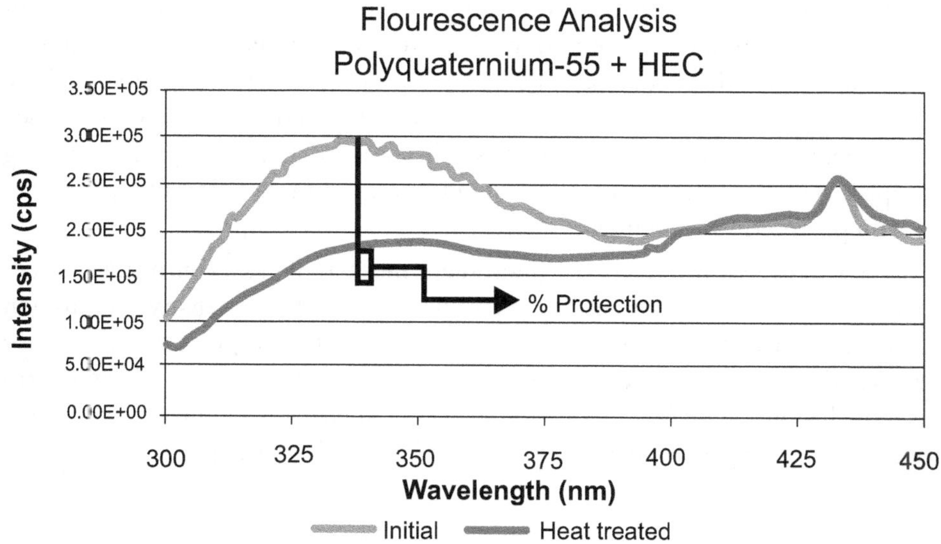

Figure 34: Fluorescent spectrum of tress treated with a polymeric pretreatment

In practice, since tryptophan levels usually decrease from root to tip from normal weathering processes, the hair tress is usually placed into a frame so that measurements are made in one specified location window. Multiple readings are then taken in this one location so as to form a statistical basis for the results.

As mentioned before, fluorescence measurements of hair chromophores were utilized to show hair photodegradation and damage from thermal styling appliances. The utility of this method was also utilized in demonstrating the protective effects of particular ingredients. It was shown, for example, that dodecyl dimethylaminobenzamidopropyl-dimethyl ammonium tosylate, a substantive photofilter, decreased tryptophan degradation, especially when applied from a hair conditioner. This was supported by other methods such as mechanical combing analysis [110, 111]. The photofiltering effect was due to this compound absorbing primarily in the UVB region of the spectrum, thus protecting the hair protein from degradation.

Fluorescent measurements were also utilized to demonstrate the thermal protective effects of VP/DMAPA Acrylates Copolymer and Quaternium-70, which were also supported with combing and textural analysis measurements [112]. VP/DMAPA Acrylates Copolymer and Polyquaternium-55 were shown to protect the hair from the more excessive heat of hot flat irons (**Figure 34**). These were additionally supported by SEM, DSC, and the quantification of fiber fragmentation using a controlled combing method [113].

Besides these techniques, further investigation for thermal protection from hot irons performed by Zhou et al. utilized Atomic Force Microscopy, Differential Scanning Calorimetry, FTIR image analysis, Dynamic Vapor Sorption, and thermal image analysis. Analyzing the date from all these methods provided evidence for the thermal-protective effects of the polymer pretreatments, as well as contributing to the formation of a proposed mechanistic explanation for the thermal degradation and protection processes [4]. The variety of methods are mentioned here as an example of how researchers utilize multiple methods to provide evidence for a particular result or theory, as well as substantiating the validity of measuring tryptophan as a viable method for assessing the alleviation of hair protein degradation with polymeric pretreatments.

To expand the utility of using fluorescent measurements even further, three-dimensional graphs, or matrices, were produced by plotting intensity of emission as a function of excitation wavelength. By so doing, the progressive increase or decrease of chromophores contained in the hair could be monitored. From the results, conclusions could be made as to the chemical changes taking place during a variety of damaging treatments on several different hair types [114].

c. Microscopy

The term "microscope" is derived from the ancient Greek words meaning "small" and "to look." It was developed in the late 16th and early 17th centuries in the era of Galileo. Because of the utility of this instrument for studying what the eye cannot see, the technology continues to advance. Instruments are now available to see beyond what visible light can discern by its refraction through convex lenses. Consequently, we can now observe objects on a nanoscale level as well as the micron and submicron level. This is an ideal situation for studying hair and its hierarchical structure of components. For example, not only can we observe cuticles on the hair surface, but also the deposition of polymers and the effects of damage, such as cracking and pore formation. These observations allow for the diagnosis of the effects of stresses on the hair as well as providing essential information on the protective and cosmetic effects of deposition agents. As a consequence, the literature abounds with photomicrographs of many of the different states of the hair to support scientific hypotheses and conclusions. Some of the results of microscopy, as they relate to hair science and specifically hair damage and its protection and repair, will serve as examples of this most important field.

1. Optical Microscopy

The optical microscope is indispensible in many disciplines in the physical and biological sciences. A few examples of its use in cosmetic chemistry alone include assessing emulsion stability, interaction between polymers and surfactants, and identification of microbes. However, one particular drawback in studying a hair fiber with conventional optical microscopy is the narrow depth of field, where the plane of focus perpendicular to the direction of the vertical line of view does not encompass the whole specimen. This prevents the entire fiber from being viewed with total clarity. As the microscope focus is adjusted, the plane of focus is adjusted through different parts of the hair fiber so that different parts of the fiber come into clear view. Also, light that is coming from under the stage is transmitted through the fiber and prevents the observation of details on the surface.

However, this narrow depth of focus can be advantageous in assessing the degree of thermal damage inside the cortex. A hair fiber taken from a tress that was exposed to the heat from a hot iron was shown to have micropores localized within the cortex of the hair. These were observed as the plane of focus was shifted towards the center of the hair fiber. The micropores were actually seen as white dots due to diffuse light scattering contrasted with the consistency of the cortex. Through digital photography and image analysis, the pore count was quantified with respect to their distance from the surface to the center of the fiber [115]. Using this technique, Gamez-Garcia was able to demonstrate that a corresponding increase in pore count was observed as the number of hot iron cycles and the temperature of the iron were increased. This result suggests an increase in thermally induced cortical hair damage. Also, polymeric pretreatments, such as applying a solution of vinylpyrrolidone methacrylamide/vinyl imidazole copolymer, were able to reduce pore count substantially in both Asian and Caucasian hair.

Gamez-Garcia also utilized optical microscopy to detect damage to the cuticle. This was accomplished by observing light interference patterns using a Hi-Scope digital optical microscope. When a stress was applied to the hair, such as tensile stress, it was observed that iridescent color patterns of light were observed where the cuticle had lifted. The theory of why this occurs entails the phenomenon of thin film interference, such as the phenomenon observed in soap bubbles [116]. The degree of cuticle lifting was quantified by digital image analysis. Observations on thermally damaged hair indicated that there was an increase in cuticle lifting. In contrast to the control, when a protective polymer pretreatment was applied prior to hot ironing there was a reduction in cuticle lifting [115].

Other advancements in optical microscopy include the use of a mechanical z-stage to make a composite of multiple transverse layers (multiple images) of the fiber based on the plane of focus to produce a composite image in which all of the elements are in focus (this eliminates depth of field effects). To overcome the drawbacks of a standard transmission microscope, where the sample is between the light source and the optics, a light source above the image (epi-reflectance) allows light to be reflected off of the surface of the specimen to provide more surface detail as is naturally found in a hair fiber's cuticle.

2. *Microfluorimetry*

When a material absorbs and subsequently re-radiates light, fluorescence or phosphorescence occurs. Fluorescence, as was noted in the section on Spectrofluorimetry, occurs almost instantaneously (in the time frame of a microsecond), whereas phosphorescence consists of a longer lifetime emission after the excitation light has been cut off. If a material has the natural ability to fluoresce, termed primary or autofluorescence, or can be made to fluoresce when treated with a fluorophore (a chemical capable of fluorescing), then the specimen can be studied with fluorescent microscopy, or commonly termed microfluorimetry.

From an optical standpoint, a fluorescent microscope works the same as the optical microscope, with the exception that a fluorescent microscope is augmented with a series of light filters and an excitation lamp (e.g., Hg lamp). With the exception of a very narrow band corresponding to the absorption wavelength, the incident radiation used to illuminate the specimen is blocked. The wavelength band that is transmitted through this filter is selected depending on the excitation wavelength of the molecule in the specimen under study. Various filters can be chosen and the selection depends on the wavelength under consideration. The electrons in the fluorescent molecule of the specimen jump to a higher orbital and release a photon when relaxed to its ground state, with the resultant emission of light typically shifted to a lower wavelength. There is then another filter that excludes the wavelengths used for excitation and transmits the emission spectrum of the fluorescent molecule of the specimen so that this fluorescent effect can be observed either by eye or by a digital camera. An example of a filter system consists of blocking light except in the excitation band of 545 +/– 15 nanometers (green part of the visible spectrum). The filter system also only allows a characteristic emission spectrum of 620 +/– 22.5 nanometers (orange part of the spectrum). In this case, a fluorescent molecule that either makes up the structure of the specimen, or has a compound added chemically as a tag that has an excitation and emission in the specifications of this filter system can be quantified by the intensity of the fluorescent effect which in this emission range is orange.

Human hair has the property of autofluorescence since it contains within its protein structure aromatic and heterocyclic amino acids. This property of hair was utilized by Ruetsch and Weigmann [117] to study the effect that tensile stress has on hair. In their method an individual hair fiber is mounted on a frame that is adapted with a device that can stretch the fiber in a longitudinal fashion (controlled strain). The frame is placed under a fluorescent microscope and the autofluorescence of the hair as observed by the presence of a diffuse blue-white light. The fluorescence in the hair is produced by illuminating the specimen by filtering all light except in the UV region of 340–380 nm. It was observed that as the hair was stretched more fluorescence was observed, especially at the cuticle scale edges. The authors hypothesized that as the scales of the cuticle moved by each other during stretching, the endocuticle would no longer be protected by the upper layers of the cuticle cell where the higher disulfide cross-linking would quench the fluorescent effect. As the hair is continually stretched, the degree of scale lifting was categorized into ràndom scale lifting, common scale lifting, and extreme scaling lifting, which is close to the point of fiber failure. It was found that it took less deformation of the fiber to cause scale lifting at the tip versus the root sections of the hair fiber, indicating that the hair was more damaged as you proceed down the length of the fiber. From the results of this fluorescent technique, in combination with Scanning Electron Microscopy (SEM), the authors proposed a mechanism of scale edge lifting that consists of stresses in the stretch-induced endocuticle and results in structural failure of the cuticle layers. Alternatively, increased fluorescence intensity upon stretching could also be due to a change in the fluorophore's immediate environment (e.g., if it had more degrees of motion). This is a known effect in the study of other substrates.

Rhodamine B has been used as a fluorescent tag in many studies to show the effect of damaging treatments to hair. Since it is cationic (see structure in **Figure 35**), it will preferentially bind to anionic sites of hair. Since damaged hair has more cysteic acid, the anionic byproduct of disulfide bond cleavage, it is expected that there will be a higher deposition of Rhodamine B to hair as indicated by a higher level of fluorescence. This was observed experimentally where it was found that a higher level of fluorescence intensity was directly related to the time of exposure to 6% hydrogen peroxide during a bleaching treatment [118, 119]. It was also shown that fluorescence was evident on untreated fibers mostly along the scale edges. This would suggest that this part of the hair morphology carries an anionic charge, which relates to the behavior of cationic polymer deposition [118].

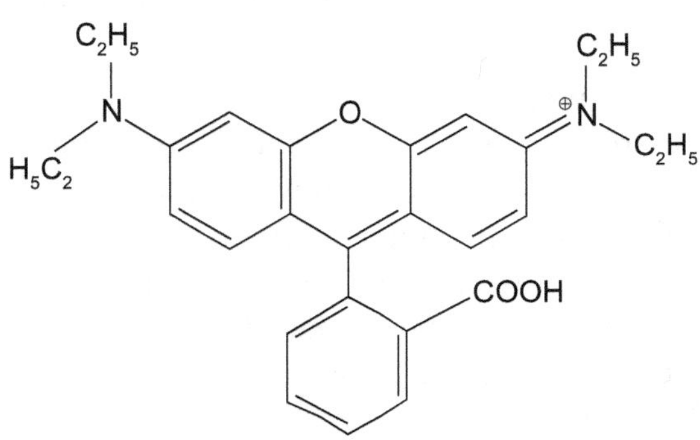

Figure 35: Structure of Rhodamine B

Microfluorimetry has been used to provide evidence of the deposition of compounds on the hair surface. There are two ways a fluorescent tracer can be utilized for this. The first is a non-covalent binding, where the tracer has an ionic attraction for the compound in question, such as an anionic fluorophore being attracted to a cationic polymer. The other is when the molecule being studied can be modified chemically such that it will have an intrinsic ability to fluoresce when exposed to a certain wavelength of light. In the case of polymers, there are two synthetic routes to do this. Polymerization can be performed where one of the constituent monomers has a fluorescent tracer bound to it. Also, a fluorophore can be grafted onto a preformed polymer as long as one of the polymer's functional groups is reactive with the fluorophore. It is important to consider whether the addition of the fluorophore to the polymer affects the fluorescent effect of the molecule, or the substantivity of the polymer.

An example of a non-covalently bound tracer is found in studies by Weigmann et al. in which the sodium salt of fluorescein, also known as uranine, an anionic fluorophore, was added to solutions of cationic cellulosic ethers. By experimenting with various treatment schedules, the deposition behavior of this cationic polymer to the hair was characterized [120].

Polymer deposition was also characterized by fluorescein-labeled polyquaternium-10. Here the fluorophore was covalently linked to the reactive sites on the parent polymer. The synthetic pathway and initial deposition results are described by Goddard and Winnik [121]. As indicated by microspectrophotometry, fluorescent deposits could be seen on a hair fiber, as indicated by the presence of a bright green color on top of a dark background after it was immersed in a 0.1% solution of the labeled polyquaternium-10. Deposition was especially concentrated near the cuticle edges. Since this polymer is applied to hair from a shampoo system, where the mechanism of deposition is quite different from that of the solution, Gruber utilized the same labeling technique for polyquaternium-10 and studied deposition from a model surfactant system [122]. Different molecular weight and charge density variants of tagged polyquaternium-10 were investigated. The study was done quantitatively, by measuring the amount of fluorescence from digested hair samples, as well as by observing the qualitative fluorescent photomicrographs. Quantitative results indicated that polymer molecular weight, polymer charge density, number of washes with the shampoo, and the location of the sample of hair taken on the tress were important variables in polymer deposition. Qualitative photomicrographs were similar to those taken by Goddard, where the green fluorescence on the hair especially along the cuticle edges indicated polymer deposition.

Additional details concerning optical microscopic techniques can be found online on the Nikon and Olympus websites [123, 124]. Despite recent advancements in optical microscopy, it still has limitations in magnification, for example, and the lack of sub-microscopic detail limits the understanding of the mechanism of a damaging process or the effect of compounds frequently formulated for the hair's protection or repair. In hair damage research, efforts focus on obtaining high-resolution images on the nanoscale as opposed to the micron scale. This is done with Scanning Electron Microscopy (SEM), and also Atomic Force Microscopy (AFM), which are discussed in the following two sections.

3. *Scanning Electron Microscopy (SEM)*

This technique has been utilized extensively in hair research. Technical articles abound with high-resolution SEM photomicrographs of the surface of hair. These have illustrated, for example, characteristics of surface morphology for forensic evidence, surface damage through the effects of chemical treatments, and demonstrating the deposition of polymers through rinse-off conditioning products. The basic operation of the SEM consists of focusing an electron beam on the specimen surface. As this incident beam rasters back and forth over a particular area of the surface, it results in the emission of low-energy secondary electrons from the atomic elements on the surface. With the use of a detector and other components of the SEM, the emitted electrons are translated into a three-dimensional topographical image of the surface. Besides the high resolution, another advantage of the SEM is the high depth of focus, which gives the three-dimensional aspect to the photomicrographs. This is exemplified in the SEM image in **Figure 36**, where a hair fiber is magnified 11,000X to show the morphological character of the cuticle.

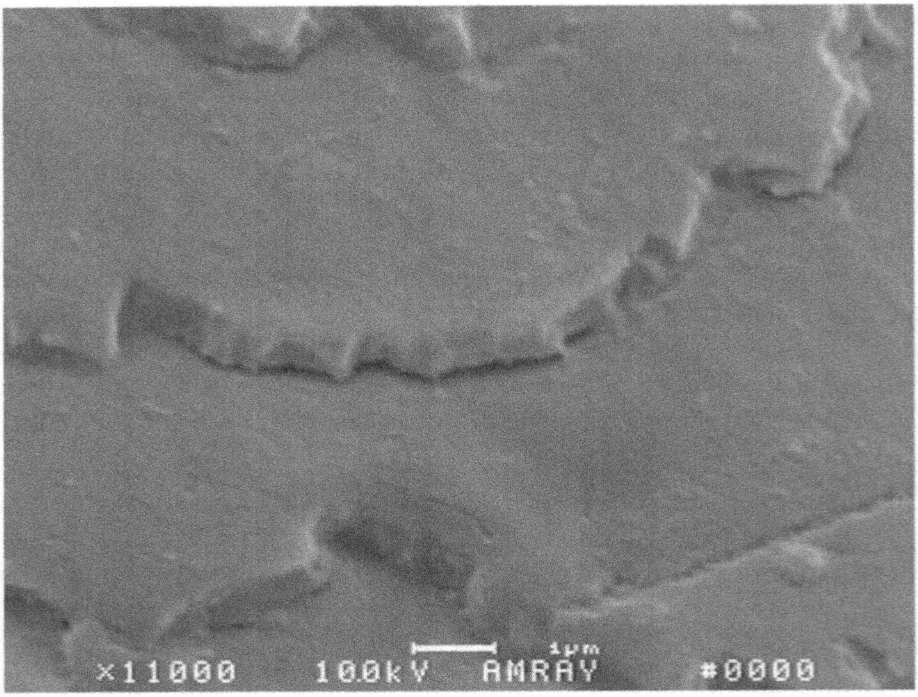

Figure 36: High magnification of the cuticle using SEM (B. Thompson, Ashland Analytical Dept.)

SEM has shown great utility in capturing various types of hair damage. Brown and Swift have used it as a diagnostic tool to show hair damage from various straining experiments (39). Examples of some of the different types of hair damage are portrayed in **Figures 37** through **40**. Protein denaturation is shown in the cuticula after exposing to the heat from a hot flat iron (**Figure 37b**). Cuticular lifting, transverse fractures, and a split end fiber in **Figures 38, 39,** and **40**, respectively were produced from mechanical or a combination of thermal and mechanical stress. An undamaged fiber in **Figure 37a** can be used for comparison.

a) b)

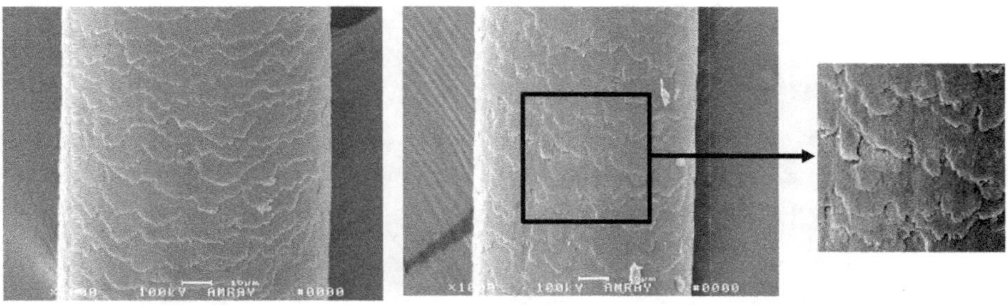

Before Heat Treatment After Exposure to 12 minutes of Hot Flat Ironing (205 °C)

Figure 37: SEM of a) undamaged fiber; b) heat treated fiber (B. Thompson, Ashland Analytical Dept.)

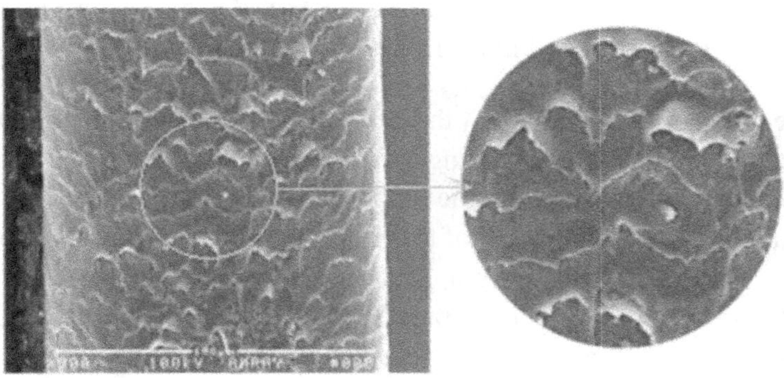

Figure 38: SEM of cuticular lifting (B. Thompson, Ashland Analytical Dept.)

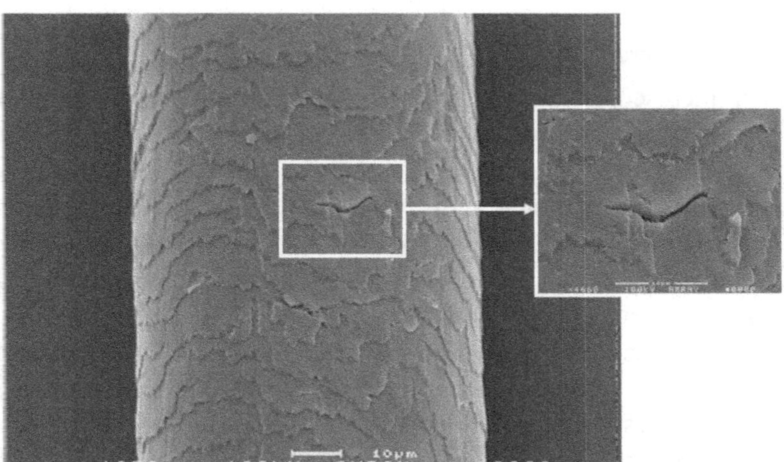

Figure 39: SEM of a transverse fracture (B. Thompson, Ashland Analytical Dept.)

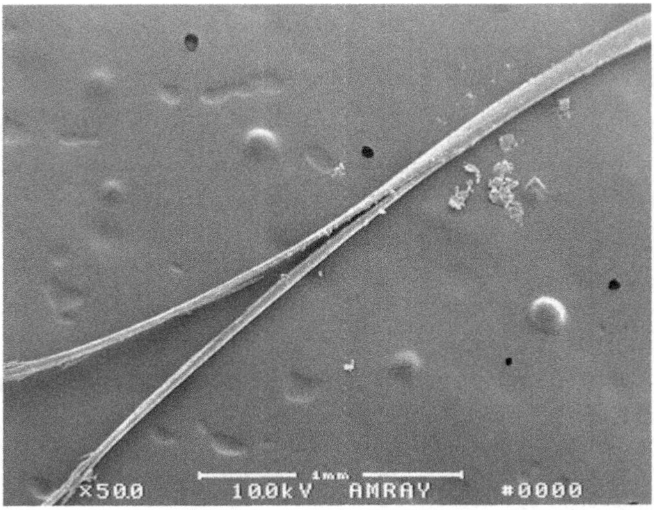

Figure 40: SEM of a split end fiber (B. Thompson, Ashland Analytical Dept.)

Despite the quality of detail that the SEM affords, the experimenter must proceed with caution in making overriding conclusions. It is important for the microscopist to take many pictures along the length of the fiber and to choose those that are most statistically representative of the damaged state. Swift put it very precisely: "To put it into context, a photograph of a single hair, even at the relatively low magnification of 1000X from the average SEM, samples only a mere one hundred millionth of the total surface of the hairs on the average scalp" [125]. Therefore, SEM pictures provide only partial evidence for a particular damaging or protective effect. Typically, as can be seen in the technical literature, it is substantiated by results from other methods such as those portrayed in this chapter.

4. Atomic Force Microscopy (AFM)

Unlike other microscopic methods, this technique does not employ any part of the electromagnetic spectrum. Instead, the AFM consists of a conical or pyramidal shaped probe that has a very sharp submicron diameter tip. The probe is scanned back and forth over an area that is in the realm of square nanometers or microns. As the probe rasters across the surface it analyzes the surface for spatial characteristics that can produce topographical images of the surface as well as provide a host of mechanical characteristics. The method has distinct advantages in that the specimen is not usually sacrificed in its analysis so that treatments can be assessed both before and after their application. This makes the technique ideal for hair protection and repair studies. Another advantage of AFM is in studying the surface when exposed to different humidity levels. In fact the surface can be analyzed in water, which is an obvious advantage for certain hair treatments. The capability of AFM and its utility in the personal care industry has advanced over the last two decades and it is anticipated that this trend will not change.

As the sharp tip traverses and interacts with the surface of the specimen there is a mechanism that the equipment employs for data collection. This is accomplished by having the probe attached to a cantilever. As the tip interacts with the surface it deflects the cantilever and the deflection is followed by a laser beam focused on the surface of the cantilever. This deflection is converted to an electrical signal that then moves the location of the mounting stage to keep the cantilever in its normal position. The movement of the stage in the vertical direction is combined with the coordinates of the back-and-forth movement of the stage as the probe rasters across the surface. This data are then converted with the help of a computer to produce a topographic map of the surface. If the sample contains a soft surface, such as a polymeric film, then tapping instead of a contact mode is used [126]. Other modes are available to detect the adhesion properties of the surface through torsional deflection of the probe on the surface, as in Lateral Force Microscopy (LFM) [127]. Another capability is nano-indentation that examines the surface for its micromechanical properties such as hardness and elasticity [128]. Following is an introduction on some of the major areas of the utility of AFM techniques in hair care.

Structural characterization—In some of the early work by Goddard and Schmitt, polymer and polymer-surfactant complexes were identified on mica surfaces. This substrate was chosen since it presented the probe with a flat and anionic surface to study deposition of cationic polymers from rinse-out systems. A preliminary study showed that contact of the sharp edge of the cantilever as it moved across the surface would tend to perturb the polymer coating as exhibited by a loopy structure. This was later rectified by utilizing the tapping mode of the instrument. J. Smith utilized AFM to demonstrate the high-resolution topography of the hair surface [129]. A 20 × 20 um area was scanned and the resultant profile not only showed the cuticle cells but also the subcellular endocuticle, exocuticle, and A layers of the cuticle cells. In another series of experiments this author was able to identify surface deposits such as the microgranular texture of zinc pyrrithione (anti-dandruff active) on the cuticle surface. When analyzed in the wet state with a specialized environmental chamber, the particles were removed. Also, rough surface deposits in unwashed hair were removed by washing with a conditioning shampoo. McMullen et al. showed that damaged hair, especially hair that has gone through the process of solvent extraction, exhibited nanometer-sized micropores, which the author believed was due to the dissolution of surface lipids and subsequent exposure of the proteinaceous fiber surface. He also found that damaged hair treated with the cationic polymer, VP/MAPTAC copolymer, contained surface deposits. Evidence suggests that this polymer binds to the micropores, the affinity being based on the negative charges of the micropore having a higher affinity for the cationic charges of the polymer. To prove that these micro-structural effects impact the cosmetic behavior of hair, combing work done with a Dia-Stron miniature tensile tester indicated the level of damage and was reduced almost to the level of undamaged hair when treated with a cationic polymer [127].

An example of the surface characterization of the hair by AFM is shown in **Figure 41**. On the left is an illustration of hair in its undamaged state. It can be observed that there is an intact undamaged cuticle. The picture on the right is taken from a fiber that has suffered from a damaging heat treatment. In this case, the cuticle appears less smooth and the cuticles edges are more jagged. Another indication of damage is the presence of small holes or cavities, which may affect the water management of hair as well as its color wash-fastness.

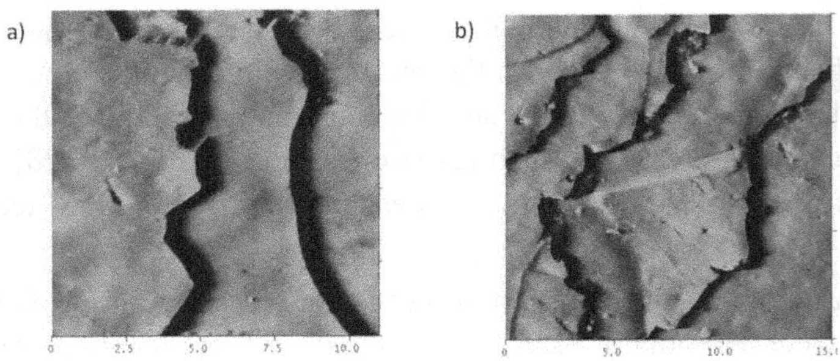

Figure 41: AFM images a) undamaged hair, and b) thermally damaged hair (G. Zhang, Ashland Material Science Dept.)

Tribology—Friction is an important attribute in characterizing the cosmetic behavior of hair. Friction is not just evident between the sensory aspects of the skin and hair, as in the case of the conditioned feel of hair, but friction between individual fibers contributes to the cosmetic behavior of hair and negatively affects combing properties. There are three factors that characterize the frictional properties of hair. These include the surface roughness, frictional force, as measured by the coefficient of friction (COF), and adhesive forces. All three of these micro-tribological characteristics can be measured by AFM and can be useful in making conclusions, along with more macro-tribological tests, in assessing fiber damage and the efficacy of conditioning and protection treatments.

Friction is measured synchronously with surface roughness using contact mode AFM (i.e., LFM). The torsion that the cantilever experiences due to friction as it scans the surface is monitored by the angle of deflection of the laser beam as it is reflected off of the cantilever surface [127]. As with topography, frictional force maps can be constructed to show areas on the hair surface of varying friction. COF of the surface is derived by measuring frictional forces as the probe rasters across the hair surface. A different mode of measurement is used for adhesion. Here the stage that the hair is mounted on is lowered and the force that is required to separate the probe from the surface is measured. Many measurements are made in a nanoscaled region of the hair surface to produce an adhesion map of the area [130].

From these three types of measurements, La Torre et al. were able to study the effects of various conditioning treatments. It was found that cationic surfactants in a fatty alcohol base preferentially deposited at the cuticle edge as revealed by the lower frictional forces and higher adhesion forces. The increase in adhesion was due to the meniscus effect between the probe and the deposits on the hair. Adding PDMS to the conditioner system does not show an increase in adhesion to the same extent due to both a lower coefficient of friction, as well as a decreasing meniscus effect due to its higher mobility on the hair surface. Amodimethicone was also shown to not deposit uniformly on the hair surface [130].

Mechanical Properties—This technique can determine the nanomechanical properties of a surface. The deflection of the probe is monitored as it is pressed into the surface with a set amount of load, usually in the mN range of force. From these data, hardness, elastic modulus, and creep of the surface against a particular load can be measured. The indentations are usually performed adjacent to each other on the same fiber. Again, since this is not a destructive technique, the indents can be done both before and after various treatments on the same fiber.

Nano-indentation was utilized by Wei et al. to study the different micromechanical properties of Asian, Caucasian, and African hair and the response to damaging and conditioning treatments. Some important findings as outlined in the conclusion are:

- The hair cuticle was found to have a higher hardness and elastic modulus than the cortex.
- The hardness of the different layers of a particular cuticle cell decreases and correlates well with cross-link density.
- Asian hair has higher mechanical properties than both Caucasian and African hair.
- The depth to which the damaging or conditioning treatment is effective can be determined by measuring the mechanical properties of the surface at various depths. In this study, the treatments had an effect to a depth of 1.5 um, which equates to 3–4 cuticles thick. The conditioning effects were not uniform on the surface.

These conclusions show that morphological differences can be observed with different hair types, in addition to their response to different treatments. This suggests that AFM can be utilized to further study the nature of hair damage and the effects of protective and repair treatments.

Reutsch found that multiple treatments of hair fibers with a cationic conditioning polymer, Polyquaternium-10, reduce the surface hardness of the cuticle face.

The reduced surface hardness was indicated by an increase in indentation from 49.4 ± 5.6 nm to 61.9 ± 8.8 nm for unconditioned and conditioned measurements respectively. The mechanism behind the softening effect of the conditioning agent may be due to the hydrophilicity of the polymer [131].

d. Mechanical Properties

1. Tensile strength

The historical method for evaluating the mechanical properties of hair is tensile strength testing, as indicated by the early publication dates of some of the technical articles in the personal care literature and wool industry [132, 133]. Tensile strength is defined as force per cross-sectional area (e.g., g/cm^2) and requires two key measurements in its calculation. First, an average diameter of the fiber is measured so that cross-sectional area (πr^2) can be calculated. Then the force in grams is measured as the hair fiber is strained in a longitudinal fashion; see insert in **Figure 42a**. Here we are controlling the rate of strain (deformation) and measuring the stress. The resultant stress-strain curve for hair is very characteristic compared to other fibers. The profile shows an elastic, yield, and post-yield region prior to breakage and is due to the composite nature of fibrous proteins and the morphological components residing in the cortex. **Figure 42b** depicts a typical stress-strain curve of human hair. The tensile properties are affected by humidity since the cortex of the hair imbibes water and swells. As can be seen in **Figure 42b**, hair at lower humidity has a lower tensile strength and higher elongation before breakage. Clearly, the contrasting results of the water content on the mechanical properties of the fiber convey the impact.

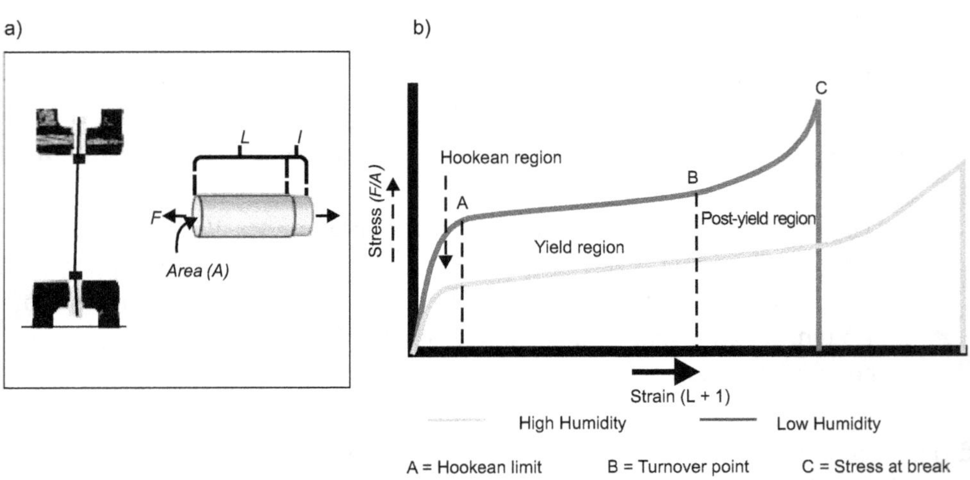

Figure 42: a) Instron imparting a controlled strain on a hair fiber and a description of units in the stress-strain curve. b) Stress-strain-behavior of human hair at high and low humidity as well as the nomenclature of the various regions in the stress-strain curve.

Tensile strength is a destructive method in that after the hair breaks it cannot be used again to see the effect of a damaging treatment or a protective pretreatment. Therefore, a population of fibers is measured from a hair tress or series of hair tresses. These data are then compared statistically to a population of fibers taken from a second experimental series of tresses, or a control. Usually, on approximately one hundred fibers are used for each experimental campaign to form a statistical basis for the conclusions.

It has been argued by several researchers that the tensile strength test does not provide a fair assessment of the state of the hair with respect to its strength or weakening since the strain on hair is in a one-dimensional longitudinal direction [134, 135, 136]. There are many other factors that contribute to mechanical stress, especially during the combing process, which have been mentioned in the previous section on simulating the damaging effects to hair. Other methods have been developed to better understand the effects of these strains on hair and include Impact Loading, Flexabrasion, Fatigue Analysis, Torsion, Texture Analysis, and Dynamic Mechanical Analysis (DMA).

2. Impact Loading

One proponent of the theory that hair breakage during the mechanical action of combing is due to more than just a one-dimensional linear deformation of the fiber was the late Clarence Robbins. Providing evidence for this is a four-part series of articles where he formulates conclusions from the results of a series of simple but convincing tests [135, 138]. One experiment included what he termed impact loading where he simulates one hair fiber impacting and being compressed against another during the combing process. This impacting event during combing is most prevalent when the teeth of the comb hit a snag so that fibers not only hit each other with a high rate of velocity, but also hit the comb tooth, which is an event that cannot be simulated by the limitations of tensile load experiments. To more realistically simulate this strain on hair, Robbins designed a test that consisted of making a circular loop with one hair fiber that has a weight attached to one end. Another hair fiber is threaded through the loop and held in a taut horizontal position. The weight of the fiber loop is lifted and then dropped in such a fashion that the fiber of the loop impacts the fixed horizontal fiber. In another test, the fiber loop is also made to impact in the same way on a fixed comb tooth. The number of impacts that the fiber can withstand is then quantified. One conclusion from this study was that hair fiber loops break more readily over other fibers as opposed to the comb tooth. From a physical standpoint there is more stress per unit area on a single fiber than on a comb tooth due to the difference in diameter (Stress=F/A).

In another series of experiments, Robbins conducted fiber fragmentation during combing. Quantification of broken fibers was assessed by classifying them by size. From the fiber fragmentation and impact loading results, Robbins concluded that short fiber fragmentation, those fibers that are less than 2.5 cm in length, and long fiber fragments break during combing by different mechanisms. The shorter fiber fragments are formed from the ends of the fibers, which is the weakest part of the hair. These hair ends wrap around themselves and around the comb tooth, which produces multiple stresses resulting in breakage. Longer fiber fragments are a result of impact loading of hair fibers against each other and against the comb tooth, especially when hitting a snag.

Although stress response behavior of hair fibers as they are deformed in a longitudinal direction, as in classical tensile strength studies, has its place in studying hair damage, it is obvious that the stresses that hair fibers are subjected to is more complex during the combing process. Although extension is one strain that hair is subjected to, the experiments by Robbins' show that impacting one hair fiber over another or over the teeth of the comb as well as compression and abrasion are other factors in the stress of combing as well.

3. *Flexabrasion*

Another proponent of the theory that hair breakage during combing occurs by more than just extensional strain is Alan Swift. He designed a method where a single hair fiber with a weight on one end is draped over a horizontal wire. The fiber is then moved back and forth over the wire that simulates the dynamic bending that occurs especially during combing. The number of cycles required to break the fiber is a measure of evaluating hair strength [139, 140]. Again, this method requires a statistical analysis of populations. Swift has argued that this is an improved method to assess the strength of a hair fiber since the hair fiber is never subjected to an excessive strain in a longitudinal direction that will subject the hair to enough stress that it will break. In fact the hair will most likely be removed from the follicle before breaking. Breakage occurs when hair is bent in a dynamic fashion; that is, the bend propagates from root to tip, and it is the shear stresses taking place in the interior of the hair that are responsible for breakage [141].

4. *Fatigue analysis*

In most cases, the force required to break a fiber is higher than the force that it takes to extract it from the hair follicle in the scalp [142]. Therefore, during the styling process, hair fibers will actually experience a variety of stresses below those that produce total fiber failure. Based on the magnitude of the deformation, hair fibers could experience stresses in various parts of the stress-strain curve that result in different levels of permanent damage. When hair is deformed in a longitudinal direction, as in tensile strength testing prior to the onset of the yield region, it will typically recover to its normal state since deformation is within the Hookean or elastic region of deformation. Here chemical bonds or morphological structures are not broken. However, when hair is deformed beyond the yield region, a permanent structural change occurs that tends to weaken the hair and to lower its resistance to withstanding successive deformations. The fiber will ultimately break, depending on the number and severity of these successive deformations. During grooming, especially during combing or brushing, the strains on individual hair fibers are random and are based on the nature of their interactions as they weave in a complex fashion with each other. The purpose of the fatigue experiment is to explore the effects of repeated mechanical insults to fibers in a more controlled fashion by standardizing the cyclical level of deformation or stress imposed on the fiber.

To assist in this type of experiment, an instrument normally used for tensile strength testing can be utilized. Instead of having the equipment set up to deform or stretch the fiber and monitor stresses through the point of break, it is instead used to deform the fiber a certain percentage of its total fiber length, or to a certain degree of stress. These controlled deformations or stresses are repeated and the number of cycles is monitored until the fiber fails. A population of fibers from a given tress with a particular treatment serving as a control can then be compared to a population with an experimental treatment to see if there is an effect on its alleviation of the weakening of hair due to the repeated cycles. Instruments have been designed with adaptations to specifically test for fatigue behavior. Dia-stron has developed the Cyclic Tester, which repeatedly applies a user-defined cycling force at a particular rate of deformation [143]. Since the fiber cross-sectional area is measured before cyclical testing, the stress that the fiber is subjected to is also known. The number of cycles to break is recorded, after which the equipment automatically installs a new fiber for the next trial. Further, stress-strain curves can be generated for each measured fiber so that the experimenter knows what region of the stress-strain curve the fiber is being subjected to.

Using the Dia-stron CYC800 equipment, Evans treated his resultant fatigue data in a statistical manner to produce survival probability plots that could be used to predict the number of cycles to break a fiber based on a controlled and repeatable applied stress [144]. He first produced what he termed S-N curves, which are constructed by plotting applied stress (g/um2) versus cycles to failure. The trend showed that the higher the imposed stress on the fibers, the lower the number of cycles it took before the fibers broke. Based on regression analysis of the data, it was possible to determine the average number of cycles to break a fiber as a result of a specifically applied stress. Exponential distributions of survival probability versus cycles, or survival probability plots, are constructed from mathematical treatment of the data using the Weibull function. The analysis using this equation includes the shape factor that indicates whether the failure rate increases or decreases with the number of cycles. One result the author used to demonstrate the utility of these survival probability plots was to show the lower survivability of hair fibers stressed at 60% versus 20% relative humidity, confirming that water plasticized and weakened the fibers due to the humidity in the atmosphere.

The implications of the fatigue experiments, where greater survivability is shown at lower levels of stress, are clear when the mechanism of how hair conditioning agents work is considered. These ingredients act primarily as lubricating agents, such that there is less friction of the comb or brush traversing the assembly of fibers during grooming. Since the fibers are subjected to less cumulative stress, their survivability is greater.

5. Torsional strain

It can clearly be envisioned how combing or brushing leads to fracture and breakage through both tensile and bending stresses. The tensile stress imparted by a one-dimensional longitudinal strain caused by combing cannot be argued. Neither can the two-dimensional strain of bending in an x-y plane. However, hair shape is in three-dimensions and stresses need to be considered in the x, y, and z planes. To accomplish 3-D analysis, the factor of torsional strain has to be considered. A model for visualizing this is the mechanical behavior of a helical coil or spring that is subjected to an axial load as per equation 15 [145]. An illustration of the torsional components applied to hair tresses is illustrated in **Figure 43**.

Obviously the deflection of the coil is directly dependent on such factors as the load (P), but it is inversely related to the torsional modulus of the fiber itself. That is, the harder it is to deform the fiber through twisting, the less the coil will be deflected. It is also interesting to note that deflection is very much dependent on the diameter of the fiber, considering the d^4 in the denominator of the equation, which partly explains why hair morphology has an influence in hair styling; see equation 15 in **Figure 43**. As curls are brushed and consequently stretched they are subjected to torsional strain. Torsional stresses are also involved in combing straight hair since the fiber entanglements that are present in the advancing front of the comb are also three-dimensional.

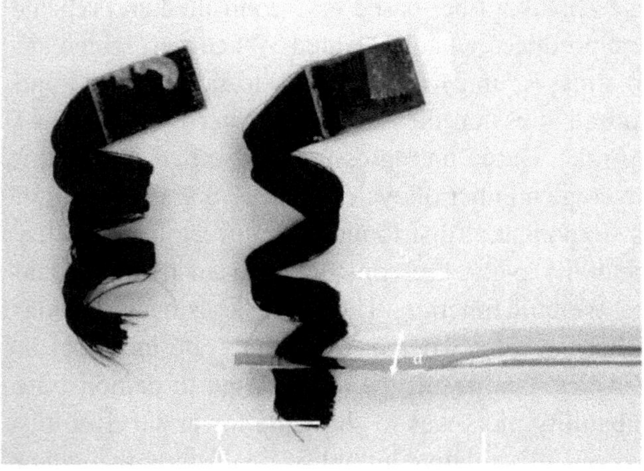

$$\Delta = \frac{KFr^2n}{Gd^4} \qquad (15)$$

where:
Δ = deflection
K = constant
F = axial load
r = radius of spring
n = number of coils
G = shear or torsional modulus
d = diameter of spring

Figure 43: Deflection is inversely related to the fourth power of the spring diameter.

Hence, measuring the fiber torsion modulus (G) may prove to be as useful as tensile and bending strains. How do the various damaging effects as well as environmental and cosmetic factors affect G? Bogarty mentions several references in the textile industry for the use of the torsion pendulum method and was one of the first to apply it to study of hair fibers. The torsion pendulum method in essence is based on suspending a hair fiber using a weight suspended from its free end. The mass is then put into rotational oscillation. The fiber torsional modulus is then calculated from Eq. 16

$$G = \frac{128\pi Il}{T^2 d^4} \tag{16}$$

Where:
I = moment of inertia of the suspended weight
l = fiber length
T = period of oscillation
d = fiber diameter

Torsion pendulums designed by Bogarty as described in his paper in 1967 were effective in measuring the fundamental relationships in this physical equation. The first apparatus allowed the operator to measure the amplitude of the fiber oscillations through a reflective device on the suspended weight. This permitted calculation of the dampening effect due to the state of the hair fiber. This is described by Eq. 17.

$$S = \frac{2.3}{n} log_{10} \tfrac{a_1}{a_n} \tag{17}$$

Where:
S = logarithmic decrement
a_1 = displacement on the first cycle
a_n = displacement on the nth cycle

Another adaptation by Bogarty was to house the fiber in a bell jar so that the torsion modulus and dampening could be measured as a function of humidity. Since then, more advanced torsion pendulums have been designed, including an apparatus built at TRI, where the oscillations of the pendulum weight are monitored by the reflection of a white strip by a light detector [146]. Recently, high-throughput measurements of hair fiber torsional properties were made possible by the use of an automated device designed and manufactured by Dia-Stron Ltd. [147].

There are various morphological features of hair that affect the torsional modulus of the fiber. When a fiber is twisted one can visualize that the section of hair that suffers the most from the torsional deformation is the outer circumference of the fiber and that this stress progressively decreases towards the middle of the fiber. Ultimately, in the exact middle of the fiber, the stress is negligible. This would be a simple physical situation if the fiber were a monofilament that does not react with water, such as a fishing line or an electrical copper wire. However, hair has a complex structure, both on the micro- as well as the nanoscale level. Since the circumference of a fiber suffers from the most stress during torsion, it is reasonable that the cuticle plays a large role in the torsional properties of hair. There are several findings that prove this. When torsional modulus of hair is measured at 65% relative humidity, there is an inverse relationship between the torsional modulus and diameter. As the diameter of the fiber decreases, the torsional modulus goes up. This is due to the fact that as hair diameter decreases, the cuticle to cortex ratio increases; see illustration of cuticle to cortex ratio in **Figure 44**. In larger-diameter hair that has the same approximate thickness of cuticle as fine hair, the cuticle to cortex ratio goes down with a corresponding decrease in torsional modulus [146]. To prove the role of the cuticle, Harper and Kamath [148] decuticled hair and found a significant reduction in the torsional modulus over the untreated control that had an intact cuticle.

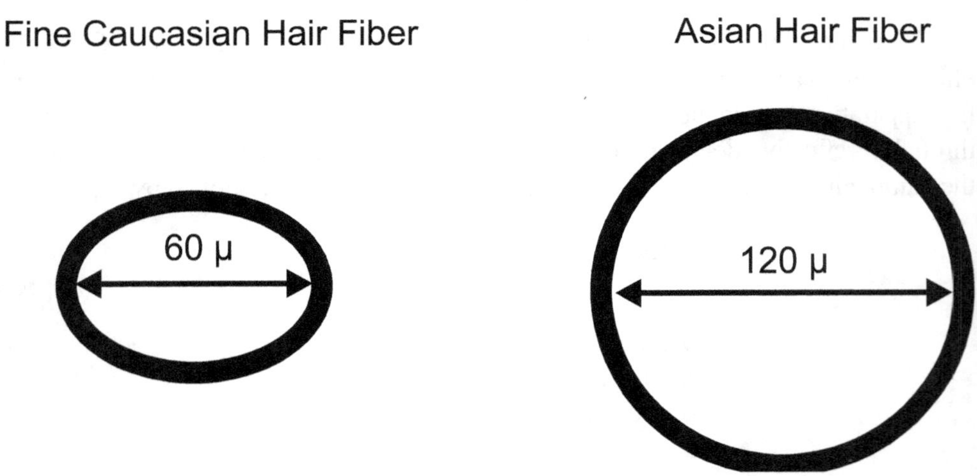

Figure 44: Cross-section of hair fibers from Caucasian and Asian hair types illustrating the relative differences in cuticle width to cortex diameter ratio. The ratio is higher for Fine Caucasian hair compared to Asian hair, a difference that influences torsional properties.

When measurements are taken with wet hair, the torsional modulus decreases compared to hair measured at 65% relative humidity [146]. Hair tends to absorb water, especially the lower cross-linked endocuticle layer of the cuticle. This tends to plasticize the cuticle and to reduce its torsional modulus. The bulk of the hair is also weakened when hair gets wet since water penetrates into the cortex easily and reacts with the intermediate filament associated proteins (IFAPs).

This situation is aggravated by hair damage, especially through chemical treatments such as bleaching. Here, disulfide bonds that are important for the integrity and strength of the hair are broken and in their place cysteic acid groups are formed that increase the hydrophilicity, or increase hair's ability to interact with water. Consequently, when bleached hair is wet or is subjected to high humidity, the torsional modulus is severely reduced. Interestingly, however, the shear modulus increases with decreasing humidity since the predominance of cysteic acid in the absence of water will form intermolecular salt linkages that increase torsional modulus higher than that of the unbleached state [148]. It can be concluded that torsional measurements can be utilized to assess the damaged state of hair, and whether a treatment composition can alleviate the extent of damage. One such compound found to fortify hair, as measured by torsional analysis, is cetrimonium bromide (CETAB) [148]. A proposed mechanism involves penetration of the low-molecular-weight compound into the endocuticle and the keratin associated proteins of the cortex. As Harper and Kamath describe, the penetrated CETAB molecules form salt linkages through the association of the cationic charge of the quaternary nitrogen and the negative charges of the hair's protein, while the hydrophobic portions of the CETAB line up in parallel. The whole structure forms a physical cross-link between the proteins of the hair that strengthen the cuticle and cortex. The result is a fortification of the hair as measured by a higher torsional modulus.

6. Texture Analysis

Hair-styling polymers are designed to provide certain mechanical properties to the hair to help set the hair in place and to contribute certain cosmetic effects to the behavior of hair while maintaining the desired properties under the stress of humidity and mechanical deformation. The initial set is indicated by the hair's stiffness and its cosmetic effects are exhibited by more advanced hair attributes such as volume, body, fiber alignment, shine, smoothness, and the like. Many of these attributes are evaluated from a sensory point of view, where panelists judge the stiffness of the applied resin on a hair tress; or by a trained cosmetologist who can assess more subtle performance effects, such as hair body, that can only be adequately perceived on a live subject. Although the sensory aspects of quantifying hair styling are important, scientists have attempted to measure these effects instrumentally. For this, texture analysis has been employed [149, 150]. Besides styling, the texture analyzer has also been used to measure the change in the mechanical properties of hair after the damaging effects of styling regimens, as well as how ingredients can affect these mechanical properties. These mechanical property changes are driven by changes in the fine structure of the hair, such as the conformation of the fibrous proteins in the microfibrilar region of the cortex, as well as other subcellular structures of the cortex and cuticula.

The texture analyzer is a force-measuring device. As with the tensile tester, it has a load cell that is designed to measure the force required to deform an object, such as a hair tress, and to measure the resultant forces during the compression cycle. As can be seen in **Figure 45**, a probe attached to the device slowly compresses a hair tress. When a threshold force is reached, the instrument will measure the force as a function of compression to produce a stress-strain curve, **Figure 46**. The two types of tress configurations depicted in the figure are the omega loop and three-point bending ribbon. These configurations have been used to assess the mechanical properties of polymer-treated hair such as initial stiffness, stiffness durability, elasticity, and plasticity [151].

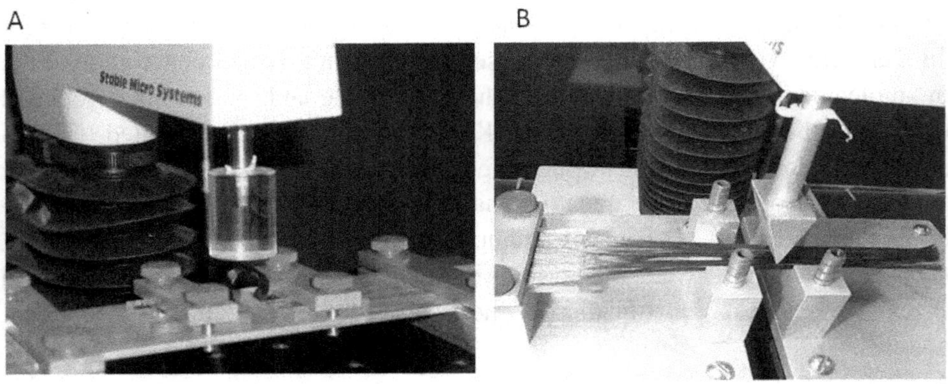

Figure 45: The texture analyzer measuring the mechanical properties of polymer-treated hair using a) the omega loop method; b) three-point or cantilever bending method. The whole apparatus is housed in a humidity-controlled box and is used to measure stiffness, flexibility, elasticity, hold, work of adhesion, and dry times of products on hair. Products may be tested at various humidity conditions to understand the product's response to humidity.

An example of how hair damage affects the mechanical properties of polymer-treated hair using the texture analyzer is provided in a study by Jachowicz and Yao [150]. Several hair spray polymers were applied to omega loops made from both virgin undamaged dark brown hair and triple-bleached hair. Mechanical properties were then measured and the results reported as the stiffness ratio, which is defined as the ratio of the maximum force measured during compression of polymer-treated hair to untreated hair. A stiffness ratio above one indicates that there is an increase in the stiffness of the fiber assembly. For each polymer tested, the stiffness ratios for bleached hair were significantly higher than for virgin brown hair. The authors hypothesized this behavior was due to the altered state of the bleached damaged hair. Since this type of hair is more hydrophilic, the wettability of the surface is higher than undamaged hair, which is more hydrophobic. Consequently, polymer solutions interpenetrate the fiber assembly to a greater extent and form more inter-fiber bonds resulting in enhanced stiffness [150, 152]. Also, because of the higher surface energy of the more hydrophilic damaged hair, the hydrophilic polymers wet more easily and adhere better to the substrate.

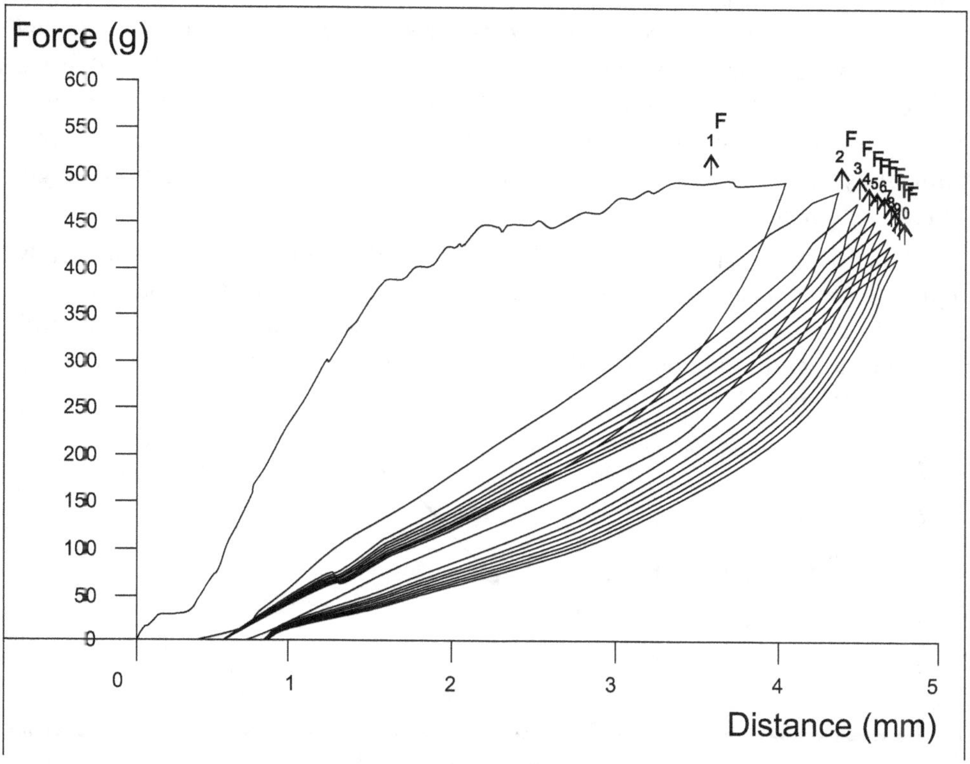

Figure 46: Typical stress-strain curve produced by a Texture Analyzer

Texture analysis was also utilized to demonstrate the protective effect of polymer pretreatments after exposure to heat from hot curling irons [112]. Hair tresses were exposed to a regimen of shampooing, application of polymer, and then heating with a hot curling iron such that the hair was given a total of 4, 8, and 12 minutes of total heat exposure. Besides mechanical combing and spectroscopic analysis, the textural properties of the hair tresses were assessed using the three-point cantilever bending test. It was found that after the hair was shampooed and dried to remove the residual polymer pretreatment, hair tresses that did not contain a protective ingredient had a stiffness ratio above 1, indicating that the unprotected hair exhibited damage. In contrast, hair that contained a thermal protective pretreatment had a stiffness ratio of one, indicating that stiffness did not change compared to the initial state of the hair. McMullen infers that the increase in stiffness in unprotected hair is due to an increase in the hair's crystallinity as a result of the exposure to high temperature.

7. Dynamic Mechanical Analysis (DMA)

Perhaps the basis for the perception that rheology is an esoteric discipline is related to the unavoidable link between rheological jargon and higher-level mathematics. In simplest terminology, however, rheology is the study of how materials flow. But, perhaps more appropriate to investigating the flow properties of treated hair fibers, rheology has also been described as the study of the flow of materials that behave in an unusual or interesting manner [153]. In extension, and pardon the pun, envisioning the prospects of *solid-like* components of a stretched hair fiber flowing is not very intuitive; however, faith in the philosophy that preaches that sufficiently coaxed solids will ultimately flow, may add clarity to the seemingly odd mental image.

Dynamic Mechanical Analysis (DMA) entails the application of a sinusoidally applied force to a sample of known dimensions, and subsequent evaluation of the material's oscillatory response [154]. For a solid material, properties such as stiffness and energy dissipation are calculated from the sample recovery and phase lag responses (**Figure 47**).

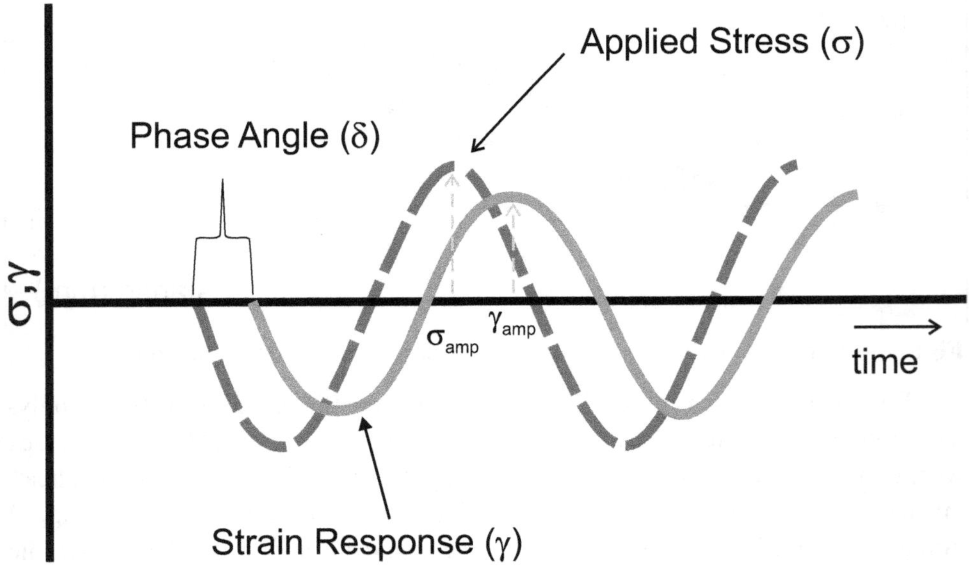

Figure 47: Response of a viscoelastic material to an applied stress. In the linear viscoelastic range the material responds to the sinusoidal stress (σ) oscillation by yielding, or straining (γ), sinusoidally. The phase angle (δ) is the difference in phase between the dynamic stress and dynamic strain and relates to the level of elasticity in the sample; and σ_{amp}, and γ_{amp} refer to the applied stress and resultant strain amplitudes, respectively. The measurement response is a function of applied stress, time, frequency, temperature, and humidity.

The stiffness is reported as the *elastic (or storage) modulus (E')*, and the energy dissipated as heat is described by *tan δ*; where tan δ is the ratio of the *viscous (or loss) modulus (E")* to the elastic modulus (see **Figure 48**). A perfectly elastic response will have no phase lag (i.e., δ = 0) between the response and the applied sinusoidal stress, or strain; whereas a solely viscous response will be out of phase (δ = 90°). The phase lag for *viscoelastic* materials lies between the two extremes (i.e., 0° < δ < 90°). Steel is an example of a perfectly elastic material. Honey is a completely viscous fluid, and dried hair-styling polymer films are typically viscoelastic—meaning that hairspray resins dissipate some of the initially applied strain as heat rather than storing the energy for a completely elastic response. In other words, after removing the deformation force applied to a viscoelastic material, the material will not immediately spring back to its original position. Important to all analogies and to all definitions is the following: all of the fancy rheological measurements are related to *reversible* deformations. That is, all applied strains and forces must be small enough to retain structure memory. Adequate "back forces," which are related to the integrity of the chemical structure and its wish to return to a lower energy state, must be preserved to enable restoration of the original structure. In analogy, imagine two styled hair tresses composed of polymers with differing moisture-dependent glass transition temperatures. Tress 1 is set using a hydrophilic, stiff and brittle polymer, whereas Tress 2 is styled with a hydrophobic and flexible polymeric resin. On application of a small sinusoidal force at low humidity, Tress 1 responds elastically and the stress response wave immediately follows the shape of the applied strain wave (δ≈0). However, Tress 2 yields slightly as the deformation energy incites molecular rearrangements in the softer, flexible film that releases energy as heat. The lost energy, in the form of thermal dissipation, delays the inevitable return of the material to its original position—a delay that can be visualized by watching upward trends in *tan δ*. Fear not—not all of this is bad news! By *damping* the applied energy, Tress 2 may ultimately be able to survive greater deformation strains than the stiffer Tress 1. Now, imagine that low-pressure system suddenly moved into your region and brings sufficient precipitation. At higher ambient humidity, the more water-loving Tress 1 absorbs water vapor and the polymer film is subsequently plasticized; the moisture-induced plasticity of the film then renders a delay in the expected stress response, which can be viewed in a decrease in *E'*, and associated increases in *E"* and *tan δ*. In contrast, at higher humidity, the performance of Tress 2 is less influenced as its chemical structure is relatively more hydrophobic. Hence, by analogy, trends in *tan δ* may be used to monitor the assault of external strains, such as temperature, humidity, and chemical treatment, on the energy-absorbing physicochemistry tied to the stiffness and softness of treated hair composites.

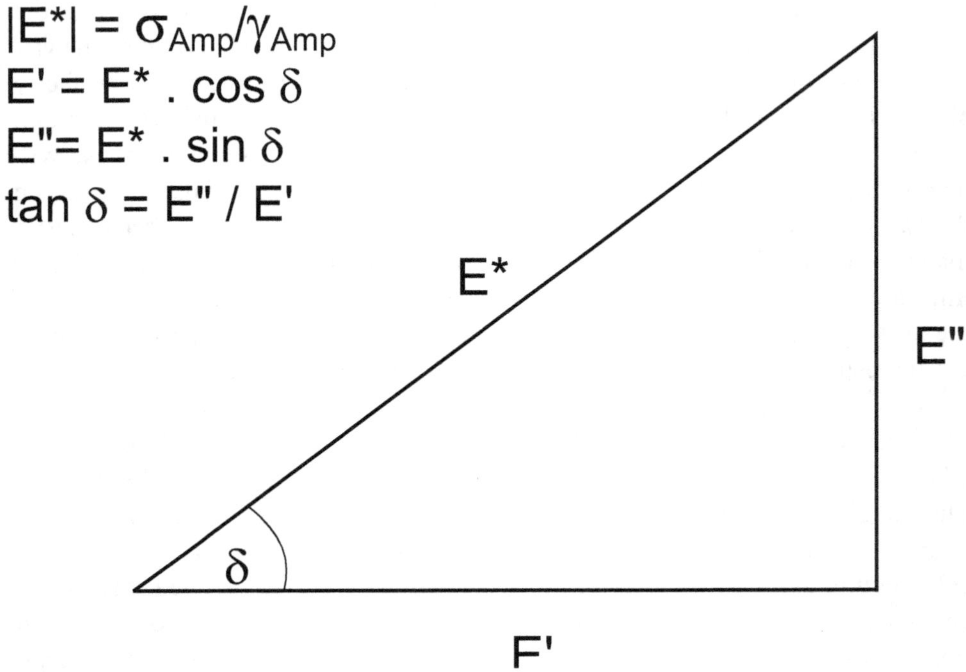

Figure 48: Argand diagram relating the real axis (E') to the imaginary axis (E"). Hence, the complex modulus (E*) has both elastic and viscous components, meaning E* is a mechanical blend of a Hookean spring and a viscous fluid.

Using DMA techniques, Gao et al. investigated the viscoelastic response of single fibers as a function of relative humidity and applied cosmetic treatment [155, 156]. Single fibers were challenged by DMA in tensile mode and compared to Young's modulus data acquired from traditional stress-strain testing. **Figure 49** shows the correlation of the Young's modulus with *E'* data acquired from DMA testing. The profiles suggest that the two modulus methods produce proportional magnitudes of stiffness data; however, the virgin sample has a different sensitivity (i.e., slope) and a lower R^2 than the bleached samples. Because the stiffness data were acquired at different isohumes, it is probable that the noted slope differences are related to oxidative fiber damage. At higher humidity levels, **Figure 50** echoes the same trend. Higher *tan δ* levels are related to the ability of a material to dampen the stressed structure via molecular rearrangements and internal friction—that is, the effects of chemical oxidation reduce the covalent cross-link density and introduce more molecular freedom. At higher humidity levels, a more rapid influx of water vapor interferes with the electrostatic attraction of the new ionic cross-links and allows the chemically compromised hair structure to dissipate the tensile strains by thermal means.

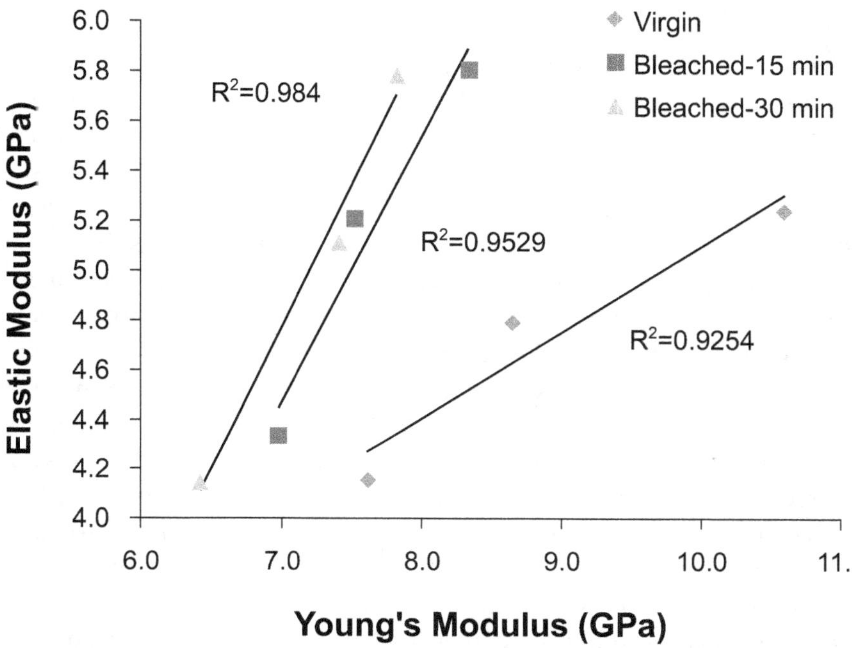

Figure 49: Correlation of Elastic Modulus with Young's Modulus data for virgin European brown, 15 min bleached European brown, and 30 min bleached European brown single hair fibers (adapted from Gao et al. [155, 156]).

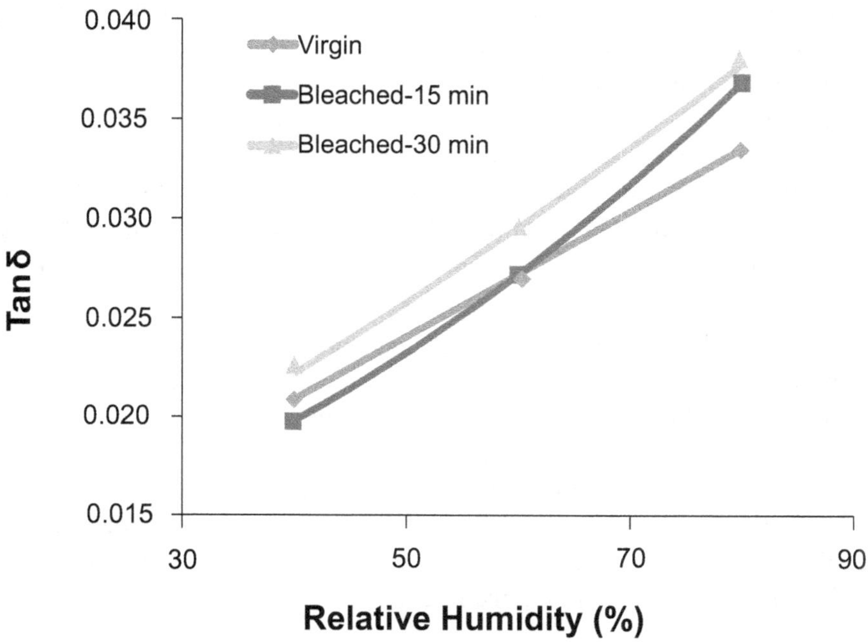

Figure 50: Damping data (tan δ) for virgin and bleached single fibers as a function of relative humidity (adapted from Gao et al. [155, 156]).

e. Image Analysis

The process of seeing by eye consists of the excitation of millions of nerve endings in the retina housed inside of the eyeball. These nerve impulses then travel by way of the optic nerve to the brain where this information is processed into a visual image. The visual image perceived by the brain is a representation of what exists in the outside world. The fundamental unit of seeing is a nerve impulse. Although this process is still being worked on by neuroscientists, the point here is that an image in the mind is not produced by one nerve impulse, but rather by millions taken collectively. Using this as an analogy to describe the nature of digital photography, the fundamental unit is the pixel and when hundreds of thousands of them are put together, which is not unreasonable given the advancements in digital cameras, they produce an image resolution that is only limited by the number of pixels making up the picture. With the help of computers and appropriate software, these pixels can be analyzed to provide information about the image. Quantification is performed with respect to the distribution of light and dark pixels, or the color distribution of pixels. Other applications exist, with the help of image analysis software, including counting particles and analyzing light and dark patterns. Based on the fact that digital cameras, as well as computer hardware and software, are continually advancing, this trend will surely continue.

There are three basic steps involved in image analysis [157]. These include the capture of the image with a digital camera, segmentation of the part of the image that needs to be analyzed, and finally with the help of appropriate software, the analysis of the digital image. Digital image analysis has been used for such things as quantifying hair luster, volume, fiber orientation, curliness, and color such as color fading or wash-fastness [159]. Although the human eye is a very good judge of these cosmetic qualities, there are times when the qualitative assessments generated from, for example, panel studies need to have the quantitative backing of instrumental data given by the image analysis technique. Following are examples of the use of this technique to illustrate its ever-increasing utility for hair damage and protection studies.

Hair shine or luster is one attribute of undamaged hair, as it provides the hair a healthy appearance. When hair becomes damaged there are two factors that contribute to its dullness or reduction in shine. The surface topography of damaged hair is rougher and accounts for a greater degree of diffuse, as opposed to specular, or mirror like reflection. Also, the way individual fibers of the assembly align themselves accounts for the degree of shine on hair. Usually damaged hair, especially at the ends, has more of an unmanageable appearance and looks dull irrespective of how shiny the individual fibers are.

Quantification of the level of shine has been achieved through image analysis [159, 160]. In this method, hair is positioned on a semi-cyclindrical barrel. A specular band of light is observed when a polarized beam of light is directed at the hair tress at a particular angle. A digital picture is then obtained. The apparatus is entirely housed in a dark box. With proper image analysis software, a plot of luminance versus distance along the hair tress is produced. Inspection and calculation of various parameters of the resultant plot will indicate if a particular treatment of the tress has resulted in either an increase or decrease in shine. Hair that has an increase in shine will be portrayed by an increase in intensity of the specular band, and a decrease in the level of diffuse light. From this apparatus, McMullen was able to show different factors that were responsible for hair luster and dullness. It was found that hair luster is proportional to the level of pigment in the hair such that dark brown hair for example was shinier than blonde hair. Addition of oils to the hair, especially phenyltrimethicone, as well as certain hair spray and styling polymers increased shine. Also, reduction in hair luster was evident in the deposition to the hair of either micronized ZnO or sebum [159].

Image analysis can also be used to assess the fiber configuration of the hair assembly. For example, an assembly of hair that has proper fiber alignment will be perceived as shiny due to the exhibition of specular bands. Frizzy or unmanageable hair will be perceived as dull due to the absence of these bands. Therefore, analyzing luminance along the length of the fiber assembly for the intensity of the specular bands will be not only an assessment of an increase in hair shininess, but also how a styling polymer can control unmanageable hair. More sophisticated techniques can be used to assess very curly hair such as hair that comes from African descent [160].

Image analysis can be used to assess the color changes in hair. This could be applicable in such areas as how dyed hair changes color due to shampooing, heat treatments, or UV exposure, as well as measuring effects of protective ingredients. One way to accomplish this is to take digital pictures during the treatment schedule. The hair tress or surface has to be held flat to present a uniform surface to the camera lest there be interfering effects of shadows due to external effects. Sections of the pictures are cropped to the same coordinates and analyzed with appropriate image analysis software. Data analysis is performed with the use of histograms. Since a digital picture is made up of pixels, there are populations of pixels of either a particular color (red, green, or blue, commonly referred to as RGB) or shade in the black-and-white or gray scale. How the pixel density and distribution changes during the treatment schedule provides an indication of the effect of either the damaging or protective treatment. For example, if hair is dyed red with a permanent hair dye and subjected to multiple stripping shampoo cycles, the tress will exhibit fading of its original color. A histogram can be produced in the red scale to show how the population of dark red pixels shifts to a higher proportion of lighter red pixels. Also, the pictures can be converted to black and white with, for example, Adobe Photoshop and a histogram produced to show the population of light and dark pixels. Hair color fading would be indicated in this case by a higher population of lighter pixels.

An example of this is shown in **Figure 51**. A digital picture of three hair tresses is taken and is represented in **Figure 51a**. The hair tresses were treated in the following way. Dark brown hair tresses were bleached and then dyed red with a commercial oxidative hair dye. The tress on the left is the control or reference tress that did not go through any subsequent treatment. The middle tress was shampooed ten times with a nonconditioning system and a leave-in color protection treatment was added after every shampoo prior to drying. The tress on the right was treated with ten cycles of shampooing and drying. A rectangular section of the digital image is segmented from each of the images of the tresses as shown in **Figure 51b**. These sections are used to perform image analysis. A histogram is produced of the distribution of pixels in each of the sections. It can be seen in **Figure 51c** that the tress treated with just the shampoo has faded relative to the reference tress since the majority of pixels are lighter (it is more to the left in the histogram). The protected tress, although more to the left than the reference tress, demonstrated shown color protection since there is less fading compared to the negative control. The images can be analyzed in other ways such as for color shift or luminance with respect to distribution along the length of the tress.

a) b) c)

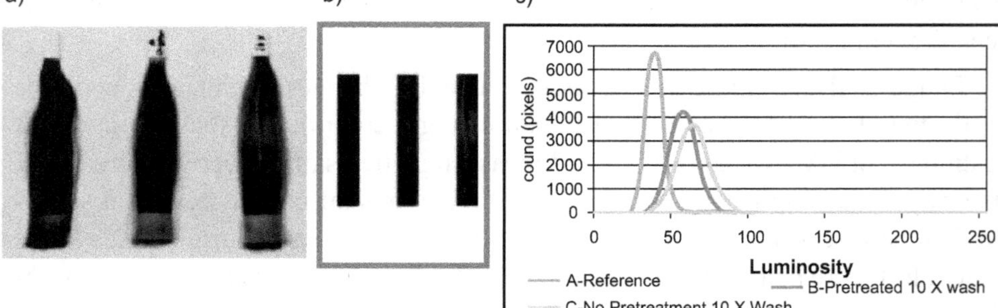

Figure 51: a) image capture; b) segmentation; c) image analysis

f. Infrared Thermography (IRT)

IRT uses thermal imaging cameras that detect emitted radiation in the infrared region of the electromagnetic spectrum. The usefulness of IRT in quantifying heat depends on the quasi-relationship between the emitted infrared radiation (λ=3–15 μm) and the magnitude of the surface temperature. Subsequently produced digital images, or *thermograms*, consist of two-dimensional image grids with temperature measurements plotted on a third axis using a relative color image scale. In the human body, heat is lost from the surface by conduction, convection, evaporation (e.g., respiration, perspiration), or radiative processes [161]. Convection transfers heat between the body and the air or liquid interface. Conduction occurs between two solid surfaces in direct contact, whereas radiative heat transfer takes place between two solid surfaces that are not physically touching.

Figure 52 invokes the Stefan-Boltzmann law, which is the mathematical connection between the maximum attainable emissive radiation across all wavelengths, Q, and the fourth power of the absolute surface temperature, T, of a material. For a solid black body radiator, which is a nonrealizable ideal, Q reaches its maximum because the *emissivity* (ε) equals unity. The emissivity, which is a measure of how much radiation a material emits relative to a black body radiator, ranges between 0 and 1, where higher magnitudes are indicative of more efficient radiators. Explicitly, if you placed a thermocouple on the surface of a black body and compared the value to the radiative energy emitted by the black body across all emitted wavelengths, the power of the radiation (Q) would correlate to the fourth power of the measured absolute surface temperature of the solid (see **Figure 52**). In effect, the human body has an emissivity similar to that of a black body—meaning that ε approaches unity and Q is nearly proportional to T^4; for example, the ε of water and human skin are 0.96–0.98 [162], and the ε for human hair is 0.91 [163]. Hence, at thermal equilibrium, human hair and the hair-water composite are intrinsically available for very efficient absorption and emission of thermal radiation.

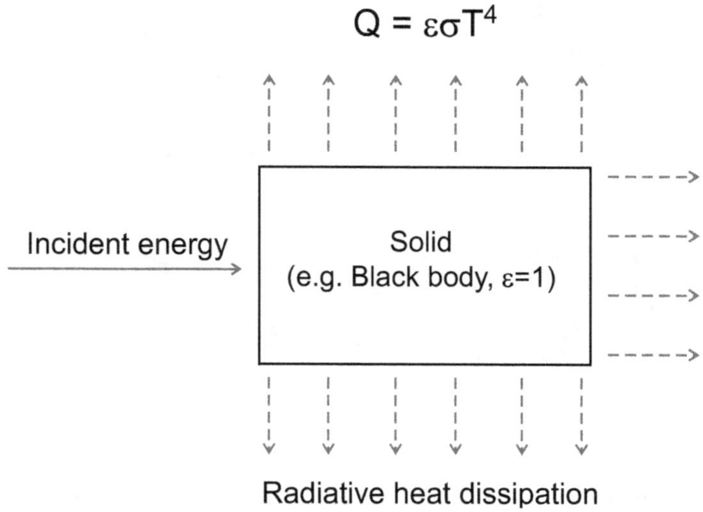

Figure 52: The Stefan-Boltzmann law describes the relationship between the observed radiation intensity (Q) and the absolute temperature (T), where σ is the proportionality, or Stefan-Boltzmann constant. Black body radiators have emissivity (ε) values equal to unity, whereas real materials radiate less than perfectly and $\varepsilon < 1$.

To gauge the impact of thermal insult on the radiative decay properties of human hair, a virgin hair tress and a previously flat-ironed hair tress were simultaneously evaluated after exposure to a convective heat source. A dark brown virgin hair tress was thermally treated with a 175°C flat iron for an exorbitantly long 5-minute period. During treatment the flat iron was repeatedly swept from root to tip at a rate of 0.6 in/min. After the 5-minute treatment protocol, the untreated virgin and thermally insulted tresses were subsequently set aside for 24 hours (20–22°C, 32–35%RH) to facilitate proper equilibration with ambient water vapor—which should impart approximately 6% water to the untreated virgin tress [95]. One end of a length of adhesive tape was applied to the PMMA tabs on the tress, and the other end of the tape was looped around a 12-inch wooden rod. The wooden rod was then fastened to the apex of two 10-inch glass bottles such that the two tresses were freely hanging from the horizontal rod. To maintain fiber alignment and control the thickness of the fiber bundles, large binder clips were then clamped to the ends of the dangling tresses. Next, a portable space heater was positioned behind the tresses and powered on high for 5 minutes. The heater was then removed and an IR camera was used to immediately monitor the radiative emission of heat from the tresses as they cooled from ~70°C to ambient. **Figure 53** captures the decay as a series of sequential thermograms and clearly suggests that the virgin tress (left) cools to room temperature more slowly than the previously flat-ironed tress (right).

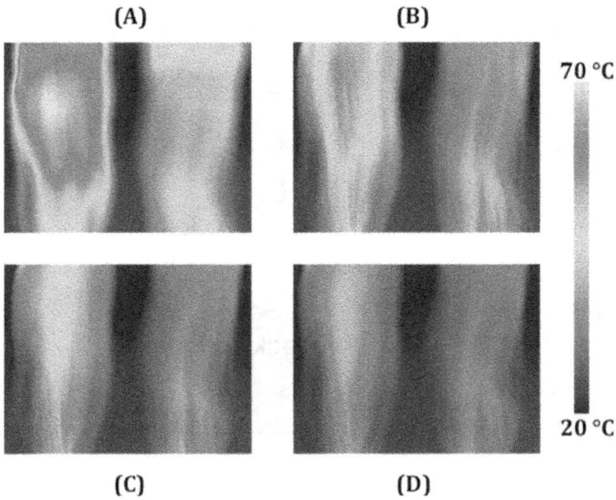

Figure 53: Thermograms showing the radiative dissipation of heat from virgin (left) and hot flat-ironed (right) hair tresses as a function of time. Images were sequentially collected 5 s (A), 15 s (B), 25 s (C), and 35 s (D) after removing the heat source from the tresses. Prior to experimentation, the thermally insulted tress was equilibrated for 24 hours at ambient humidity and temperature (32–35%RH; 20–22°C). Note that the glass supports (ε=0.93, internal control) next to each tress each reached maximum temperature, suggesting even heating across both samples.

Although it is not possible to postulate an accurate structure-property relationship for the data in **Figure 53** without supporting measurements, it is clear that excessive thermal treatment impacts the rate at which hair ultimately dissipates applied heat. Using DVS experiments, Zhou et al. [4] acknowledged the impact of excessive heat on the moisture regain of hot flat-ironed (232°C) virgin hair and indicated that the thermal response and water management properties of virgin hair are quite different than those of thermally treated fiber bundles [4]. One chemical change may be attributable to the formation of diisopeptide (amide) crosslinks, which have been reported to occur at approximately 165°C in keratin [164, 109]. Extensive amide cross-linking may lead to a reduction in swell volume, thereby limiting the maximum water regain of thermally damaged fibers. Hence, one possible explanation for differences in the radiative decay rates for virgin and thermally damaged hair is that excessive thermal treatments affect the core fiber structure and, subsequently, the intrinsic water-binding, hydrogen bonding, and thermal capacity systems of the hair.

11.4.5 COLOR PROTECTION

a. Color Wash-Fastness of Oxidative Hair Color from Shampoo Stripping

A common practice for consumers is to permanently color their hair with the use of oxidative hair colorants. This is done to cover gray or to change the color for cosmetic reasons. Many consumers realize that permanent hair color is not so permanent, and not just because the hair grows out from the roots, requiring periodic touch-ups. Rather, the initial color changes due to washing, putting the hair through various styling regimens, and weathering through exposure to the elements. From this stress, the hair becomes lighter and the hue and chroma, or saturation of the color, changes many times for the worse. For example, a bright vibrant red color will slowly change to an unnaturally looking shade of orange-red. There have been many attempts to help preserve this color. One strategy is to prevent leaching of hair color with continued exposure to washing, or to improve color wash-fastness. Another idea is to protect the hair from UV damage, which is an indirect way of preserving the color from wash-out; after the hair's integrity has been compromised, there is less of a barrier to prevent the dyes from being leached during the repeated washing cycles. Whatever the case may be, methods need to be employed to assess the original color of the hair and to monitor subsequent changes.

The human eye is an excellent instrument in detecting small differences in hair color changes both with respect to intensity and hue. An individual's opinion is very important even if instrumental methods show more precision in their discrimination of color shifts. Of course, the consumer is the final judge in deciding whether the change in color intensity or hue is acceptable. Therefore, panel testing is a necessity due to the importance of consumer perception. Nevertheless, instrumental techniques have their place in quantifying color changes in that they provide quick feedback to researchers in determining the efficacy of their raw material or formulation development efforts. However, data generated from instrumental measurements have to be correlated to real-life situations; therefore, questions in color change include determining the minimum difference measured by the instrument that can be detected by the human eye. If this correlation is not well established then panel testing results are required.

1. Colorimetry

The most common way to monitor color changes is by measuring Hunter L, a, and b values with a HunterLab colorimeter (HunterLab Ultra Scan). In this system, various aspects of color are reported, namely lightness (L), and chroma (a and b). These components come from a three-dimensional color space model created by the International Commission on Illumination (CIE) and can be monitored alone, but more commonly ΔE and ΔC are utilized to follow color changes. These are defined as follows (Eqs. 18 and 19):

$$\Delta E = ((L_t - L_o)^2 + (a_t - a_0)^2 + (b_t - b_o)^2)^{1/2} \quad (18)$$

$$\Delta C = ((a_t - a_0)^2 + (b_t - b_o)^2)^{1/2} \quad (19)$$

Where:

L = luminance
a = red to green shift
b = blue to yellow shift
ΔE = Total change in color including lightness
ΔC = Change in color

L_o, a_o, b_o; and L_t, a_t, b_t are measured Hunter L, a, b color parameters before and after treatment, respectively. The reader is encouraged to explore this more in depth by referring to www.hunderlab.com.

Using the values of E and C in comparison to an appropriate control can be calculated from equation 20.

$$\%\ Color\ Retention = \%\Delta E_{improvement} = \frac{\Delta E_{treatment} - \Delta E_{control}}{\Delta E_{control}} \times 100 \quad (20)$$

Attempts have been made to prevent color fading in hair by investigators working in the personal care industry. For example, by utilizing ΔE and to a lesser extent, ΔC, it was shown that products containing Polyquaternium-55 reduced the color change due to shampoo stripping [165, 166]. The Polyquaternium-55 was tested in different regimens of shampoo, conditioner, and leave-in treatment, with favorable results compared to appropriate controls. It was theorized by Zhou et al.

that the color wash-fastness was due to both the cationic nature of this polymer as well as its degree of hydrophobic modification, which forms biocompatible films on the hair and prevents the leaching of color during subsequent shampooing.

Another example where color indexes were utilized to show color effects entailed the use of Multi Lamellar Vesicles (MLV) made up of phosphate esters. When these were added to the dye base, the lamellar structure produced by these types of surfactants could be observed using optical microscopy equipped with cross-polarizers. The birefringence was used as an indicator of lamellar structure formation. It was theorized that the dye intermediates would be entrapped by the lamellar structure and slow down its reaction with hydrogen peroxide. This would give the intermediates a chance to absorb into the cortex of the hair before reacting with hydrogen peroxide. From this it was found that less dyeing time was necessary to achieve the same color index compared to longer dyeing times with lower MLV structures. Also, color wash-fastness through shampoo cycling was increased as well. Most of the work to show efficacy was through the monitoring of color indexes and their change with different dyeing times and shampoo cycles [167].

One must be careful in making conclusions in regard to ΔE and ΔC, as well as percent protection. By considering the equations to determine ΔE and ΔC, one may take note that the color difference takes into consideration multiple color indices. If, for example, ΔE and/or ΔC do not change, that does not necessarily mean that there is no change in color. It could be that the increase of one color index may increase and may be nullified by the decrease in another. Therefore, it is important to separately look at the data for L, a, and b both before and after the treatment regimen to see exactly which indices are changing most dramatically. From this perspective, it may make more sense to indicate the results with Δa, Δb, or ΔL individually. For example, Gao monitored Δa, which is a change in the saturation of red, for different red hair colors containing different levels of phosphate esters.

It should be mentioned that percent protection needs to be used with caution when claiming color protection. For example, a large percent protection can be calculated from very small changes of ΔE of the experimental treatment versus the control, which may not be consumer perceivable.

2. Image Analysis of Digital Photographs

Determining the color wash-fastness of a hair dye on a human subject is quite difficult. To compare two treatments, one product with a protective ingredient needs to be on one side of the head and a placebo on the other. This may be practical in the salon, but becomes difficult when the panelist is asked to do this at home, especially with rinse-off products. Usually, these types of tests are performed on tresses and mannequin heads made with natural human hair. Hair tresses can be treated with a protective ingredient and then subjected to a series of wash and dry cycles to see the change in color compared to the color change of a tress serving as a control. Of course the regimen can be designed by the experimenter to simulate practical conditions. Measurements of color changes are monitored after washing cycles using techniques such as colorimetry or image analysis. Instrumental measurements should be supported by panel studies.

Utilizing a mannequin head, the color wash-fastness effect of a hydrophobically modified cationic polymer was demonstrated by incorporating it into a regimen of products consisting of shampoo, conditioner, and leave-in treatment. The mannequin head was dyed red with a commercial hair color. One side of the head was treated with a commercial shampoo and conditioner containing a color-protective claim. The other side was treated with the color-protective regimen. After ten cycles the hair was dried in a straight style so the fibers would present a flat surface for taking digital pictures. This is an important step since, if the style of the hair has texture, it will present to the camera dark and light patches (shadows and highlights) that will interfere with true color measurements of the fiber assembly. Photographs of both sides of the head were taken in strategic areas and cropped to specific proportions as can be seen in **Figure 54**. The image analysis data can then be compared as shown in the histogram of luminance. The quantity of pixels is plotted as a function of luminosity with low luminosity values corresponding to dark shades and higher values to lighter colors. In the example, the data indicate that the side of the head treated with products with the protective polymer has a population of pixels that are darker than the control side, indicating less color loss or more color wash-fastness [165]. The mannequin head also facilitates visualization of the color differences of the two sides of the head by a panel to confirm the data generated from the digital image analysis. Also, panelists viewing a mannequin head can perceive the three-dimensional aspect of the head where specular bands due to curvature are evident and have an effect on the perception of color.

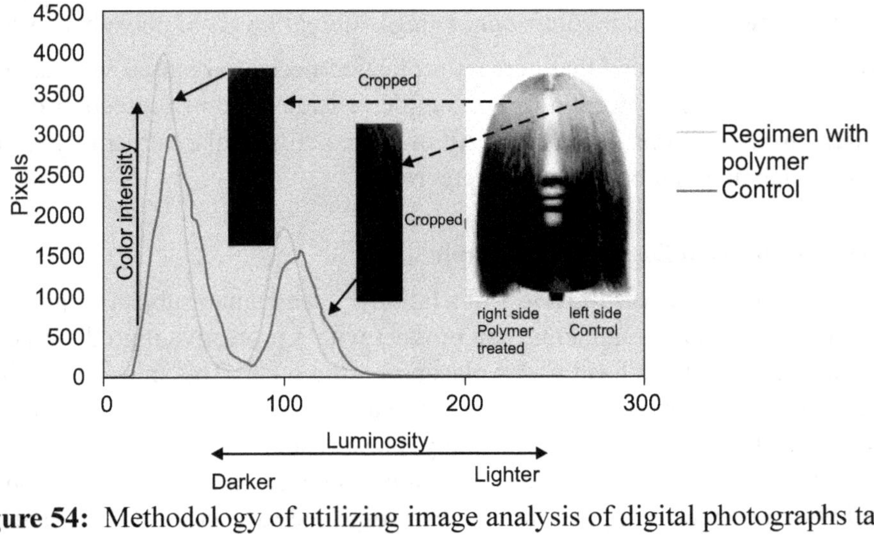

Figure 54: Methodology of utilizing image analysis of digital photographs taken from a half head evaluation on a mannequin head

b. Color Protection from UV-Induced Fading

Besides the continual washing that hair is normally subjected to, hair also fades from exposure to solar radiation. There are many factors that put a level of complexity in its study. Sunlight is composed of a spectrum of wavelengths, where the shorter the wavelength the higher its energy and level of stress that it imparts to the hair. From highest to lowest energy, the electromagnetic spectrum incident on hair from solar radiation is UVB (280–320 nm), UVA (320–400 nm), visible (370–780 nm), and IR (750–2800 nm). Besides wavelength, the length of time and intensity of the radiation has to be considered as well, usually reported as J/hr-cm^2. Another factor that makes this area complex to study is the nature of the substrate. Some hair types have a different type and level of melanin, which is hair's natural defense against photodegradation. Hair is also treated with permanent artificial hair colors that have their own sensitivity to light exposure. These oxidative hair colors are made up of a complex blend of dye intermediates that react inside the hair shaft with hydrogen peroxide to form the desired color. Therefore, in this area of study, the experimental design with respect to the treatment regimen (e.g., shampooing and light exposure cycles), exposure conditions, and hair type, need to be carefully controlled and specified in the material and methods section of the study.

Melanin, which is present in the cortex of the hair as fine granules, provides natural protection to hair from sunlight as it surrounds the keratin intermediate filaments. This level of protection depends on the type of hair with respect to the level and type of melanin. For example, dark brown hair with a high level of eumelanin affords more protection to the proteins of the hair as opposed to natural blonde or bleached hair. Artificially colored hair affords less protection to the hair since these compounds are more sensitive to decomposition by sunlight. Hence, naturally colored hair retains its color longer than artificially colored hair. It has been shown that UVA and visible light predominantly fade artificially colored hair [168]. What aggravates fading of artificially colored hair is a combination of both irradiation and shampooing [169]. The breakdown of protein or lipids on the hair surface from UV irradiation makes hair more porous; and because hair dyes are water soluble, especially those based on pyrazole dyes contained in some red colors, the dye leaches out more readily during shampooing and rinsing. Therefore, it would be beneficial to know the nature of the solar breakdown of hair proteins in order to select the correct UV absorber system to provide maximum protection.

As studied by Hoting and Zimmerman, each part of the solar spectrum has a different propensity to fade dyed hair. UVB radiation is the most damaging to hair followed by UVA, visible, and finally infrared light. These relative frequencies are illustrated in **Figure 55**. However, it should be reemphasized that the visible and UVA region of the spectrum are most degradative with respect to hair pigment. The reason is that the relative intensities of different parts of the solar spectrum are different. As measured by Locke, the ΔE values of photo-faded hair were 8.5,

3.8, 0.95, and 0.84 for visible, UVA, UVB, and IR light irradiation, respectively [169]. These relative intensities are also illustrated in **Figure 55a** for comparison. The visible and UVA portions of the spectrum account for a major share of the total photo-fading effect with UVB having a more minor role. Based on theoretical calculations, Locke and Jachowicz calculated the fraction of light absorbed at each wavelength by a given quantity of UV absorber on the hair. As expected, UVB absorbers only absorbed a fraction of the UV absorbed on the hair since the UVB only accounts for a fraction of the total amount of UV radiation. In choosing a UV filter for photoprotection, the wavelength of light that the ingredient is designed to absorb is most important. Although filters in the visible range may have a negative cosmetic effect on hair (i.e., these filters are also visible by eye), increased photoprotection can be realized by using a filter that has UVA as well as UVB properties. Other factors that the formulator must keep in mind are the extinction coefficient or the amount of radiation absorbed by the filter at a particular range of wavelengths, the photostability of the absorber after a certain degree of radiation, and the cosmetic effects when added to a hair treatment and ultimately on hair. If the product is used in a rinse-off application, such as a shampoo or cream rinse, then a mechanism must be considered to deliver the UV absorber onto the surface of the hair. Examples to consider are dilution deposition as is found in conditioning shampoos or, intrinsic features of the ingredient such as having a quaternary group that would allow substantivity of the absorber during rinse-off.

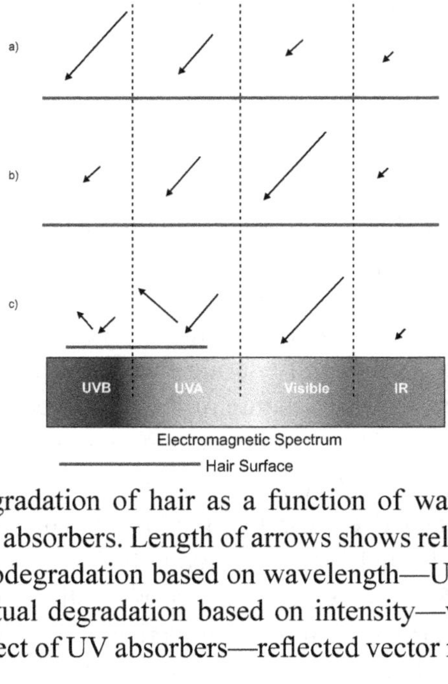

Figure 55: Photodegradation of hair as a function of wavelength, exposure to hair, and effect of UV absorbers. Length of arrows shows relative effect. a) relative effectiveness of photodegradation based on wavelength—UVB is the most degradative; b) relative actual degradation based on intensity—visible and UVA have the most effect; c) effect of UV absorbers—reflected vector represents blockage of UV by absorbers.

11.4.6 REPAIR TECHNIQUES

Thus far, we have described hair damage and various ways it can be protected from the various stresses that it is subjected to. What is more challenging is its repair. Claims abound in the market for products that strengthen and repair damaged hair. Since hair is a complex structure, there are different aspects of repair and, as a consequence, the term needs to be defined appropriately. The definition can be explained by analogy. Consider a brick wall that has a crack as by some uneven distribution of the weight of the structure that it supports. The process of repair is simply to excavate the crack so that it can accommodate mortar to fill in the crack; the chemical nature of the brick is still the same. On the other hand, if you observe a brick that has been weathered by the elements, the actual molecular structure of the brick has been compromised to the point where it will not bear a load without crumbling. At this point the brick can no longer be repaired. These two aspects of damage and the repair process are included in the term "hair repair." The first aspect of hair repair includes repairing the broken subassemblies of the fiber through a physical-chemical process. The chemical interactions associated with this would be salt linkages, hydrogen bonding, and hydrophobic effects. Since the energy to break these bonds is low, the resultant repair is temporary or at best, semi-permanent. The more intimate bonding of the molecules in hair for a permanent repair would entail covalent bonds. There are examples of each of these aspects of repair in the literature.

Repair can also be considered from a morphological point of view by observing how treatments repair the subassemblies of the fiber. Compared to synthetic fibers, such as is present in polyester or nylon fabric, human and animal hair fibers have a complex structure. Swift coined it appropriately as a hierarchical composite [125]. There are many book chapters [3, 125, 170] as well as detailed technical articles [45] on the subject that the reader is encouraged to refer to for an explanation of the complex structure evident in human hair. It should be mentioned that in going from low to high magnification in the description of the fine structures found in hair, we start with the cortex being built by smaller longitudinally shaped cortical cells which house macrofilaments. These then are composed of well-organized intermediate filaments (IF) surrounded by intermediate filament associated proteins (IFAPs) embedded in an amorphous matrix. These proteins have a specific primary, secondary, and tertiary conformation and association with each other that gives hair its physical properties, such as strength and elasticity, which then translate into cosmetic attributes such as hair body. When hair is under stress, it is damaged at its various hierarchical levels, namely from the molecular level to the subcellular level, and ultimately to the cellular level present between and amongst cortical and cuticle cells. True hair repair would bring these structures back into their normal states such that: 1) intermediate filaments that have been severed have been re-fused together, that is, broken peptide bonds that make up the backbone of the molecule are re-formed; 2) also, this would include restoration of the organized structure of the complex lipid structures found in the cell membrane complexes between cortical and cuticle cells; 3) the complex three-dimensional conformations of the IF and IFAPs are restored to their pre-denatured state; 4) damage to the cells such as micropores formed in the surface of the cuticle cells, and fibrillation of cortical cells. It is indeed a high calling to have this definition of hair repair since not only chemical bonds need to be restored, but also the complex three-dimensional structures prior to their denaturation as well. The effect is the same as descrambling an egg. In this respect there are very few treatments that will achieve such results. Rather, the effects either are cosmetic or at best have a certain durability of effect to retain the cosmetic effect of hiding the damage by keeping intact important hair attributes. However, there have been attempts to repair hair on a more molecular level. In this section examples are given on those hair repair techniques that range from temporary effects to those are more permanent.

a. Protein Hydrolysates

One realizes very quickly when studying compendiums on the chemical composition of hair that it is primarily made up of proteins [3]. Some proteins are fibrous, such as the intermediate filaments, and contribute to the supporting structures of hair. Others are more amorphous, such as those found surrounding the microfibrils. The structure of these proteins on a primary conformational level is made up of the various amino acids characterized by different functional groups. These functional groups consist of acid, base, aromatic, heterocyclic, aliphatic, and sulfur containing proteins. The higher-level secondary and tertiary structures are dependent on the sequence of amino acids in the protein's primary structure [171]. Also, the reactivity of the protein is dependent on the nature of the functional groups of the protein. In hair the sulfur-containing proteins are most important in that it is the nature of the disulfide bond to give hair its strength through molecular cross-linking. Other bonds, again dependent on the side groups, take part in hydrogen bonds, salt linkages, and hydrophobic interactions both on an intra- as well as intermolecular basis. From this standpoint, it would make sense that the addition of proteins to hair would allow them to interact with the proteins of the hair through similar chemical bonds. The end result is to provide a restructuring of the damaged proteins and to help bring back the condition of the hair to its natural state.

Since protein is a result of biosynthesis in a living organism, it can be derived from either plant or animal sources. Based on consumer demand, vegetable-derived proteins are more popular today due to the shift away from animal-derived products and towards more green and environmentally friendly sources. Although these proteins are naturally derived, they do experience processing and chemical modification prior to their addition to a hair or skin care product. One reaction includes the hydrolysis of the peptide bond with either an alkali or enzyme in order to reduce molecular weight, primarily done to increase water solubility. Functional groups are also added to proteins to increase their interaction with hair as well as their performance. Examples of this include quaternization for hair conditioning, and reaction with a silanol group. Therefore, the conformational and chemical variations that proteins can assume are quite large.

There is evidence that proteins that have been hydrolyzed by various means to lower molecular weight can absorb into the interior of the hair as well as on its surface. As mentioned above, they then can interact with the fibrous proteins of the hair with the same bonds that are found both on an intra- as well as intermolecular basis of the native proteins. Various methods have been utilized to show their substantivity to hair. ^{125}I-labelled collagen was used to determine substantivity from a surfactant system. This study also revealed the important factors governing substantivity such as molecular weight, isoelectric point of the protein, and formulation variables [172]. Radio-labeling techniques using ^{14}C-labeled amino acids produced from the complete hydrolysis of wheat proteins showed penetration from shampoo and conditioner [173]. Another method consisted of removing protein from treated hair using a high-temperature salt solution and then analyzing the resultant extract using gel filtration and fluorescent techniques [174]. Diffusion of hydrolyzed wheat proteins into hair was detected using fluorescently labeled peptides, analyzing the hair using laser-scanning fluorescent microscopy [175]. The details of the methods and results will not be described here, but rather serve as examples of the substantivity of proteins.

Proteins have been formulated into rinse-off and leave-in hair products for many years based upon their interactions with hair protein and their consequent cosmetic effects. Although some claims may be sometimes exaggerated, there is documented information that substantiates their benefits. Teglia and Secchi [176] state explicitly that proteins are proven to increase the hair's tensile strength, elasticity, body, softness, repair of split ends and cuticular damage, and protect against insulting treatments such as detergents and chemical treatments. References are also cited by the authors stating that protein hydrolysates and those that are derivatized such as with quaternization, reduce the loss of tensile strength caused by anionic surfactants. It would be worthwhile here to mention that these compounds may have a resurgence of use due to their natural origin and appeal for sustainability in addition to its functional attributes.

b. Cuticle Decementation and its Repair

There is ample evidence showing that the tensile properties of hair are due primarily to the cortex and not to the cuticle. Robbins proved this with the use of diperisophthalic acid, which oxidized the cuticles of the hair. It was shown that despite the damage incurred to the surface of hair as assessed microscopically, the tensile properties of hair were not affected [177]. Another important conclusion from this work was that tensile properties alone could not totally assess hair damage since cuticular damage can occur without being detected by changes in tensile strength. This was indeed the case, as demonstrated by Ruetsch and Weigmann, where cuticular damage was shown using both SEM and microfluorescence. Here, hair was extended in a longitudinal fashion. It was observed that the degree of cuticular lifting was greater for a given extension percent as hair samples were tested from root to tip. The weathering of the tip sections of hair resulted in a higher degree of cuticular lifting and a lower percent extension. Although the mechanical properties would be reversible as detected by tensile forces in the yield region, the reversion of the cuticulae was not. It was theorized that as the hair was being stretched, shear forces in the endocuticle, the least cross-linked area of the cuticle, would suffer the most stress and fracture. The cuticle would then lift and expose the fractured endocuticle.

Gamez-Garcia studied this phenomenon of cuticle decementation further and found that cuticle lifting increased with the number of applied tensile cycles and was sensitive to moisture, whereas at lower humidity levels it took less strain and/or fewer cycles to initiate cuticle lifting [178]. The mechanistic explanation for this is twofold. At high humidity the endocuticular region of the cuticle is plasticized and is more pliable. It is able to hold more moisture due to its lower cross-link density. Also, when the cortex is swollen with water there will be less of a Poisson contraction, which normally puts stress on the cuticular envelop during strain. By putting certain polysiloxane-modified compositions on hair with lifted cuticles, a recementing would take place in that the cuticles would not lift with subsequent strain. This was not the case with several other ingredients. The phenomenon could be easily observed by knotting a hair fiber and observing the lack of cuticular lifting as seen by SEM. The recementing of the cuticle by these compounds was shown to entail cross-linking as shown by measuring the rate of solubility of dried films. The dried films of these compounds formed insoluble films despite the drying conditions, providing evidence for cross-linking [179, 180].

c. Repair of Split Ends

One of the manifestations of damaged hair is the presence of split ends, which are perceived as longitudinal splits in the end of the fiber. They form through the shear stresses at work as a comb or brush is pulled through the hair and eventually produces the longitudinal fracture [134, 141]. Once enough of them form they become noticeable. This is usually accompanied by other manifestations of damage such as ends being unmanageable during styling, hard to comb through, and lacking shine.

To repair split ends and restore hair to its normal state, a technology is available that consists of a polyelectrolyte complex that is able to semi-permanently mend the damaged ends. The semi-permanence here is defined as having the durability to further mechanical action such as combing [181, 182].

The method consists of tagging fibers at their root end in a typical hair tress to determine their fate during a treatment and/or styling regimen. The tress is first damaged mechanically by exposing it to a combing device, where it is continuously combed to produce split ends. Split end fibers are then located in the tress and tagged appropriately. With the use of a stereomicroscope, a small red dot is added right before the split end to act as a landmark to make sure through subsequent treatments that the breakage of the split end off of the fiber is not taken as a false positive. A picture of the damage is captured and then compared and quantified after addition of the repair ingredient. Combing after the repair ingredient has been applied tests the durability of the mend from the shear forces at work during the combing process (see **Figure 56**). The advantage of the method, although time consuming, allows the tagged split end fibers to experience typical combing forces or the stress of other designed treatment regimens. From this method it was shown that the polyelectrolyte complex mended the split end after treatment, but more importantly, was able to show durability after the post-combing process, thereby simulating normal grooming and mechanical stress for consumer relevance [181, 182].

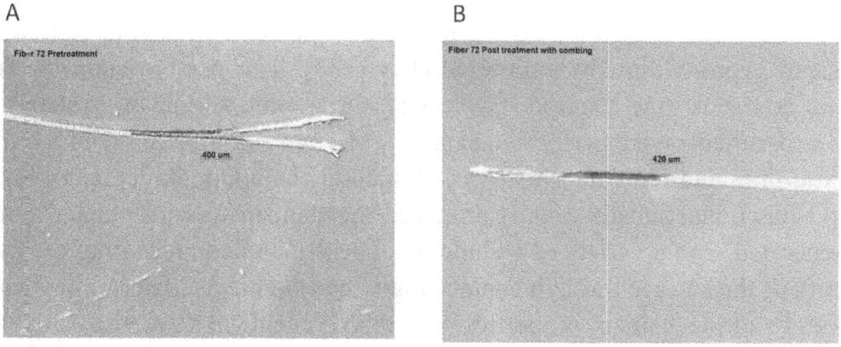

Figure 56: Spit end mending as observed under a stereomicroscope (20X), a): before treatment; b) post-treatment after the stress of combing

Mending of the split ends occurs based on the morphology and physical-chemical properties of the resultant microgel that forms as a result of the complexation. A proposed mechanism consists of the following. The microgels are characterized microscopically and are dispersed particles on the scale of one to three microns. These tend to infiltrate the subassemblies of the broken fiber. Cationically charged domains of the microgel, which are based on unassociated moieties of the cationic polymer, interact electrostatically with the cortical proteins, which are predominantly anionic. Also, anionic domains of the microgel work as an adhesive through hydrogen bonding. Based on the physical chemistry of these microgels, they act as cross-linking structures to draw together and bind the broken parts of the fiber in such a fashion that the split ends will not open up with the stress of subsequent combing.

d. Repair of the Surface Lipid Layer

The F layer located on the periphery of the hair surface is an important morphological component that is important for many cosmetic attributes such as shine, combing, feel, and overall manageability. The appearance and behavior of hair's damaged state is evident once this lipid layer is compromised by either an aggressive treatment such as bleaching or the persistent weathering of hair through UV or daily grooming practices. Rinse-out conditioners are then utilized that deposit a layer of cationic surfactant, such as behentrimethyl ammonium chloride in combination with fatty alcohols, to restore this hydrophobic layer and its resultant cosmetic effects. However, this is temporary since this layer is easily removed during the shampooing process, with the result that the hair reverts back to its damaged state. There is a need, therefore, to provide a more permanent hydrophobic layer on the surface of hair that will maintain hair health despite the weathering and damaging treatments that hair is subjected to.

A technology that provides a persistent hydrophobicity to the surface of damaged hair has been achieved by depositing a complex of 18-MEA in combination with stearoxypropyldimethylamine (SPDA) [183]. The persistence was shown over the course of one shampoo cycle with an anionic surfactant system. Controlled experiments were performed using 18-MEA in combination with a series of tertiary amines and fatty acids that varied in alkyl chain length, degree of branching, and functional substitution. A proposed mechanism was formulated through data generated with a variety of techniques. These included measuring the hydrophobicity of the surface through contact angle measurements, determining surface roughness and mechanical properties with AFM, chemical state versus depth on the hair surface with angle-resolved X-ray photoelectron spectroscopy (ARXPS), and fatty acid absorption with liquid chromatography/mass spectrometry. The model of surface lipid restoration consists of 18-MEA and SPDA being packed on the surface of the hair with the carbonyl and amide groups attaching to the surface of hair. The orientation of the lipid molecules are at an approximate angle of 35 degrees, which translates into a layer being 1.4 nm in thickness. Another factor in producing a persistent hydrophobicity is the fluid-like nature at the upper region of the lipid film caused by the anteiso branching of the 18 MEA molecule. This fluid character imparts a greater molecular mobility that contributes to the persistent nature of the film after shampoo washing [184].

e. Strategies for Permanent Mending of Hair

The major constraint in using chemical means to achieve a permanent repair to damaged human hair is the fact that it is attached to a living person. If hair was like wool sheared from its owner, or synthetic or cotton fabric that can be manipulated at extreme conditions of pH, temperature, or strength of chemical treatments, then products would be on the market that would deliver one hundred percent on its claims. As Jachowicz states in his article on hair damage and attempts at its repair, there are no methods of practical utility to achieve this; however, there are several that he cites in the literature from a general research strategy point of view [67]. The first includes reactive low-molecular-weight compounds that absorb into the hair and react with the cortical proteins.

Examples include compounds that contain alkyl groups that have the effect of reducing water swellability, resulting in a positive effect on mechanical strength. Other compounds can react with hair proteins through covalent bonds, which act as cross-linking agents. One such compound is formaldehyde, which is used in products designed to straighten the hair. This ingredient, however, has come under severe scrutiny since it is now considered a carcinogen and requires appropriate warning labels for its proper use [185]. Another category includes compounds that polymerize within the hair. Just as in an organic synthesis reaction, small monomeric intermediates such as methacrylic acid in the presence of appropriate initiating agents will react *in situ* in the hair. Although these reactions can take place *in vitro*, their practicality is quite limited. However, research may uncover someday a reactive system that can repair and strengthen hair *in vivo* without negative consequences to the consumer.

The consumer deems hair repair products efficacious from either a product-perception point of view or its actual performance. In the technical community, these products, and the key ingredients used for hair repair claims, need to be substantiated by both a sound theoretical mechanism of action as well as data from appropriate test methods. Based on this latter consideration there are not many hair repair systems currently available that provide permanent repair. Hence, there is the opportunity for innovation for new technologies as well as the accompanying test methods to show their benefits.

11.4.7 TESTS TO STUDY WHOLE HAIR ATTRIBUTES FROM DAMAGING EFFECTS AND IMPROVEMENTS WITH COSMETIC TREATMENTS

There is a data continuum inclusive of the most analytically based techniques to the more subjective, with the latter involving perception of the human senses in consumer evaluations. Instrumental techniques, although of great value in themselves for substantiation of effects, have to be correlated to sensorial attributes since this is the ultimate criterion for the success of a technology or finished product. For example, a product such as a conditioning shampoo can be shown to deposit ppm levels of silicone on the surface of hair; but if this amount of silicone does not surpass the threshold of what can be felt by the consumer with respect to combing and feel properties, then a statistical increase in silicone deposition is without merit. Showing a statistical difference in data between a control and experimental treatment by an instrumental technique has to take into account the minimum difference perceived by the senses before a conclusion is made. If you cannot see it by eye, then a statistical difference is purely a mathematical one. Another factor is working solely with hair tresses to assess the efficacy of ingredients. Although this comes closer to real-life consumer usage, it will be mentioned in more detail later that some hair attributes are only revealed by evaluation on a whole head of hair assisted by the trained eye of a cosmetologist. This section then goes into those techniques that are closer to what can be perceived in the more macroscopic view of product evaluation.

a. Panel Testing

The only industry standard utilized in panel testing with hair tresses is to use properly controlled designed experiments so that conclusions are based on a deductive reasoning of the results. Hair tresses are made to a set configuration of length, width, and net mass of hair as well as hair type that will be appropriate for testing the hair attributes under study. For example, damaged hair such as from bleaching that is eight inches in length would be most appropriate to test wet and dry combing properties from a conditioning shampoo and/or conditioning treatment. Fine hair would be most appropriate for testing volumization effects of, for example, polymers from a leave-in styling treatment. A selection of hair attributes can be evaluated that will provide information for conditioning, protection, repair, or styling type of products. It is up to the discretion of the scientist to choose the right substrate for the test that he or she has in mind for the particular hair attribute(s) that are important to the study.

There are essentially two types of designs for panel tests. One is based on an absolute and another on a relative scoring system. In an absolute scoring system, the panelist judges a particular hair characteristic against set criteria. For example, if the hair attribute is ease of combing and if the scoring consists of values between 1 through 5, where 1 represents poor combing and 5 is excellent combing, then each score value would have a particular standard that the panelist can be calibrated against. This may be done by treating a tress with a highly conditioning system that would provide excellent comb-through and having the panelist evaluate this as a standard for a score of 5. Standards can also be designed for scores of 1 though 4 in the same manner. Once the panel is calibrated against these standards they can be considered "expert" panelists and can then be human instruments to provide data on the effect of experimental treatments on tresses. This type of scoring system was utilized to show the contribution of the Silicone Quaternium-22 (INCI) for improving detangling, wet-combing, and wet-feel properties in a shampoo and conditioner formulation [186]. Here a panel consisted of ten experts that combed tresses damaged through bleaching after being conditioned by various treatments with the Silicone Quaternium-22. Bar charts are utilized to portray the positive effects over the control systems, where the individual bars represent an average of multiple measurements. Using the absolute scoring system, other hair attributes can be handled in the same way depending on the objectives of the test.

In a relative scoring system, tresses with various treatments are compared to each other without reference to a particular standard. In a simple case, two tresses are used for comparison and a group of panelists are asked to simply evaluate which tress is preferred with respect to a particular hair attribute. Although these panelists do not have to be expert in the sense that they need to be calibrated, as with absolute scoring, they do need to be trained on the proper technique of evaluating the particular hair attribute being considered. For example, it seems simple enough to comb through hair to get the perception of friction of the comb going through the hair; but results will be varied if each panelist holds the comb at a different angle. After the panelists provide their scores on the paired tresses, they are tallied to indicate which treatment is preferred for that particular hair attribute. This method was utilized to compare the conditioning properties of a hydrophobically modified cationic cellulosic polymer, Polyquaternium-67, to quaternized guar gum when incorporated into a silicone containing shampoo. A group of ten panelists were asked to judge wet comb and feel, dry comb and feel, as well as volume properties on tresses conditioned with the two treatment types, one treated with the Polyquaternium-67 shampoo and the other with the cationic guar shampoo. Results indicated that wet combing was equivalent despite the fact that the Polyquaternium-67 shampoo had one-fourth the amount of silicone, indicating the increased silicone deposition to the hair surface. These results were correlated with quantification of the silicone deposition on the hair surface using atomic absorption spectroscopy. Preferences were also seen with other hair attributes for the Polyquaternium-67 shampoo treated tresses. From a structure-performance point of view, the authors indicated that hydrophobic modification is one more intrinsic variable of the polymer that can be modified, in addition to molecular weight and charge density, to affect improved properties over its parent compound, Polyquaternium-10 [187].

Besides combing and hair feel properties, panel tests can also be used to test the color and shine of hair tresses and again can be judged by panelists in either an absolute or relative fashion. The difference is that one must control lighting conditions. Light boxes can be used and are equipped with different light sources such as incandescent and fluorescent light. A typical setup is illustrated in **Figure 57.**

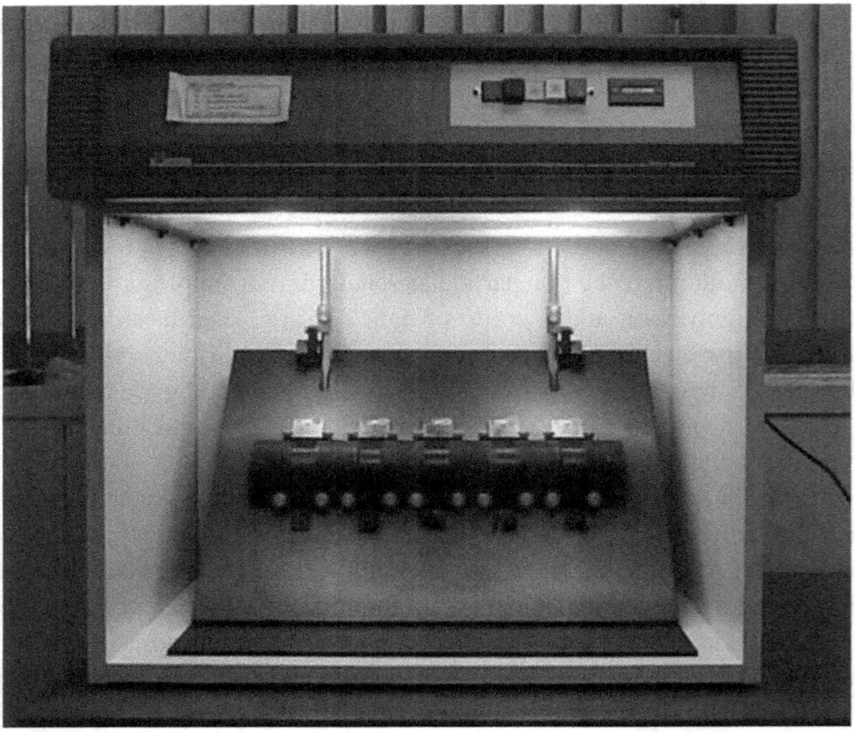

Figure 57: Light box to conduct panel studies to assess such hair attributes as color and shine.

b. Fiber Fragmentation Techniques

Combing methods—Breakage through combing imparts many mechanical stresses to hair. Test methods have been employed where hair is combed by hand in a controlled fashion or combed with a mechanical device and the number of fibers that have broken from the hair are quantified. The number of fibers, when compared against appropriate controls, is an assessment of the degree of damage or the alleviation of weakening by a pretreatment [4, 113, 137, 188]. Normally, these tests are conducted so that there is a statistical basis to the conclusions from the test due to the very nature of the variables inherent in the combing process.

c. Mechanical Combing

As a comb is passed through hair it can be observed in the advancing end of the comb that the fibers appear to be weaving among each other in a random fashion. Hair that is undamaged is relatively easy to comb through because of the intact lipid layer that is present on the surface of the cuticles. This provides a lubricating action so that fibers can pass over each other as well as through the teeth of the comb easily during the combing process. Another factor is the greater pliability of undamaged hair. The undamaged proteins in the cortex have more elasticity and can take the stress of bending with more ease and without the propensity to fracture and break. Damaged hair does not have these advantages and as a result, passing a comb through hair is a lot harder due primarily to higher frictional forces. A measure of hair damage and the effect of treatments on alleviating damage is through measuring combing forces and the work it takes to pass a comb through the hair. This can be done by hand, and in fact is utilized in sensory testing techniques. Instruments are available that can quantify combing forces in particular the Dia-Stron, Instron, or texture analyzer, which are adapted with a mechanical comb device. Because the comb traverses through the hair at a constant rate and the resultant stress is measured by force in grams, the testing technique is then a strain-controlling device. The data are portrayed as a combing curve and with the help of computer software, the work involved in passing the comb through the hair is calculated (e.g., in grams/cm). Comparing the combing work of a tress treated with a conditioning treatment will result in a reduction in combing work, and usually a percent reduction in combing is reported [189, 190].

Combing work, as measured by mechanical combing devices, has been used to not only determine the conditioning effects of shampoos and conditioners, but also with respect to this chapter, the protective effects of pretreatments to factors that damage the hair. Locke studied the reduction in combing work observed by applying a substantive photofilter to hair prior to a controlled solar irradiation and treatment regimen [111]. McMullen utilized combing work measurements to show the protection of hair from curling irons with the use polymeric pretreatments in the treatment regimen [107, 112]. Comparing polymeric treatments to appropriate controls, there was found to be less of an increase in combing after successive applications of the heat from a curling iron. In this case the iron was applied to one particular spot for a set period of time creating an area of the tress that would suffer damage as indicated in an increase in combing work. As seen in **Figure 58**, the section of hair that was exposed to eight one-minute cycles of the curling iron, the window of exposure, had higher combing work values as compared to the area after four one-minute cycles. This increase in combing work appears in this window of the full profile of the combing curve, where the area under the curve in the window is a measure of the combing work to pass the comb through that part of the tress.

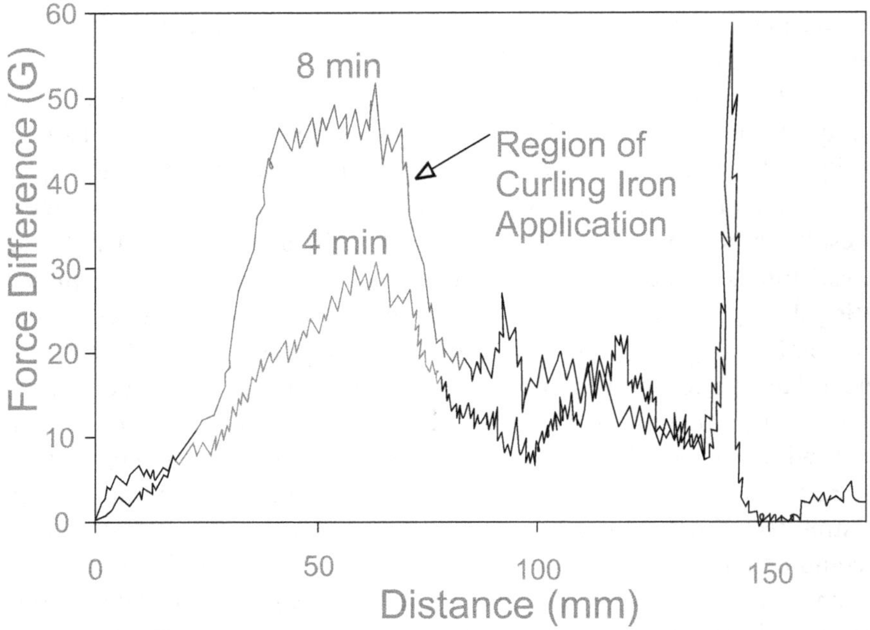

Figure 58: Increase in damage from heat damage of hair as evident from higher combing forces in the window of damage.

The advantage of the window technique in combing tests is that the combing work can be compared directly both before and after treatment on the same tress. Comparing combing work from different tresses requires a statistical base of samples since there is a high variability of combing forces from one tress to another. Comparisons with the windows technique can be done using one tress since it serves as its own control. This technique was developed further by Jachowicz and Helioff in a method they termed spatially resolved combing analysis [110]. In this method a tress is enclosed by a frame that allows only a certain part of the tress to be exposed; the other parts of the tress are covered by the housing of the frame (see **Figure 59**). Two variants of the procedure can then be employed. In the first procedure the tress is contained in the frame and only the window section(s) of the tress is damaged, such as can be done with a bleach or permanent wave. After rinsing, the tress is then removed from the frame and a combing curve is generated showing an increase in combing work in the windows from the damaging treatment. The tress is then put through a conditioning regimen to show the reduction in combing work, especially in the windows section. In a modified version of the method, the whole tress is exposed to a damaging treatment and combing forces then measured. The tress is then enclosed in the frame and a conditioning treatment added to the window section. The resultant combing curve will show a reduction in combing work just in the area of the window showing the conditioning effect. Besides conditioning of damaged hair, this method has also been employed in showing the protection of hair from UV light with a photofilter [191] and polymeric pretreatment on thermal protection [107, 112].

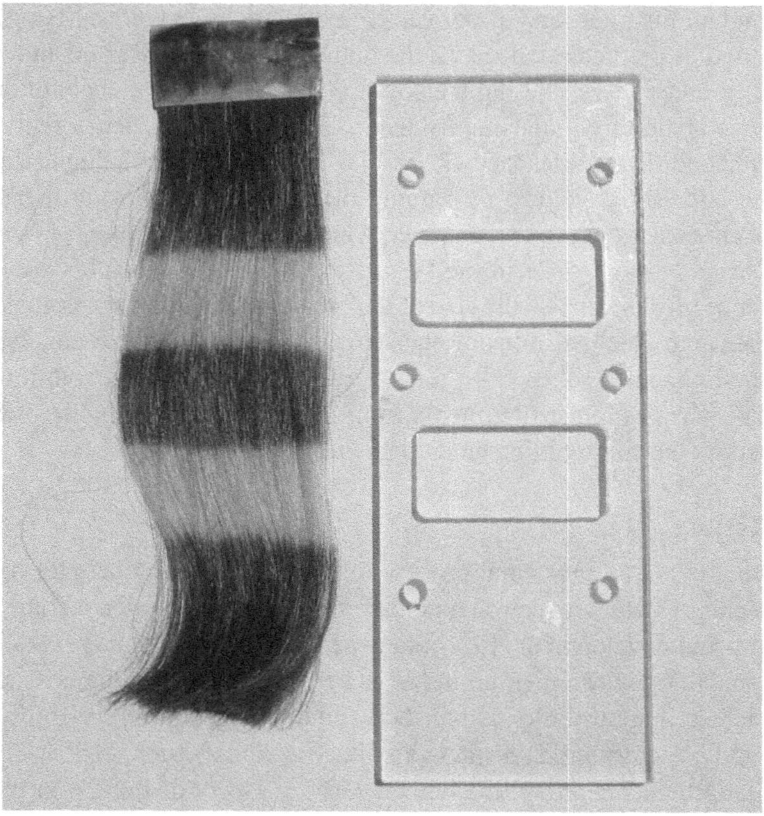

Figure 59: Spatially Resolved Combing Analysis; treated tress where exposed areas of tress were bleached and specialized frame for treating tress

Continual brushing and combing of hair imparts various levels of stress to individual fibers of the hair assembly. For the most part, these stresses are not strong enough to break the hair; but with repeated application of smaller stresses, eventually fibers become fatigued and break. Here the stresses are applied over hundreds of fibers during a stroke of a comb. Evans saw that this was similar to his fatiguing experiments using single fiber studies and applied the same type of statistics to analyze breakage data to construct survival probability plots [192].

A mechanical combing device is constructed to help understand the variables involved with hair breakage or prevention of breakage and consists of a hollow rotating drum containing four brushes or combs attached on its outer circumference. As the drum rotates, the combs traverse a hair tress so that it experiences 50 strokes per minute. Broken fibers begin to fall out on a plate on the bottom of the apparatus after many strokes of the comb. In experiments conducted by Evans [192], fibers were collected from eight tresses after every 1,000 strokes up to 10,000 strokes. The resultant data were then subjected to Weibull statistical analysis to determine survival probability plots, and its converse, failure prediction plots. Major findings were reported as predicted failure vs. the number of strokes. Results indicate that the failure prediction vs. the number of strokes were lower for conditioned vs. unconditioned hair, virgin undamaged hair vs. bleached, bleached conditioned vs. bleached unconditioned, bleached vs. 3X bleached, and lower vs. higher humidity. One of the interesting features of running the Weibull statistics on the breakage data is the characteristic shape parameter, which indicates whether the majority of breakage occurs early or late in the fatigue experiment. By quantifying not only the number of breaks but also the size of the broken fibers, Evans was able to theorize the breakage mechanism using the shape parameter. Here he concluded that small fiber fragments broken from the tip end of the fiber form from a wear-out mechanism, whereas longer fragments form from a premature failure most probably caused by the comb hitting entanglements [192].

d. Salon Testing

Salon testing is not an incidental process in the testing of products for hair damage and repair. Albanese makes a good case for the value of salon testing in product research and development [193]. Many advanced hair attributes, which only a trained cosmetologist can pick up in his or her evaluation, will be missed. These include such styling attributes as hair body and manageability, stylability during brushing and blow drying, and subtle auxiliary attributes such as fiber alignment and curl definition. Therefore, the human sensory aspect of results on the whole hair attributes on panelists have to be included with subjective panel testing on tresses and in objective and detailed instrumental analysis.

Advice from an experienced cosmetologist is important for the experimenter in designing the treatment scheduled as simulated on hair tresses in the laboratory. For example, in exposing hair tresses to the heat of a hot flat iron, the rate of descent of the iron along the hair tress, the amount of heat applied as controlled by the thermostat, as well as the pressure of the jaws of the iron on the hair are all important variables to consider. Other damaging regimens such as relaxing, perming, oxidative hair coloring, and the like also have their own subtle, yet important variables to consider.

Unlike conditioning and styling products, hair protection and repair product testing in the salon is somewhat limited. This is due to the simple fact that no one would like their hair purposely damaged, whether it be a whole-head study where candidates have their hair damaged, where half of the panelists have a protective pretreatment, or half-head study where one side of the head has the control formula and the other the product with the experimental protective ingredient. The best course is simulating the damage in the lab on tresses or possibly a mannequin head that are based on human hair that have a treatment schedule as realistic as possible.

CONCLUSION

If cannot be stressed too much that hair has a complex structure and that because of this it responds to stresses induced by external factors in various ways. Changes occur at different levels consisting of the molecular, the nanoscale, subcellular, and the micron-size cellular level. Damage on each of these levels produces effects that contribute to the decrease in the cosmetic behavior of hair and ultimately can be perceived by a person during their normal grooming routine. To help study this multifaceted array of variables and effects, there are many instrumental techniques, each designed to give a clear picture of the changes incurred to the different hierarchical components of hair. One must, therefore, know exactly what the instrument measures and the consequent conclusions that can safely be made. When a damaging process has multiple effects on hair, such as surface as well as cortical damage, then various techniques need to be employed, where one reinforces the conclusion of the other. As in a legal argument, one must make a case to prove through appropriate evidence that the data link cause-and-effect relationships. The planning and execution of the experimental design, such as the practicality of the treatment schedule and employing the proper measuring techniques, are part of this process as well.

ACKNOWLEDGMENTS

The authors would like to thank those individuals who helped with the manuscript. Guojin Zhang contributed the AFM images and Bill Thompson the SEM photomicrographs. Don Koelmel lent his expertise on Differential Scanning Calorimetry. Dan Burnett of Surface Measurement Systems Ltd provided information on the DVS and IGC methodologies, and Paula Clark of Tascon USA patiently distilled thoughts relating to ToF-SIMS and XPS. The manuscript was peer reviewed by Larry Senak, Roger McMullen, Linda Foltis, and Manuel Gamez-Garcia. The authors also give thanks to the many authors who have diligently kept up with their research and who are mentioned in our 193 references to this work. Finally, we thank Ashland, Inc. for the opportunity and the resources to even consider starting this endeavor.

REFERENCES

1. Ratnapandian, S., et al., Photodegradation of human hair, J. Cosmet. Sci., 49, 309-320 (September/October 1998)
2. Feughelman, M., The physical properties of alpha-keratin fibers, J. Soc. Cosmet. Chem., 33, 385-406 (December 1982)
3. Robbins, C. R., *Chemical and Physical Behavior of Human Hair*, 3rd edition, Springer-Verlag, 1994.
4. Zhou, Y., et al., The effect of various cosmetic pretreatments on protecting hair from thermal damage by hot flat ironing, J. Cosmet. Sci., 62, 265-282 (March/April 2011)
5. McMullen, R. and Jachowicz, J., Thermal degradation of hair. II. Effects of selected polymers and surfactants, J. Cosmet. Sci., 49, 245-256 (July/August 1998)
6. J. Cosmet. Sci. 2013; 64: 119-131.
7. Lee, W. S., Integral hair lipid in human hair follicle, Journal of Dermatological Science, 64 (2011) 153-158
8. Hoting, E.,et al., Photochemical alterations in human hair. I. Artificial irradiation and investigation of hair proteins, J. Soc. Cosmet. Chem., 46, 85-99 (March/April 1995)
9. Nogueira, A. and Joekes, I., Hair melanin content and photodamage, J. Cosmet. Sci., 58, 385-391 (July/August 2007)
10. Hoting, E., and Zimmermann, M., Sunlight-induced modifications in bleached, permed, or dyed human hair, J. Soc. Cosmet., Chem., 48, 79-91 (March/April 1997)
11. Locke, B. and Jachowicz, J., Effect of formulation on the hair protective efficacy of a substantive photofilter, Cosmetics and Toiletries Manufacture Worldwide, 2001, pgs. 161-167
12. Signori, V., Review of the current understanding of the effect of ultraviolet and visible radiation on hair structure and options for photoprotection, J. Cosmet. Sci., 55, 95-113 (January/February 2004)
13. Grossman, D. M., Know Your Enemy: The Weather and How to Reproduce it in the Laboratory, Q-Panel Lab Products, Technical Bulletin LU-0821

14. Zhou, Y., et al., Protection of oxidative hair color fading from shampoo washing by hydrophobically cationic polymers, J. Cosmet. Sci., 60, 217-238 (March/April 2009)
15. http://www.perkinelmer.com 2010: 1-16.
16. J. Struct. Biol. 2012; 177: 553-560.
17. J. Therm. Cal. 2005; 79: 289-293.
18. Biopolymers 2005; 81 (5): 371-375.
19. Proc. R. Soc. B 2013; 280 (1750): 20122158.
20. J. Cosmet. Sci. 2007; 58: 621-627.
21. J. Appl. Polym. Sci. 1993; 48: 137-150.
22. PhD Thesis, Aachen University, DWI (Germany) 2001.
23. J. Cosmet. Sci. 2007; 58: 311-317.
24. J. Cosmet. Sci. 2007; 58: 311-317.
25. Biopolymers 2008; 89 (7): 311-317.
26. Biopolymers 2006; 83 (6): 630-635.
27. J. Photochem. Photobiol. B 2010; 101 (3): 1011-1344.
28. Springer-Verlag, NY, USA; 2002.
29. Butterworth-Heinemann; Oxford, UK; 1992.
30. IFSCC Monograph 2004: 94.
31. Wiley-Interscience; New York, USA; 1992.
32. John Wiley & Sons; New York, USA; 1997.
33. J. Colloid Interface Sci. 1979; 71 (2): 283-92.
34. J. Appl. Polym. Sci. 2006; 102: 5255-65.
35. J. Appl. Polym. Sci. 1984; 29: 1011-26.
36. J. Soc. Cosmet. Chem. 1977; 28: 273-84.
37. J. Colloid Interface Sci. 2001; 237: 40-6.
38. American Chemical Society, Washington D.C., USA; 1964.
39. Langmuir 2010; 26 (10): 7365-9.
40. J. Colloid Interface Sci. 2004; 269: 329-35.
41. J. Colloid Interface Sci. 2007; 306: 34-40.
42. Industrial and Engineering Chemistry 1949: 2014–15.
43. Journal of Applied Polymer Science 2001; 79: 1054–61.
44. Lipids 1988; 23 (9): 878–81.

45. Chem. Soc. Rev. 2007; 36: 1282–91.
46. University of New South Wales Press; Sydney; 1997: 22-7.
47. Thermochimica Acta 2010: 33–9.
48. Clarendon Press; Oxford; 1966.
49. J. Am. Chem. Soc. 1936; 60: 309-19.
50. Agricultural University, Wagingen, the Netherlands; 1981.
51. J. Sci. Food Agric. 2005; 85: 1805-14.
52. J. Therm. Anal. Calorim. 2010; 102 (1): 43-8.
53. J. Cosmet. Sci. 2011; 62: 109-20.
54. J. Cosmet. Sci. 2004; 55: 13-27.
55. Allured Business Media; Carol Stream, IL; 2012.
56. IFSCC Magazine 2007; 10 (4): 317-20.
57. J. Cosmet. Sci. 2007; 58: 135-45.
58. J. Cosmet. Sci. 1998; 49: 141-53.
59. J. Cosmet. Sci. 1998; 49: 223-44.
60. J. Am. Acad. Dermatol. 1994; 30: 54-60.
61. J. Cosmet. Sci. 2004; 55: 437-47.
62. Biomacromolecules. 2006; 7: 3499-504.
63. Colloids Surf. B: Biointerfaces 2004; 39: 39-43.
64. J. Cosmet. Sci. 1998; 62: 191-202.
65. An. Dermatol. 2011; 23 (4): 455-62.
66. J. Struct. Bio. 2012; 177 (2); 553-60.
67. J. Cosmet. Sci. 2004; 38: 263-86.
68. United States Patent US 5,452,233 1995.
69. J. Soc. Cosmet. Chem. 1994; 45: 309-36.
70. ASTM International 2013.
71. Mikrochimica Acta 2000; 132: 259-71.
72. Spectroscopy Europe 2005; 43 (5): 25-7.
73. J. Cosmet. Sci. 2004; 55: 265-79.
74. J. Cosmet. Sci. 2005; 56: 323-30.
75. J. Cosmet. Sci. 2001; 52: 169-84.
76. Appl. Surf. Sci. 2006; 252: 6786-8.
77. Sci. Total Environ. 2005; 338: 213-27.

78. Surf. Interface Anal. 2011; 44: 736-9.
79. Surf. Interface Anal. 2010; 43: 410-2.
80. Surf. Interface Anal. 2009; 43: 298-301.
81. Langmuir 2010; 26 (21): 16434-41.
82. Eur. Cell. Mater. 2012; 24: 60-73.
83. J. Cosmet. Sci. 2012; 56: 65-77.
84. 2013.
85. J. Cosmet. Sci. 2009; May-June, 60, 337-345
86. Chromatographia 1989; 28 (11): 588-92.
87. J. Coatings Technology 1999; 71 (893): 53-60.
88. Chromatographia 1989; 28 (9): 469-72.
89. Intl J Pharm 2012; 422: 238-44.
90. J. Soc. Cosmet. Chem. 1971; 22: 839-50.
91. J. Soc. Cosmet. Chem. 1999; 50: 23-47.
92. J. Soc. Cosmet. Chem. 1989; 40: 173-89.
93. J. Cosmet. Sci. 2000; 51: 15-25.
94. Surf. Interface Anal. 2011; 44: 736-9.
95. Springer-Verlag, NY, USA; 2002.
96. Allured Business Media; Carol Stream, IL, USA; 2012.
97. Biochem.Biophys. Res. Comm. 2002; 299: 857-62.
98. J. Cosmet. Sci. 1998; 49: 213-22.
99. Biomacromolecules 2006; 7: 3499-504.
100. J. Cosmet. Sci. 2011; 62: 191-202.
101. Int. J. Cosmet. Sci. 1979; 1 (6): 317-28.
102. J. Soc. Cosmet. Chem. 1994; 45: 85-94.
103. Neonatal Network 1994; 13 (2).
104. FLIR Systems 2011.
105. 2002 Adv. In Bioengineering 2002; 53: 1-2.
106. Appl. Polymer Symp. 1971; 18: 175.
107. J. Cosmet. Sci. 1998; 49: 223-244.
108. Pande, C. M, and Jachowicz, J., Hair photodamage-Measurement and prevention, J. Soc. Cosmet. Chem., 44, 109-122 (March/April 1993)

109. McMullen, R., and Jachowicz, J., Thermal degradation of hair. I. Effect of curling irons, J. Cosmet. Sci., 49, 223-244 (July/August 1998)

110. Jachowicz, J., and Helioff, M., Spatially resolved combing analysis, J. Soc. Cosmet. Chem., 48, 93-105 (March/April 1997)

111. Locke, B., and Jachowicz, J., Effect of Formulation On The Hair Protection Efficacy By A Substantive Photofilter, Cosmetics and Toiletries Manufacture Worldwide, Publisher Year pgs 161-167

112. McMullen, R., and Jachowicz, J., Thermal degradation of hair. II. Effect of selected polymers and surfactants, J. Cosmet. Sci., 49, 245-256 (July/August 1998)

113. Rigoletto, R., et al., Quantification of fiber fragmentation of hair through combing as a measure of thermal protection, J. Cosmet. Sci., 60, 578-579, (Sept/Oct 2009), pgs

114. McMullen, R., et al., Spectrofluorescent characterization of changes in hair chemistry induced by environmental stresses, J. Cosmet. Sci., 62, 191-202 (March/April 2011)

115. Gamez-Garcia, M., Heat Damage to the Cortex and Cuticle Sheath of Human Hair Produced by Hot Appliances, Cosmetic Science Technology, 2011, pgs 119-127, Caroline Johnson Publisher

116. Gamez-Garcia, M., Patterns of light interference produced by damaged cuticle cells in human hair, J. Cosmt. Sci., 58, 269-282, (July/August 2007)

117. Ruetsch, S.B., and Weigmann, H-D., Mechanism of tensile stress release in the keratin fiber cuticle: I, J. Soc. Cosmet. Chem., 47, 13-26 (January/February 1996)

118. Tate, M.L., et al., Quantification and prevention of hair damage, J. Soc. Cosmet. Chem., 44, 347-371 (November/December 1993)

119. Ruetsch, S.B., Kamath, Y. K., Change in the Surface Chemistry of the Cuticle of Human Hair by Chemical and Photochemical Oxidation, IFSCC Magazine, vol. 7 no. 4/2004

120. Weigmann, H.-D., et al., Characterization of surface deposits on human hair fibers, J. Sco. Cosmet. Chem., 41, 379-390 (November/December 1990)

121. Goddard, E. D., Winnik, F. M., Fluorimetry: A Useful Tool in Cosmetic Research, Vol. 114, No. 11/November 1999

122. Gruber, J. V., et al., Examining cationic polysaccharide deposition onto keratin surfaces through biopolymer fluorescent labeling, J. Cosmet. Sci., 52, 119-129

123. www.microscopyu.com, Nikon, The Source for Microscopy Education

124. www.olympusmicro.com, Olympus, Microscopy Resource Center

125. Swift, J. A., Fundamentals of Human Hair Science, Cosmetic Science Monograph Number One, Micelle Press,

126. Schmitt, R. L., and Goddard, E. D., Investigation into the Adsorption of Cationic Polymers, Cosmet. & Toil., 1994, 111, 57-65

127. McMullen, R., et al., Correlation of AFM/LFM with Combing Forces of Human Hair, IFSCC Magazine, Vol. 3, No. 3, July/September 2000

128. Wei, G., et al., Nanomechanical characterization of human hair using nanoindentation and SEM, Ultramicroscopy, 105 (2005) 248-266

129. Smith, J. R., Use of atomic force microscopy for high-resolution non-invasive structural studies of human hair, J. Soc. Cosmet. Sci., 48, 199-208 (July/August 1997)

130. LaTorre, C., et al., Nanotribological effecs of silicone type, silicone deposition level, and surfactant type on human hair using atomic force microscopy, J. Cosmet. Sci., 57, 37-56 (January/February 2006)

131. Ruetsch, S. B., et al., Effects of conditioners on surface hardness of hair fibers: An investigation using atomic force microscopy, J. Cosmet. Sci., 54, 579-588 (November/December 2003)

132. Menkart, J., et al, Caucasian Hair, Negro Hair, and Wool: Similarities and Differences, *J. Soc. Cosmetic Chemists*, 17, 769-787, (1966)

133. Beyak, R., et al., Elasticity and Tensile Properties of Human Hair. I. Singe Fiber Test Method, J. Soc. Cosmetic Chemists, 20, 615-626 (Sept. 16, 1969)

134. Brown, A. C., and Swift, J. A., Hair Breakage: the scanning electron microscope as a diagonostic tool, J. Soc. Cosmet. Chem., 26, 289-297 (1975)

135. Robbins, C., Hair breakage during combing. I. Pathways of breakage, J. Cosmet. Sci., 57, 233-243 (May/June 2006)

136. Robbins, C., Hair breakage during combing. II. Impact loading and hair breakage, J. Cosmet. Sci., 54, 245-257 (May/June 2006)

137. Robbins, C., and Kamath, Y., Hair breakage during combing. III. The effects of bleaching and conditioning on short and long segment breakage by wet and dry combing of tresses, J. Cosmet. Sci., 58, 477-484(July/August 2007)

138. Robbins, C. and Kamath, Y., Hair breakage during combing. IV. Brushing and combing of hair, J. Cosmet. Sci., 58, 629-636 (November/December 2007)

139. Swift, J. A., Flexabrasion: A Method for Evaluating Hair Strength, Cosmetic & Toiletries Magazine, Vol. 116. No. 12/December 2001, pgs 53-57

140. Jones, D.L.C., et al., Flexabrasion hair strength – a comparison of two commercial actives,

141. Swift, J. A., Mechanism of split-end formation in human head hair, J. Soc. Cosmet. Chem., 48, 123-126 (March/April 1997)

142. Brown A. C., and Swift, J. A., Hair breakage: the scanning electron microscope as a diagnostic tool, J. Soc. Cosmet. Chem., 26, 289-297 (1975)

143. Hornby, S., et al., New Technique to Capture Viscoelastic Changes in Hair Induced by Mechanical Stress, IFSCC Magazine, Vol. 5, No. 2, 2002

144. Evans, T. A., Fatigue testing of hair-A statistical approach to hair breakage, J. Cosmet. Sci., 60, 599-616 (November/December 2009)

145. Bogarty, H., Torsional Properties of Hair in Relation to Permanent Waving and Setting, J. Soc. Cosmet. Chemists, 18, 575-589 (Sept. 16, 1967)

146. Persaud, D., and Kamath, Y. K., Torsional method for evaluating hair damage and performance of hair care ingredients, J. Cosmet. Sci., 55, (Supplement), S65-S77 (2004)

147. Bell, F. I., et al., Advantages of a high-throughput measure of hair fiber torsional properties, 63, 81-92 (March/April 2012)

148. Harper, D. L., and Kamath, Y. K., The effect of treatments on th shear modulus of human hair measured by the single fiber torsion pendulum, J. Cosmet. Sci., 58, 329-337 (July/August 2007)

149. Jachowicz J., and Yao, K., Dynamic hair spray analysis. I. Instrumentation and preliminary results, J. Soc. Cosmet. Chem., 47, 73-84 (March/April 1996)

150. Jachowicz, J., and Yao, K., Dynamic hair spray analysis. II. Effect of polymer, hair type, and solvent composition, J. Cosmet. Sci., 52, 281-295 (September/October 2001)

151. Jachowicz, J.,and McMullen, R., Mechanical analysis of elasticity and flexibility of vergin and polymer-treated hair fiber assemblies, J. cosmet. Sci., 53, 345-361 (November/December 2002)

152. Jachowicz, J., Dynamic hair spray analysis. III. Theoretical considerations, J. Cosmet. Sci., 53, 249-261 (September/October 2002)

153. SOR Rheology Bull 2004; 73 (1).

154. CRC Press, NY, NY 1999.

155. J. Cosmet. Sci. 2007 Annual Sci. Seminar 2007; 584-85.

156. IFSCC Magazine 2010; 12 (2): 93-8.

157. McMullen, R., et al., Image analysis to quantify histological and immunofluorescent staining of ex vivo skin and skin cell cultures, International Journal of Cosmetic Science, 2010, 32, 143-154

158. McMullen, R., Image Analysis Tools to Quantify Visual Properties of Hair Fiber Assemblies, Chapter 9, Practical Modern Hair Science, Edited by T. Evans and R. Randall Wickett, Alluredbooks, 2012

159. McMullen, R., and Jachowicz, J., Optical properties of hair: Effect of treatments on luster as quantified by image analysis, J. Cosmet. Sci. 54, 335-351 (July/August 2003)

160. McMullen, R., and Jachowicz, J., Optical properties of hair-Detailed examination of specular reflection patterns in various hair types, J. Cosmet. Sci., 55, 29-47 (January/February 2004)

161. Neonatal Network 1994; 13 (2).

162. FLIR Systems 2011.

163. 2002 Adv. In Bioengineering 2002; 53: 1-2.

164. Appl. Polymer Symp. 1971; 18: 175.

165. Zhou, Y. et al., Protection of oxidative hair color fading from shampoo washing by hydrophobically modified cationic polymers, J. Cosmet. Sci., 60, 217-238 (March/April 2009)

166. Zhou, Y., et al., Protection of Oxidative Hair Colour Fading from Shampoo Stripping by Styleze W-20, Cosmetic Science Technology, 2008

167. Gao, T., et al., Multilayer Lamella Vesicles in Oxidative Dye Formulations: Characterization and Performance, Cosmetics & Toiletries magazine, Vol. 121, No. 5/May 2006

168. Hoting, E., and Zimmermann, M., Sunlight-induced modifications in bleached, permed, or dyed human hair, J. Soc. Cosmet. Chem., 48, 79-91 (March/April 1997)

169. Locke, B., and Jachowicz, J., Fading of artificial hair color and its prevention by photofilters, J. Cosmet. Sci., 56, 407-425 (November/December 2005)

170. Swift, J. A., The Structure and Chemistry of Human Hair, Chapter 1, Practical Modern Hair Science, edited by T. Evans and R. Wickett, Allured Books, 2012

171. Lehninger, A. L., Biochemistry, 2nd edition, 1975, Worth Publishers, Inc.

172. Turwski, A., Adelman-Grill, B.C., Substantivity to hair and skin of 125I-labelled collagen hydrolysates under application simulating conditions, International Journal of Cosmetic Science 7, 71-84 (1985)

173. Jones, R. T., Chahal, S. P., the use of radiolabelling techniques to measure substantivity to, and penetration into, hair of protein hydrolysates, International Journal of Cosmetic Science, 19, 215-226 (1997)

174. Mintz, G. R., et al., Relationship between collagen hydrolysate molecular weight and peptide substantivity to hair, J. Soc. Cosmet. Chem., 42, 35-44 (January/February 1991)

175. Swift, J. A., et al., Investigations on the penetration of hydrolyzed wheat proteins into human hair by confocal laser-scanning fluorescence microscopy, J. Cosmet. Sci., 51, 193-203 (May/June 2000)

176. Telia, A., Secchi, G., Proteins in Cosmetics, Chapter 9, Principles of Polymer Science and Technology in Cosmetics and Personal Care, edited by Goddard, E.D., Gruber, J.V., Marcel Dekker, Inc., 1999

177. Robbins, C.R., and Crawford, R.J., Cuticle damage and the tensile properties of human hair, J. Soc. Cosmet. Chem., 42, 59-67 (January/February 1991)

178. Gamez-Garcia, M.,The cracking of human hair cuticles by cyclical thermal stresses, J. Cosmet. Sci., 49, 141-153, (May/June 1998)

179. Crodasone W, Croda, Inc., February 14, 2013

180. Crodasone Cystine, Croda, Inc., October 28, 2011

181. Rigoletto, R., and Zhou, Y., Polyelectrolyte Complex for Mending Damaged Hair, Cosmetics and Toiletries Mag. Vol. 124, No.3, (2009)

182. Rigoletto, R., Zhou, Y., Foltis, L., Semi-permanent split end mending with a polyelectrolyte complex, J. Cosmet. Sci., 58, 451-476 (July/August 2007)

183. Tanamachi, H., et al., Deposition of 18-MEA onto alkaline-color-treated weathered hair to form a persistent hydrophobicity, J. Cosmet., Sci., 60, 31-44 (January/February 2009)

184. Tanamachi, H., et al., A role of the anteiso branch of 18-MEA in 18-MEA/SPDA to form a persistent hydrophobicity to alkaline-color-treated weathered hair, J. Cosmet. Sci., 60, 509-518 (September/October 2009)

185. Valdez, A., Brazilian Hair Straightening, Cosmetiscope, Summer 2011, Vol. 17 No. 6

186. Herrwerth, S., et al., Silicone Quaternium-22: New Silicone Technology for Premium Hair Conditioning with Additional Benefts, SOFW Journal, 6-2009

187. Drovetskay T. V., et al., New high charge density cationic hydrophobically modified cationic HEC polymers for improved co-deposition of benefit

agents and serious conditioning for problem hair, J. Cosmet. Sci., 58, 421-434 (July/August 2007)

188. Haake, H-M, et al., Hair breakage-How to measure and counteract, J. Cosmet. Sci., 60, 143-151 (March/April 2009)

189. Garcia, M. L., and Diaz, J., Combability Measurements on Human Hair, J. Soc. Cosmet. Chem., 27, 379-398 (September 1976)

190. Kamath, Y. K., and Weigmann, H-D, Measurement of combing forces, J. Soc. Cosmet. Chem., 37, 111-124 (May/June 1986)

191. Jachowicz, J., et al., Photodegradation of Hair and its Photoprotection by a Substantive Photofilter, Drug and Cosmetic Industry, December, 1995

192. Evans, T. A., and Park, K., A statistical analysis of hair breakage. II. Repeated grooming experiments, J. Cosmet. Sci., 61, 439-455 (November/December 2010)

193. Albanese, J., The Value of Salon Testing, Spray Technology, May 2005, pgs. 39-40

www.ingramcontent.com/pod-product-compliance
Lightning Source LLC
LaVergne TN
LVHW011110300926
849160LV00008B/332

9780820604053